The Longevity Kitchen

For Christopher

Nourishing Thoughts

Rebecca Katz

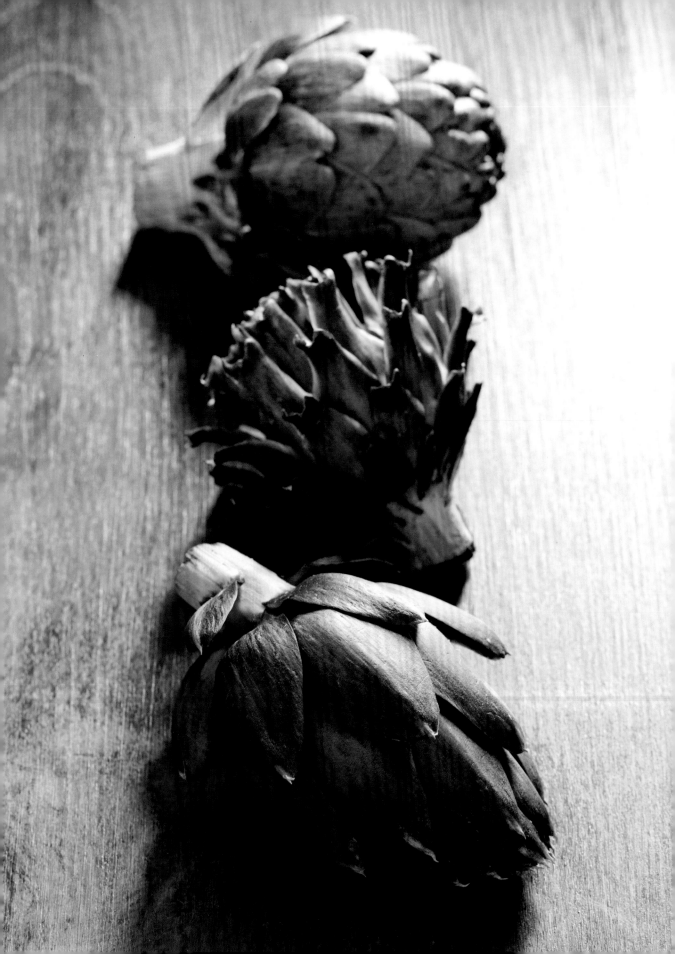

The Longevity Kitchen

Satisfying, Big-Flavor Recipes
Featuring the Top 16
Age-Busting Power Foods

Rebecca Katz with Mat Edelson

PHOTOGRAPHY BY LEO GONG

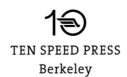

TEN SPEED PRESS
Berkeley

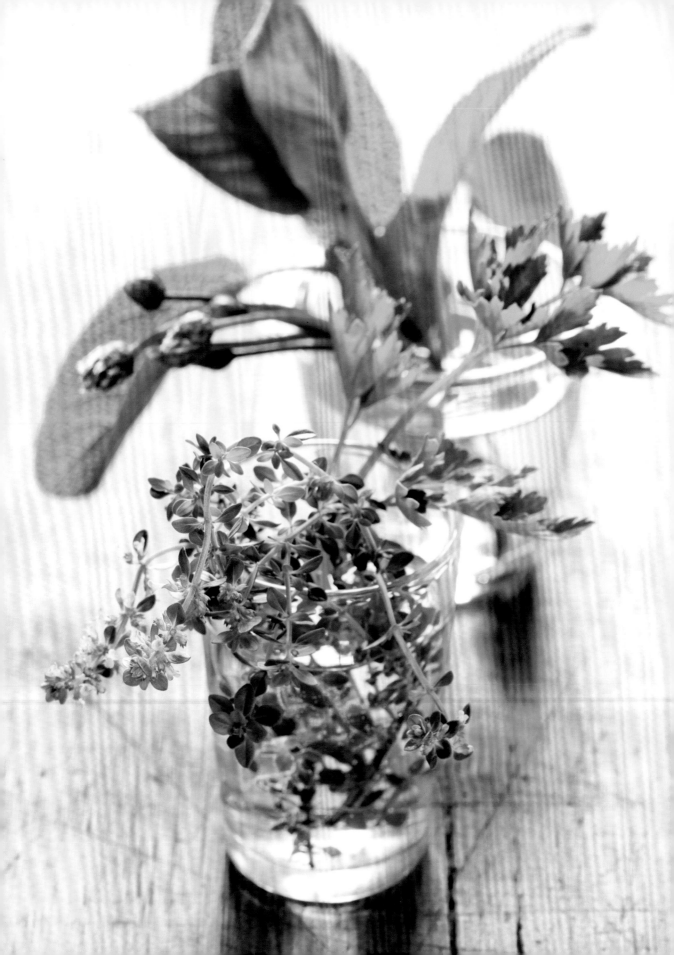

Contents

Foreword

I want to take a moment to tell you about two
of the most important healing tools I rely upon:
my garden and my kitchen.

I make it a priority to spend time in both of them, no matter how busy I am. As a physician, I believe we live in perilous times, especially with regard to aging gracefully—that is, with strength and vitality keeping pace with our internal calendar. In the last hundred years, medicine has taken us farther, chronologically, that at any time in human history. If you had been born in America in 1900, your life expectancy would have been just over forty-eight years. Jump forward a century, and a tiny bundle of male joy born on the first day of the second millennium can expect to live to reach seventy-five, while his twin sister can expect to reach eighty!

It should be a time of celebration, but for many people, the expectancy of those extra twenty-five to thirty years is tinged with trepidation. Medicine may have given us years, but it has also disconnected us from all that gives us personal control over how *well* we age. What's happened to us, including an increasing sense of helplessness as we age, is a conglomeration of unintended consequences. Longer lifespans led to longer work lives, greater stress, less time for self-care—such as a nourishing, home-made meal—and less societal patience for those who would "indulge" in such things as family over work. Our dependence on modern medicine has led us to abdicate responsibility for our own personal maintenance.

Our parents—and our grandparents even more so—ran their own kitchens, had their own workshops, and were generally more self-reliant. Medicine was originally rooted in nature, drawing on the healing powers of herbs, spices, and food. Both the Latin and Greek roots of the word *physician* relate to knowledge of nature, while the Latin word for "doctor" means "teacher." You've heard the phrase "Physician, heal thyself!" Most likely it was an admonition to physicians to inspire their patients to take care of themselves by setting a good example.

We are at a critical moment in terms of societal health. I'll be blunt: we've reached the top of this rollercoaster ride, and if we don't relearn how to really take care of ourselves, the plunge towards chronic illness is not only going to be steep, but will begin earlier in life. It's one thing to consider a long, vital life with a quick denouement, another to face the reality of ten, twenty, or thirty years or more of chronic impairments. It's already beginning; lifespans are on the verge of shortening, with obesity and type 2 diabetes now threatening the entire population, including the very young.

But this doesn't have to be our collective fate. With my long experience in the garden, I've devoted much of my professional life to educating people about how they can use great foods, *deliciously prepared*, to create a sense of well being that they can enjoy every day and nurture them across a lifetime. It is a philosophy that my colleague and kindred spirit, Rebecca Katz, embraces with her heart and soul, and whose essence is imprinted in every page of this inspiring, informative cookbook. Rebecca and her co-author, medical writer Mat Edelson, have delectably fused together a blend of taste and science that is irresistible to the palate and the mind.

Rebecca's enthusiasm is impossible to miss; it makes you want to jump over the countertop and get behind the stove. Reading this book, you get the very real sense that she's right beside you with a smile of encouragement. Those new to the kitchen will love her embracing style, while veteran home cooks—and I can say this, being one of them—will marvel at her easy-to-learn techniques to enhance taste and flavor.

In a time of crisis—the vast majority of Americans no longer know how to cook—Rebecca's book is literally a lifeline to longevity. It meets readers wherever they are along the cooking/nutrition spectrum. That's the key to creating a rapport. The delight in these pages is that for those who just want to eat delicious and healthy food, any recipe in this book will accomplish that. But inevitably, that first encounter will draw you in deeper. Believe me, the experience of your taste buds and the way your body feels after eating this way create a soul-level desire to know more. The information is all here, written in entertaining language accessible to both the layperson and wellness professional. I appreciate the depth of scientific information in this book—every ingredient's link to longevity and wellness is covered—and its presentation in a way that is incredibly accessible.

Rebecca has a phrase that encapsulates the message I've always used to encourage people to eat well. She says, "Great nourishing food and great taste *can* joyfully coexist at the dinner table." I say, "Good health begins in the kitchen." Life is too short—and eating too regular—to not make every meal both healthy and delicious. You can learn to live and thrive this way, throughout all your years.

All you have to do is peer inside this book.

Andrew Weil, MD
Tucson, Arizona

Acknowledgments

The Longevity Kitchen was graced by a community of people who gave fully of their time and talents to make this book all that it could be. Together we'd like to thank:

Andrew Weil, MD, you have our eternal gratitude and appreciation for your support and encouragement during this project and for your inspirational foreword.

Joseph Pizzorno, ND; Cynthia Geyer, MD; Colleen Fogarty Draper, MD, RD; Kathie Swift, MS, RD, LDN; Dale E. Bredesen, MD; Stephen Sinatra, MD; Jeanne Wallace, PhD; and Annemarie Colbin, PhD. We are blessed and grateful for your singular and cumulative expertise, which have informed and enhanced these pages.

Jeremy Katz, our wonderful agent and friend who provided savvy guidance during all aspects of this project, and his son Simon Katz for his inspiring culinary concoction.

Julie and Stan Burford, along with their pooch Josie. A huge culinary hug to all of you (and a special belly skritch for Josie) for buoying up Mat and myself with nourishing meals, wisdom, and a major dollop of moral support.

The fantastic folks at Ten Speed Press: talk about a dream team! We thank publisher Aaron Wehner and editorial director Julie Bennett for their dedication to this project; Melissa Moore, editor extraordinaire, for using her razor sharp editorial eye to sculpt the manuscript into its current form and for sheperding us through the editorial process with calm certainty; Chloe Rawlins for delivering yet another masterful and beautiful design; Toni Tajima for lending us her art director's keen eye during the photo shoot; Jasmine Star for her extraordinary copyediting; Jean Bloomquist, our proof reader, for crossing the T's and dotting the I's; Patricia Kelly, Michele Crim, Ali Slagle, and Ashley Matuzak for their sales and marketing expertise; and Kara Van de Water for her public relations wizardry.

So many people have told us how important beautiful photography is towards setting an uplifting tone. We are continuously smitten with the talents of photographer Leo Gong and his fantastic team, including food stylist Jen Straus, who created the beautiful, tantalizing, and sumptuous images that grace the pages of this book. You guys are amazing! Thanks also to Jen's assistant Alexa Hyman; Leo's wife, Harumi; and mascot Samantha the dachsund for support during the photo shoot.

If you've never heard of Gene Kranz, look him up; he brought safely home every NASA flight he directed. "Failure is not an option," was his motto, and that phrase, along with Gene's stern countenance gazing at us from a picture over our computers, gave us a muse we refused to mess with. Gene, we thank you.

REBECCA THANKS . . .

An homage to my kitchen crew including: Wendy Remer, baker *par excellence*, for digging deep into her bag of tricks to create her extraordinary confectionary contributions; Katie Biehler and Jen Dobbins, my kitchen angels, whose hard work, sense of humor, and positive attitude were essential ingredients in these recipes; Catherine McConkie, the oracle of taste, recipe tester, amazing teacher, and the most patient and gracious person I know; and Heidi Snyder, CHN, MS, NC, for her expert nutritional analysis that accompanies each recipe.

A huge thank you to my co-author Mat Edelson. This is our third book together and he continues to dazzle me with his ability to tell a story, whether it's about molecular biology or Mexican food! You are a brilliant writer no matter the genre.

A special acknowledgment to my Commonweal family: I continued to be amazed by your collective wisdom. Particular thanks to: Susan Braun for encouraging me to tap into my connections to the grandmothers who inspired me during my culinary journeys; Michael Lerner for continued support and guidance; Lenore Lefer, MS, MFCC, MFT, for her taste buds and nourishing wisdom; Waz Thomas for always being at the other end of the phone line with a sprinkle of love; Claire Heart, a true culinary alchemist; Sadja Greenwood, MD, for your science and sagacity; Rachael Remens, MD, Arlene Allsman, Kate Holcombe, Stuart Horance, Jhani Chapman, Irene Gallway, Elizabeth Evans, Jenepher Stowell, Mimi Mindel, and the rest of the Commonweal community for making it such a special and magical place for people to find healing.

Thank you to Jim Gordon, MD, founder and director of the Center for Mind Body Medicine; the staff and faculty of Food as Medicine; and Jo Cooper, dear friend, colleague, and my impresario. You are a treasure!

Thank you to recipe road testers, cheerleaders, and friends, including: Debra Cohen, Kathleen McDonough, Paul and Vicki Remer, Sandy and Harlan Kleiman, Genevieve Gutierrez, Fredi Kronenberg, Donald Abrams, MD, and Gerry Mullin, MD. Also to Cathryn Couch, founder of the Ceres Project; the ever-gracious Caroline Nation, founder of My Food My Health; Trudy Shafer, amazing chef; Eric Gower for being an enthusiastic eater and keeping my brain sharp with his incredible Breakaway Matcha; and my real BFF, Jill Leiner, for sharing many adventures and being a phone call and text away.

Super special thanks to my Ma, Barbara Katz, for her love and support throughout my journey—and her culinary expertise; my dad, Jay, for giving me his passion for food and compassion for people; my brother, Jeff, for his enthusiasm and great pep talks that helped me cross the finish line; my nephew and niece, Harry and Amelia, who are talented cooks in their own right; Bella, my muse and kitchen dog, who would do anything for a carrot or sweet potato; and my husband, Gregg Kellogg, for tasting every recipe many times over and making sure it was indeed good enough to be included in this book, for his patience and unwavering support for my work, and for always knowing when to deliver a necessary hug.

And finally, all my nourishing thoughts and gratitude to the readers, students, and teachers who have taught me along the way.

MAT THANKS . . .

Everyone who believes in writers, especially those with vested interests who (correctly) imagine there are far saner (but far less interesting) ways to make a living. Mom, Dad, you made it possible. I miss you both, every day. To my friends and family, your enjoyment of what I do, and the way I do it, makes making the donuts a whole lotta fun.

To Deb, your love and belief in me gives me strength; believe me, I can use it. Pea, you're a goofy puppy who gives me hours of joy. To everyone who spoke to me for this book, I reiterate what I've always said about interviews: if you have nothing to say, I have nothing to write. So, thanks for telling your tales . . . all of them. And, finally, to Bec, a cook who said she always knew how to pick a horse; you've taught me that picking the right oats (and preparing them properly) can really put some giddy-yup back in your step. Your work is making the world a better place, and I'm grateful to be part of it.

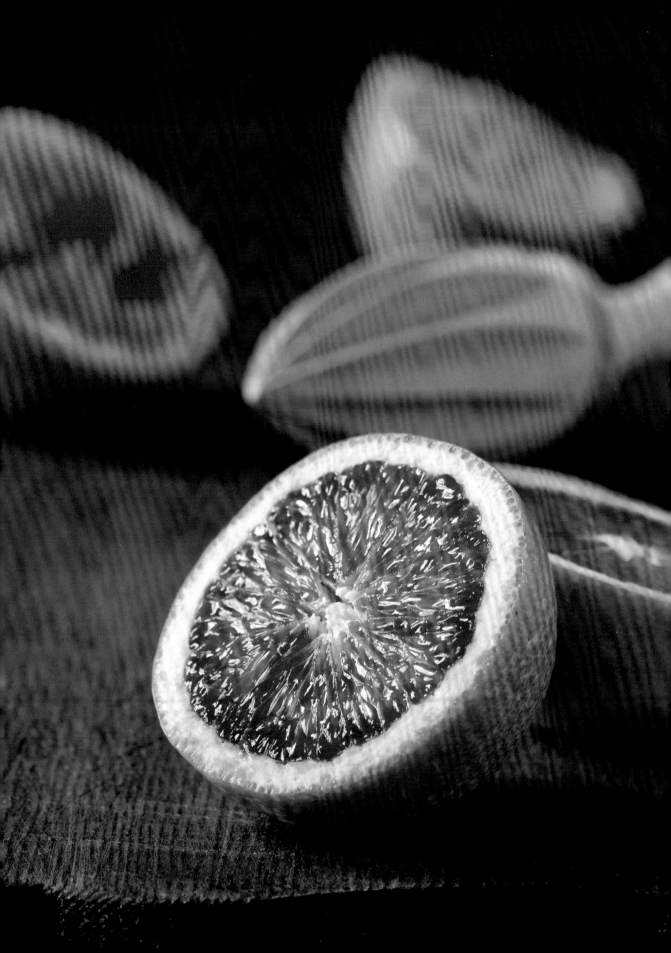

Introduction

I've spent more than a decade motivating people to eat well.

My primary tool has been flavor, as I showed people how great taste and great nutrition can joyfully coexist at the dinner table. Flavor is a fantastic, and usually essential, agent of dietary change. As a friend of mine says, "If something doesn't taste good, people won't eat it in the long run, no matter how good it is for them." All along, I knew that someday I'd have another incredibly powerful motivating force in my healing arsenal: science.

That day is here. As with any emerging field, the study of nutrition—particularly nutrition as related to longevity—has taken a few decades to reach critical mass. The fact that I'm able to now write about the links between food and longevity, relying not on speculation but on thousands of published scientific studies, gives me so much confidence that I'm practically bursting at the seams. It's as though scientists all over the world have confirmed what Grandma instinctively knew when she said, "Eat this. It's *good* for you."

It's clear to me that, as a society, we're embracing—or at least really curious about—living not just long lives, but long *healthy* lives, and doing so at least in part through the foods we eat. Just take a look at *New York Times* best-seller list over the last few years; numerous chart-busting books have delved into the topic, with writers traversing the globe in an effort to figure out why people who live in certain regions have significantly longer life spans. As it turns out, in many cases diet appeared to play a key role. While there are factors that go beyond food, including exercise, being active in the community, having a sense of purpose, and employing mind-body relaxation techniques to relieve stress, a great deal of research has looked into the interplay between food and the body. As a cook with a master's degree in nutrition, that synergy has always fascinated me.

I'll freely admit that it was flavor (and some heavenly smells) that first attracted me to the kitchen. I've been a cook since I used to sit on the kitchen countertop as a six-year-old, helping my mother make everything from brownies to soups. I remember that, even then,

I felt an instinctive sense of which foods were nourishing and which were more of an indulgence than good for me. And unlike many kids, I usually found that the most flavorful foods hit my "yes!" button. No one ever had to convince me to eat ripe wild Maine blueberries or broccoli, which I always thought looked like trees. Now, all these years later, it's extremely gratifying to hear scientists report that eating blueberries can also boost memory and broccoli can protect against cancer. Well, if you're going to twist my arm . . .

The truth is, I believe we're all born with an instinct that draws us toward the foods that nourish us best. That instinct probably evolved as a survival trait, but in modern times, many people have drifted away from this innate wisdom.

The Science of Yum!

Rest assured that I didn't rely on my kitchen-countertop wisdom for the information in this book. I spoke to numerous topflight physicians, nutritionists, and researchers who have delved deeply into the science of nutrition and longevity. Their knowledge informs every recipe—and just about word—in this book. After all, we can't truly understand how foods impact our health and wellness unless we utilize solid science, meaning rigorous, peer-reviewed studies.

If that sounds a bit dry, here's some delightful news: the most beneficial foods are those that many of us already know and love. (And if you don't love some of them now, I guarantee you will once you've tried them in the recipes in this book.) Consider what I call the Super Sixteen—foods that, nibble for nibble, offer the highest levels of antioxidants, those invaluable nutrients that help sweep the dangerous metabolic by-products known as free radicals out of the body. These ancient foods are also premier sources of healthy omega-3 fats, probiotics, and other body-boosting phytochemicals, vitamins, and minerals.

Perhaps not coincidentally, the Super Sixteen also contain a host of other health-promoting nutrients. So what are the Super Sixteen? Here they are, in alphabetical order:

- Asparagus
- Avocado
- Basil (and mint, which is in the same family)
- Blueberries (and other dark berries)
- Coffee
- Dark chocolate
- Garlic
- Green tea

- Kale
- Olive oil
- Pomegranates
- Sweet potatoes
- Thyme
- Walnuts
- Wild salmon
- Yogurt

Pretty surprising, isn't it? Contrary to popular opinion, eating the most nourishing foods isn't drudgery; rather, it will please your palate. Look at that list again. What do you see? Veggies, fruits, fish, nuts, herbs, and *chocolate*. Yes, you read that correctly: chocolate.

And that's just the top sixteen. Every ingredient you'll find in this book (well over two hundred of them) explodes with nutrition and flavor. Many of them, along with their benefits to the body, are listed in the Culinary Pharmacy (see page 21). As you peruse that section, you're likely to find that quite a few are already family and personal favorites. And if you've gotten out of the habit of cooking, that familiarity can serve as the hook for getting you back into the kitchen.

The Wisdom of Our Elders

Here's the issue in a nutshell: Every day I meet smart, motivated folks—people just like you, dear reader—who want to dive into eating well. They want to figure out how to turn the wealth of nutritional science into incredible meals, but they don't know where to start. Fortunately, I think I can provide a culinary clue: Instead of looking for some magic app or whiz-bang futuristic solution, like a meal-in-a-pill or a push-button Star Trek–type food replicator, I say we should seek the solution to our present culinary dilemma in the past. We need to consult our elders, the nanas who possess a lifetime of culinary wisdom.

It's great that science has evolved to the point where it can give us ten reasons why ginger is good for the digestive tract. But Grandma? Maybe she never got an advanced degree (not many did in the old country), but she knew that kids stopped complaining about their bellyaches when they downed a little ginger tea.

As you read and use this book, you'll see that I've sought out and presented traditional wisdom to complement the science and spice up laboratory results with the flavor of real-world knowledge. After all, science can't be the tail that wags the dog. I don't know about you, but I've never seen a list of phytochemicals that made me salivate.

To help you embrace getting behind the stove and get the most from this book, I've spoken to elders from noted longevity hotspots, including Okinawa, Greece, and Sweden, who hold generations of accrued cooking wisdom. They all grew up learning about cooking from *their* elders, usually women who saw food as something that connected their families to the earth and to wellness—a perspective that probably comes more naturally to those whose gardens and farms are their primary source of sustenance.

That ability to nurture, which can be learned and shared, is incredibly empowering. One woman I spoke with, Dorothy, told stories of her 102-year-old grandmother's reputation as a culinary healer. Every day brought another knock on the door or word of an injury or illness that needed tending. Her grandma would listen, nod sagely, and then toddle off to the stove. Before long, wonderful smells would fill the house, and eventually something soothing—homemade applesauce, strawberry and rhubarb compote, or hot tea made from cornhusks and laced with ginger and honey—would be placed in young Dorothy's hands, in a container with a bow tied around it and instructions tucked in. Her grandmother might say, "Take this to Miss Constance across the street and tell her I'll be right over," and then gently turn the youngster's shoulder toward the door with a weathered hand.

All of us have such memories in which we can see food in that healing light, and we can draw on them when we need to. For Dorothy, eating well became especially important in times of stress—something she knew plenty about because of her job as a police chief. Long hours, lousy coffee, and poor eating came with the territory. She couldn't do much about the first two, but she refused to put up with bad food, for herself or her staff. Every time a tough case had her detectives tied up in knots, she brought in home-cooked meals. That's what I call a morale booster! And after she retired, she took up where her grandmother left off, making meals for the chronically ill and serving her "joy tea" to all of her visitors.

I've felt a similar connection and reconnection with the healing power of food, thanks to a number of grandmothers. I emphasize reconnection here because, like many Americans, when I was younger I fell into eating on the run and other poor dietary habits. My return to the kitchen wasn't planned; it was a fortuitous side effect of traveling to Italy, where I'd arranged to stay with an Italian *nonna*, Signoria Rizzo, who took in borders. I think I was more (or less) than she bargained for. She didn't speak English, and I spoke only a smattering of Italian, but when she encountered me in the kitchen, the message in her pitying eyes needed no translation: *This one can't even cook pasta.*

But instead of casting me aside as hopeless, she took me on as her science project. I became an Eliza Doolittle of sorts, but instead of having to sing or balance books on my head, I had to learn to cook. After all, from Signora Rizzo's old-world perspective, that was essential if I was ever to snare a husband. Of course, learning to cook well also meant learning to shop, and in Italy that means daily trips to the market. I was suddenly part of a posse: Signora Rizzo, a half dozen of her white-haired friends, and me. Harpo Marx would have been proud: using only pantomime, Signora Rizzo showed me how to feel up (there's really no other word for it) every piece of produce in the market. In her eyes, this wasn't a luxury; it was an economic necessity. Who had the money to waste on bad produce? At first, her friends just stood back and tut-tutted at me, the waif who had stumbled into Signora Rizzo's life. But over time—and a lot of meals—I won their confidence and found mine.

I tell you all of this for a reason. Learning to eat for longevity, and moving toward cooking healthfully (and deliciously), is a gradual process, and it benefits from positive reinforcement. It happens on almost a subconscious level. It can be really helpful to begin with foods you already enjoy, like the Super Sixteen. It's easier to use a new ingredient, say an herb or spice, when it's combined with a food you naturally crave. I know I'm always more willing to go out on a limb and try something new when the foundation is familiar fare.

As you become more conscious about your food choices, you'll discover a growing awareness of the connection between what you eat and how well you feel. That's what happened to me in Italy. The healthy, life-enhancing way of eating I'd been exposed to was expansive and exhilarating. It was a gift from the *nonnas*, who asked but one thing in return: that I share this gift with others.

Okay, they didn't actually ask that, but their way of life spoke volumes. They lived to pass on their culinary expertise, including their wisdom about the connections between food and longevity. It was perhaps the greatest treasure they possessed, and passing that torch represented an initiation into the responsibility of caring not just for oneself, but also for one's family and community.

I took their message, and their methods, to heart. When I returned home, I began cooking for others, often people who were dealing with chronic illness. Many of them suffered from cancer and had understandably grown fearful of eating due to treatment side effects. Others who were dealing with lifestyle-related diseases such as diabetes, heart disease, and autoimmune diseases had been put on restricted diets but still craved certain flavors. I began acting in a role I later came to call "culinary translator"—figuring out people's needs and then giving them healthful, delicious whole food meals that left them feeling nourished.

Over the last decade, through thousands of hours of conversation with colleagues and clients, and after writing my two previous books, I've honed my knowledge and streamlined the process of creating healthful meals. And with the growing interest in eating for longevity, it made sense to create a book that translated my experience, all of the incredible scientific findings, and the wealth of traditional wisdom into delicious, healthful meals that anyone can make and share. As you read through and use this book, I hope you'll feel as though a friendly, helpful presence is with you in your kitchen, offering ideas, support, and advice— perhaps a grandmother whose greatest wish for you is a long, healthy, happy life.

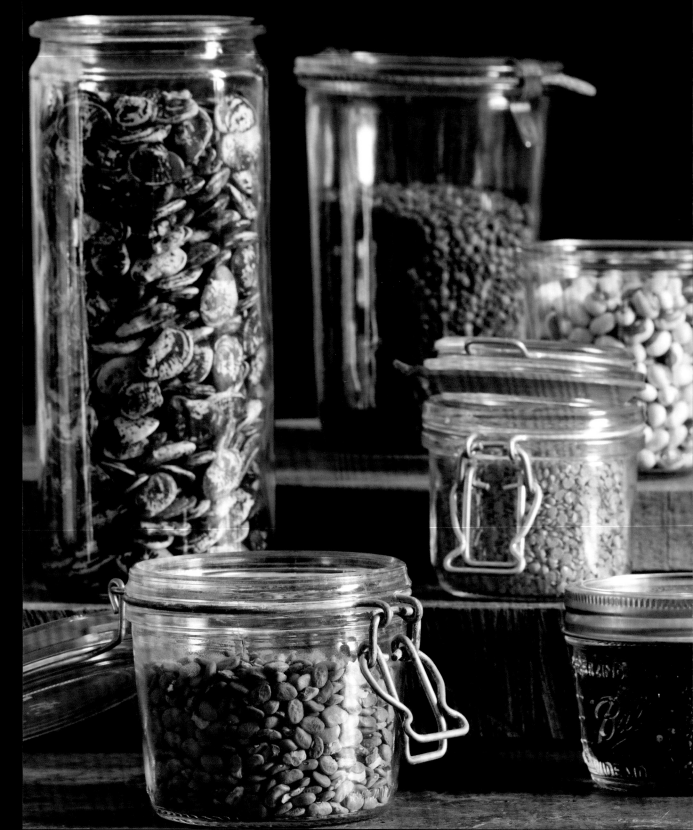

CHAPTER 1

Food, Nutrition, and Your Body

I want to take you on an incredible journey, one that involves every cell in your body and every fiber of that most magical of creatures: you.

When I first started cooking seriously, many of my fellow cooks and other colleagues in the field of wellness had the notion that great-tasting food exploding with nutrients could also act as medicine—something we believed based on our own upbringing and the way so many cultures use food for healing (hello, chicken soup!). But even though this wasn't so long ago, we didn't have much science to back up our belief.

Now we do. Since the 1980s, the number of nutritional studies published in peer-reviewed science journals has doubled each decade. In all, serious researchers at the top academic medical centers in the United States and around the world have published nearly *250,000* nutritional studies, including more than 100,000 since the turn of the millennia. From my stove-front viewpoint, this means I can point to almost any food and know that someone with a long string of credentials has studied how that food affects health and specific body systems, from head to toe, inside and out.

All of this information is empowering and allows us to more confidently choose delicious, nutritious foods that can give us a great deal of control over our well-being and, ultimately, our longevity. Do these foods *have* to be delicious? You bet. Because, as mentioned in the introduction, no matter how healthful certain foods are, if they aren't scrumptious, you won't make a habit of eating them.

I know people like playing favorable odds. And I know that you're probably wondering whether eating well can guarantee that you'll live to be a centenarian. Maybe, maybe not. But what is almost assuredly guaranteed (and backed up by science) is that no matter where you or your family are on the health continuum, what you choose to put on your plate can both improve your quality of life and extend your years.

If you're healthy to begin with, eating the right foods will keep your cellular energy high and immune system strong, helping stave off the inevitable decline of these systems due to the aging process. And if you're healthy but your family history of illness has your brow furrowed like a shar-pei's, here's a startling fact that should act like mental Botox: your genes are not necessarily your destiny. The foods you eat can affect genetic expression, the signaling process that determines which segments of DNA are translated into substances in the body. Put more simply, gene expression tells your cells what to do, like build a protein, and when to do it. Certain foods may actually inhibit the same cellular triggers that, when turned on, may have caused particular diseases in your parents, grandparents, and other family members.

But even if you or someone you care about is seriously ill, nutrition can help. The right foods can work wonders, from jump-starting the process of generating healthy cells to replacing those that are damaged or diseased to reducing the side effects of medications and improving the body's ability to detoxify medications once they've done their job.

I often conduct workshops teaching people how to reconnect with healthy foods. It thrills me to know that while I'm grabbing them by the taste buds and watching their hands create foods that make their voices sigh with pleasure, I can fill their minds with example after example of how specific foods can nourish all of their cells, organs, tissues, and other physiological systems that keep their bodies purring with contentment. That's exactly what I'm going to do in the next two chapters: show you many of the delectable connections between outstanding flavors, power-packed nutrition, and longevity. Think of it as a starting point for a culinary adventure, connecting the dots between the wonderful recipes you'll find later in the book, the delicious foods that lend them their flavors, the beneficial nutrients that abound in those foods, and their life- and health-enhancing effects.

Where to start? To understand how foods affect the body, you first need to have a good understanding of how the body works, and especially how it metabolizes food. So let's start there: with some basic information about the body's systems.

In the Beginning

When you got your start in life, you were just a single cell whose only job was to go forth and multiply. Congratulate yourself on a job well done, because at this point you consist of 100 *trillion* cells supporting ten major organ systems.

Talk about management issues! The list of nutrients the body needs to function is enormous, from macronutrients (carbs, proteins, and fats) to vitamins, minerals, and a long list of phytochemicals (beneficial compounds in fruits and veggies) from anthocyanidins to zeaxanthin. Yet somehow, for a hundred thousand years, humans got by on whatever they could forage and their bodies did a phenomenal job of adapting to whatever fuel was available.

We've come a long way from our hunter-gatherer days, and in recent decades the science of nutrition has proliferated almost as wildly as the cells in your body have since the moment of conception. In fact, that's really where we need to start: with a brief overview of the science—and specifically the science of the processes that led from your first day as a single cell to the marvelous complexity of you, in this moment, reading this book: epigenetics.

Epigenetics

The truth is, for all the studies out there on nutrition, few are focusing on investigating whether a single food or nutrient can lengthen life. The reason is simple: reality is complex. Numerous variables impact human longevity, from our genes (about twenty-five thousand of them!) to the complex environment in which those genes function and interact. For better or worse, everything in that environment, from the foods we eat to the air we breathe to the songs we sing (think stress, or the lack thereof) affects our genes, playing a role in how long we live.

The emerging field of science called epigenetics studies the factors affecting genetic expression. Although genes are the colorful fabric of our being, that fabric doesn't weave itself. Our genes are the raw material waiting, indeed, wanting, to be woven by a host of cellular processes that direct genetic behavior. Those processes determine everything from protein production to cell differentiation. They are the marching orders that say to a stem cell, "You: Go to the brain and think" versus "You: Go to the spine and feel." When you add in the fact that we're all genetically different, the idea that any single nutrient could somehow navigate and heal our unique variabilities and vulnerabilities is clearly far-fetched. There's a reason why Ponce de León never found his fountain of youth.

In any case, given that we haven't found a magic food that heals the entire body, what have we discovered? A lot. About ten years ago, we finally managed to map all of the genes in the human genome. Along the way, we've learned that almost every process in the human body, including the creation of most disease states, involves the interplay of anywhere from three to more than a dozen genes. Damage to any of those genes can wreak havoc on the entire process. It's like going to a square dance, constantly rotating partners throughout the dance to keep things humming along smoothly. Now imagine what would happen if you were to slip on a banana peel—or, more aptly, the wrapper from some sort of sugar-laden junk food: the do-si-do could quickly devolve into a do-si-don't.

Eventually, we'll tease out the interplay within these complex relationships and learn how to work the produce aisle to restore order on a systems level. But for now, we're making some good inroads. As researchers have learned more and more of the genetic, metabolic, and cellular causes of disease, they've also figured out which nutrients can turn those processes around. Take cancer, which is essentially uncontrolled cell growth. Somewhere, the numerous genetic signals that say, "Hey, cells, stop dividing!" have gotten turned off. For a long time, conventional wisdom has held that once those signals were short-circuited and tumor growth started, diet couldn't do much to impact the process.

Au contraire. Jeanne Wallace, PhD, an authority in integrative cancer nutrition notes that when a person transitions from what nutritionists euphemistically call a SAD diet (an acronym for the standard American diet, dominated by highly processed foods) toward a whole food diet featuring healthy fats, complex carbs, and veggies (particularly cruciferous vegetables) that critical signaling process seems to kick back in. She says that, when people make such changes, "if we do an analysis looking at hundreds of genes, we can see four hundred to five hundred oncogenes, the genes responsible for causing cancer, being turned off within a short period."

Wallace goes on to say, "One thing I've learned from my field that's really stood out for me is that the foods we eat communicate with our genes, and we're able through our food choices to alter our gene expression. This is surprising for most laypeople, who think you're just stuck with the genetic luck of the draw that you got when your parents gave birth to you. We've learned that this is *not* true. The expression of those inherited genes can be changed." This is just one example of the many ways in which the work we do in the kitchen can have wonderful health-promoting effects. And when you consider how delicious those foods can be, that definitely isn't a bitter pill to swallow.

So, with that introduction to how you came to be you, as you are in this moment, and how you can use food to influence who you become in the future (hopefully a very long future), let's take a look at various physiological systems within the body and how foods can influence them for good or ill. I'm going to start with some unsung heroes: the gut, liver, and kidneys.

The Gut, Liver, and Kidneys

Although the brain and the heart are always stealing the spotlight, I think the gut, liver, and kidneys should come first in any discussion of longevity. Maybe they just need a better public relations agent. Just think about it: if you don't keep your body's intake and waste management operations in tip-top shape, all the other organs will be seriously compromised. It's kind of like worrying about your car's brakes when you've got a blocked fuel line and a potato up the tailpipe. Forget the brakes, because the car simply won't run. No fuel (energy) in + no exhaust (toxins) out = no go, whether you're talking about cars or people.

The Gut

The gut, or digestive system, is where food is taken in, moved along, and broken down; nutrients are absorbed; and solids are collected for elimination. It's an incredibly long and complex system that starts at your mouth and travels through some thirty feet of gut before reaching the final frontier. It takes a sophisticated brain to control such a system, and thank goodness you have one—only it's not in your head. Located in the gut itself, it's called the enteric nervous system. ("Enteric" is just a fancy way of saying that it's centered in the intestines.) The enteric nervous system coordinates all of the gut's business.

Neurobiologist Michael Gershon, of Columbia University, refers to this Grand Central Station of digestive decision making as the second brain, and with good reason: there are as many nerve cells in the gut as in the brain, and the gut is home to many of the same neurotransmitters, as well.

You've probably heard about serotonin, a neurotransmitter that plays a role in mood, among other things. Serotonin is found in abundance in the gut, possibly to let the brain know when the belly's happy—and when it's not.

Serotonin is produced with the help of foods rich in vitamin B$_6$ (sweet potatoes and broccoli), omega-3s (wild salmon and halibut), and tryptophan (shrimp and asparagus). In a very real sense, serotonin may play an important role in keeping us connected to food, in terms of that "gut sense" of what we need to both feel nourished and *be* nourished.

How does this play into longevity? There's evidence that serotonin levels drop as we get older. Lower serotonin levels inhibit body signaling between the stomach and the brain, so the body keeps asking for a certain food it needs, but there's not enough serotonin to deliver the message to the brain clearly. (Why do I see a cartoon of sad-faced signaling molecules in my stomach looking upward and pleading, "Can you hear me now?") Keeping serotonin levels high could boost the overall signal between the two nervous systems and help maintain the balance of nutrients the body needs as a result. It may also play a role in easing some forms of irritable bowel syndrome, since serotonin helps signal muscles to move food farther down the line.

Another point of potential tummy turmoil involves hydrochloric acid, or HCl. You might remember HCl from high school chemistry class. Maybe your teacher made you dress up like a mad scientist just to handle the stuff because it's so powerfully corrosive.

When we're young, our stomachs are full of HCl, which helps break down food. But HCl levels decline as we age. As a result, the stomach may pass along food that's still too intact for optimum absorption, depriving us of vital nutrients. The culprit may be the bacteria *Helicobacter pylori*, which also causes ulcers. *H. pylori* multiplies like wayward bunnies when we don't get enough vitamin C. That massive bacterial growth spurt is what impairs HCl production, but what's cool is that food can help reverse the process.

Joseph Pizzorno, a naturopath who has served on medical advisory boards for presidents Bill Clinton and George W. Bush, says "500 milligrams of vitamin C will stop the overgrowth of *H. pylori* and, over time, promote rebuilding of the stomach lining, which helps people produce hydrochloric acid again."

As you read through this book, you'll find plenty of other examples of delicious foods that enhance gut health. But for now, let's keep this train rolling and move on to the liver and kidneys.

The Liver and Kidneys

The liver and kidneys do much of the heavy lifting of removing environmental toxins from our bodies. Their burden often becomes greater as we age, in part because they're called upon to metabolize medications, which we tend to use more often as we get older.

The liver detoxes in two phases. I won't go into the (very, very) technical details, but the key is the liver breaks down toxins—everything from pesticides to the caffeine in your morning cup of joe—and converts them into water-soluble molecules so they can be flushed from your system rather than being stuck to certain fats in your tissues and possibly staying in your body for years, wreaking havoc along the way. If the detox process is efficient, the toxins roll merrily along through the body's liquid waterways, exiting most often as either urine or bile.

There are plenty of nutrients that keep the liver and body happy, including one that you may not expect: fiber. Some of the final products of detoxification are heavy metals that mostly came from the environment. If everything is working right, those heavy metals hitch a ride out of the body with dietary fiber. But as Joseph Pizzorno notes, "If you look at our evolutionary diet, we had 100 to 150 grams of fiber daily. Now, we typically consume 10 grams. We've always been exposed to heavy metals, and the body evolved a way to get rid of them, but changing our diet made that mechanism much less effective."

By consuming more fiber, which is abundant in foods such as whole grains, beans, berries, dark leafy greens, other crunchy vegetables, and herbs like cilantro and parsley, we help our bodies haul out the liver's metabolic trash, leaving our insides cleansed.

Another important role that certain foods play is hydration. Studies show that the more water we drink, the better the kidneys flush numerous metabolic by-products. And therein lies a dilemma. I meet so many people who feel like they're hydration failures, unable to chug their way through the half gallon of water a day we need for optimal health. But where is it written that all that water has to come from straight-up water, which not everyone enjoys? There are wonderful, delicious, hydrating foods that can supplement your H_2O habit, such as broths and smoothies, and beverages like green teas. Believe me, your kidneys will be just as thrilled, and you'll get a nutritional boost, as well.

The Brain

These days, many people fear the potential mental decline that comes with aging even more than physical decline, and with good reason, given the growing epidemic of Alzheimer's disease. Memory impairment is a huge issue, as it can drastically affect both quality and length of life. Fortunately, many nutrients can help keep your mind razor sharp, most notably omega-3 fatty acids, found in foods ranging from flaxseeds and walnuts to cold-water fish.

While the link between omega-3 consumption and brain health is common knowledge these days, it turns out that other nutritional factors may also play a major role in the development of Alzheimer's disease, as indicated by some fascinating research doctor Dale Bredesen brought to my attention. Bredesen, an expert on neurodegenerative diseases at the University of California, San Francisco and the Buck Institute for Research on Aging, has been looking at the mechanisms of neurodegeneration. He notes that people with type 2 diabetes (the type associated with obesity and a poor diet) have twice the risk of getting Alzheimer's, noting that the risk increases anytime insulin, which breaks down blood sugar, is at elevated levels.

Here's a possible link: if you look at the brain of someone with Alzheimer's, you'll find large concentrations of the protein beta-amyloid. Beta-amyloid is broken down and flushed out of the brain with the help of an enzyme—the very same enzyme that breaks down insulin (which is why it's called insulin-degrading enzyme). But there's only so much insulin-degrading enzyme to go around in the body, so if your insulin levels are chronically high, the brain may suffer the consequences.

Here the food fix is twofold: move away from consuming refined carbs like sugar, white rice, white bread, and white pasta, and eat more fiber-rich foods, such as whole grains, beans, and dark leafy greens. The complex carbohydrates in these foods release their sugars into the body more slowly and evenly, and their fiber can help slow the absorption of sugar, both of which help keep insulin levels from spiking.

Bredesen also says that moving toward unsaturated fats, like olive oil, can help lower levels of LDL cholesterol, which can decrease the odds of getting Alzheimer's. And the cook in me just loves the facts that spices such as curcumin and turmeric may have protective effects as well—just one more testimony to the power of yum.

The Heart

Among the plethora of findings on the heart, which is perhaps the most researched organ, are some incredible long-term studies that have linked dietary factors with heart disease. The tenets of good heart health are so well-known they can be chanted like a mantra: "HDL good. LDL bad. Triglycerides low. Aerobic exercise high."

Mantras are great, but action is even better, which is why I always promote foods such as black beans, nuts, seeds, and wild salmon, which can help prevent heart disease. (Diet can help with three out of four of the factors in the mantra; you're on your own when it comes to taking a good walk.) But what if you've already developed heart disease? Is there any solution other than going on a slew of medications? Can food help reverse the illness and stave off a life-threatening situation?

According to Stephen Sinatra, MD, the answer is an unequivocal yes. Sinatra is an integrative cardiologist who uses nutrition as part of his healing arsenal. He practices what he calls metabolic cardiology, using nutrition to boost cardiac efficiency at the cellular level, with a focus on mitochondria.

Mitochondria are organelles within our cells that produce the cell's energy, just like power plants crank out electricity, except the energy mitochondria produce comes in the form of adenonsine triphosphate (ATP). But if the heart is damaged—as in congestive heart failure, a progressive disease in which the heart beats of out of sync, greatly impairing blood flow—the cause may be malfunctioning mitochondria. It's like a six-cylinder car trying to run on five cylinders, then four, and eventually just a cylinder or two. When that happens, less ATP is produced, and according to Sinatra, "ATP is what restores cells. All the cells in the heart can replace themselves one or two times, possibly more in a lifetime. That's why people with advanced heart disease can live for years—if you give them nutritional support to strengthen the mitochondria."

Sinatra uses what he calls the Awesome Foursome of nutrients as the base for such support: coenzyme Q_{10} (found in wild salmon, cauliflower, and oranges), carnitine (found in grass-fed red meat, sardines, and pistachios), D-ribose (found in yogurt and mushrooms), and magnesium (found in halibut, buckwheat, and artichokes). He also suggests foods rich in vitamins C and E, omega-3s, and alpha-lipoic acid (found in broccoli and spinach).

"When you build ATP, you buy time for the intrinsic stem cells within the heart to take over," says Sinatra, mirroring something I've always said about spending time in the kitchen making health-promoting foods: how many things do you make time for that actually end up giving you *more* time back in return?

The Bones and Muscles

Along with the skin, the bones and muscles may be the parts of the body that most visibly tell us things ain't what they used to be. We literally begin to disappear with age: starting at about age thirty, muscle mass begins to drop by around 1 percent per year, and losses in bone density often start appearing around age forty. In fact, a report on bone health and osteoporosis from the US Surgeon General noted that "by 2020, half of all Americans will have weak bones unless we make changes to our diet and lifestyle. . . . The bad news is that few people follow the steps known to strengthen and protect their bones."

When confronted with these stats, a lot of people, especially women, worry about hip fractures, partially because these injuries often have such dire consequences. From a longevity viewpoint, that misses the bigger picture, one that revolves around our definition of frailty. From a medical perspective, frailty is that point on life's see-saw when you can no longer bounce back from injury or illness and instead begin what is all too often a quick decline.

Researchers are finding that keeping our muscles and bones strong can help us stay vital and further away from our personal "frailty point" even as we advance into our seventies, eighties, and beyond. So be sure to eat foods that help maintain strong and healthy bones (such as kale and chicken) and muscles (such as eggs and salmon). It's also important to engage in resistance training, such as weight lifting, even if only with very light weights.

The Immune System

Discussing the immune system gives me a great opportunity to talk about antioxidants. Many cellular processes, including those of the immune system, create a certain amount of waste, some of it in the form of free radicals. If these highly reactive substances aren't neutralized, they can do some nasty things, including trigger overactivation of immune cells, burning out those cells prematurely. The immune response also causes inflammation, which is now thought to be a precursor to many conditions, including cardiovascular disease and cancer. Abundant free radicals keeping the immune system in constant four-alarm fire mode could be at least partially to blame for the increasing incidence of these diseases.

This may be why immune cells tend to carry around lots of antioxidants. If you aren't familiar with them, their name suggests their role: they're sort of like a protection posse, picking off predatory free radicals and preventing them from doing damage. That brings me to glutathione, which noted physician Mark Hyman called "the mother of all antioxidants, the master detoxifier and maestro of the immune system" in his *Huffington Post* blog.

Joseph Pizzorno agrees: "People who live the longest are the most effective at producing glutathione in the body. Certain diets will promote the production of glutathione. People on diets rich in cysteine, which is found in whey, will produce more glutathione and have more longevity." Beyond whey (the watery part of milk), foods rich in cysteine, one of the three amino acids that make up glutathione, include egg yolks, asparagus, avocados, and garlic. Those foods are sort of like Pac-Man: chasing down and devouring the free radical goblins.

The Respiratory System

It's a good thing I was just talking about antioxidants, because they're also key to good respiratory health. The science on optimal lung function and nutrition is still emerging, but what is known is that environmental toxins, either those all around you or those self-imposed (that is, via smoking) can greatly deplete antioxidants and other key nutrients, potentially leaving the lungs vulnerable to a range of diseases, including asthma, emphysema, chronic obstructive pulmonary disease (COPD), and cancer.

According to an analysis of numerous nutrition and lung health studies in the journal *Proceedings of the Nutrition Society*, "Epidemiological studies suggest that dietary habits may have an influence on lung function and the tendency to common lung diseases. . . . In particular, a diet rich in fresh fruit and fish has been associated with a salutary effect on lung health."

All in all, this seems like a pretty solid argument for eating nutrient-dense meals (and that's all you'll find in this book, where I make every calorie count), as well as keeping up your intake of antioxidants, especially vitamin C, which is abundant in bell peppers, papayas, and strawberries. One huge study followed over a thousand people, both smokers and non-smokers, and found that both groups had better lung function when they consumed fruit regularly. So let's hear it for a kiwi a day!

The Circulatory System

If you thought the gut was long at thirty feet, think again. The circulatory system is really long—really, really, *really* long, as in 60,000 miles long. That's even longer than the US Interstate Highway system (47,182 miles, last I checked). Keeping all of those circulatory byways clear and flowing is a full-time job, and we can do our dietary part by keeping our overall cholesterol, and especially our LDL, or bad cholesterol, low.

People tend to focus on the relationship between circulation and the heart, but there are other areas where circulation can impact longevity. Peripheral arterial disease, caused by obstruction of arteries in the extremities (primarily the legs) ups the risk of heart attack and stroke. The restriction of blood flow causes pain and potentially life-threatening blood clots. As you might have guessed, peripheral arterial disease becomes more common after age fifty—and as you also might have guessed, we can use food to fight this disease.

According to a study in the *Journal of Nutrition*, a combination of certain omega-3 fatty acids in fish oil and other nutrients helped dilate blood vessels and inhibit clotting, which could increase blood flow through the arteries. The researchers included the fish oil in a shake, along with oleic acid, folic acid, vitamin B_6, and vitamin E. Personally, I'd rather eat things like avocados (for oleic acid and vitamin B_6), crunchy romaine lettuce (for folic acid), and almonds (for vitamin E). But be that as it may, the results of the study were promising: in addition to lowered cholesterol levels, those who consumed the super shake could walk two and a half times farther before they felt leg pain, suggesting that their arteries had become more pliant, allowing the blood to flow more freely. That's enough to make me do my happy dance.

The Nervous System

The nervous system is more than just the brain and spine. It branches off repeatedly and extends to the farthest reaches of our limbs. There, peripheral nerves create a constant feedback loop that helps us place ourselves properly in time and space. Imagine what it would be like to weave your way down a crowded city sidewalk without your nerves constantly sensing where, *exactly*, the sidewalk is. Thank goodness we don't have to continuously look at our feet when we're walking. These same nerves warn us when we're too close to damaging cold or heat and allow us to feel the pleasure of a caress or apply just the right pressure to insert a contact lens.

Keeping these nerves in tip-top shape isn't something we should take for granted. A major player in peripheral nerve health is vitamin B_{12}. The University of Chicago's Center for Peripheral Neuropathy notes that a B_{12} deficiency "damages the myelin sheath that surrounds and protects nerves." In a way, nerves are like electrical lines, and the myelin sheath is akin to insulation of those lines. When the sheathing breaks down, electrical signals get disrupted. The result is peripheral neuropathy, which can cause problems ranging from tingling digits to pain to weakness and heightened fall risk.

The Endocrine System

The hormones in our bodies are primarily produced by eight different glands, known as endocrine glands. Hormones are the master regulators of our physiological functions, and range from thyroxine, which the thyroid gland churns out to increase metabolic rate, to somatotropin, or human growth hormone, which the pituitary gland produces to initiate growth spurts.

In terms of longevity, I'd like to talk about a hormone you're very familiar with, though you might not have known that it's a hormone: insulin. It's produced deep inside the pancreas, by endocrine cells with the coolest name in biology: the islets of Langerhans (which actually sounds more like a misty destination somewhere off the Scottish coast).

Our bodies have a love-hate relationship with insulin. It helps remove excess sugar from the bloodstream, escorting it to the liver and muscles and fat tissue to be stored as glycogen for later use. But if you dump too much sugar into the bloodstream too often and too quickly, insulin resistance can result. Then the excess sugar stays in the system and damages numerous tissues (notably the blood vessels), increasing the risk of a host of potentially life-shortening conditions, including diabetes.

Good eating habits can go a long way toward preventing insulin resistance from developing. First, as discussed in regard to Alzheimer's, replacing sugar and refined carbs with complex carbs and whole grains works wonders. Whole foods contain sugars too, but they're generally packaged with fiber, as in a whole apple versus apple juice. If sugar is a slalom skier, fiber is the moguls that pepper the course, slowing the sugar in its race from the mouth to the bloodstream. When sugars are released into the bloodstream gradually, there's less demand for large quantities of insulin in a short period of time.

If blood sugar is an issue for you or someone you care about, you may be familiar with the glycemic index, a chart that estimates how the carbohydrates in given foods will affect blood sugar levels. Glycemic load provides information that's a bit more useful, as it takes into account the quantity of given foods that are typically eaten. However, I prefer to take an overall look at the total amount of carbohydrates, protein, fat, and fiber in a meal. After all, we seldom eat foods in isolation. Sure, carrots are rather sweet and rate high on the glycemic index. But don't let that scare you away from eating them. If you include a modest amount of carrots in a salad with dark leafy greens, olive oil, lemon juice, fish, and some nuts sprinkled on top, the fiber in the greens and the fats in the olive oil and nuts will slow the release of the carrots' sugar into the bloodstream. Therefore, the glycemic load for the overall meal will be very low. I wouldn't want you to miss out on the benefits of a nutrient-rich and delicious carrot because of misplaced fear.

The Next Phase of the Journey

I hope you've enjoyed this brief tour of the body. And I know you're chomping (literally!) at the bit to get cooking. But before you dive into the recipes later in the book, there's another piece of the puzzle that's worth exploring: the delectable foods that deserve a place in every longevity kitchen. The next chapter will explore dozens of the most nutritious and healing ingredients in this book and describe their health benefits.

CHAPTER 2

The Healing Power of Food

During our tour of the body in chapter 1, you saw many examples of how specific nutrients can supercharge your health.

At this point, you may be wondering, "Why bother with seeking out the most nutritious foods and doing a bunch of this cooking? Why not just pop a supplement and be done with it?" It all comes down to the value of team play.

Why Balanced Nutrition Is a Team Sport

The interactions of the nutrients within a single food tend to make individual nutrients easier for the body to access. One theory about why this is so is that life nourishes life. Foods are components of complex living entities that require, and therefore contain, a broad spectrum of nutrients to survive, just as we do.

A case in point is beta-carotene. Diets rich in beta-carotene have been shown to fight cancer, yet in at least one study, beta-carotene supplements had the opposite effect. Cynthia Geyer, medical director at the renowned Canyon Ranch health spa in Lenox, Massachusetts, thinks she knows why: "Beta-carotene doesn't exist in food on its own. There are all kinds of carotenoids—at least seven, aside from beta-carotene. It's their synergy together that probably has the disease-fighting impact," says Geyer.

Another potential factor is the unique assemblage of nutrients in each foodstuff. So, while many foods contain vitamin C, for example, perhaps you can get all the vitamin C you need from a bell pepper, whereas my body might assimilate it better from broccoli, due to differences in our individual genetics and how we each digest foods and absorb nutrients. This is also the best argument I've heard for eating a varied diet. It's another way of tilting the odds in your favor. Since the science hasn't yet evolved to let any of us know for sure what our ideal foods are for getting the nutrients we need, bringing a variety of foods to the table will not only keep everyone's taste buds dancing, but also up the chances that each person gets the nutrients they need.

There are times when supplements are necessary or helpful, but given that I am, first and foremost, a cook, whenever possible, I lean toward delicious foods to provide life-enhancing nutrients. I think this stance is actually pretty objective, and my conversations with various doctors and nutritionists supports that. Many of them recommend supplements primarily as a stopgap measure on the road to healthier eating. Cindy Geyer says, "The more I do this, the more I come back to foods. If I have a client who is very symptomatic due to a severe nutrition deficiency, I may start with supplements first, just to help them feel better, but it's always a stopgap until we get them on more nutritious foods."

Colleen Fogarty Draper, MS, RD, an expert in nutrigenomics (the interplay of genes and nutrition), agrees. She sees food as the most efficient way to get nutrients into the system: "You've got all these bioactive compounds in foods that likely enhance the absorption of any individual nutrient. Our foods are already their own recipes. Imagine placing just one nutrient in the body. It's like having just one flavor to eat. It's not satisfying for you to eat and it's not statisftying for the body to absorb."

Why Whole Foods Are Great Team Players

As my wonderful mentor Annemarie Colbin has often said, if you want to find out why people live a long time, just ask a bunch of seriously seasoned citizens what they've spent a lifetime eating. Colbin has done just that, and along the way she's developed a number of fascinating theories on food and longevity, which she's brought to the hugely influential school she founded in 1977, the Natural Gourmet Institute for Health and Culinary Arts.

Looking at both science and culture around the world, Colbin, who has a PhD in holistic nutrition, was convinced that the interplay of numerous whole foods in the body is key to long-term health. In her view, these food synergies, orchestrated by seasonal shifts that keep an ever-fresh, ever-changing tapestry of nutrition within arm's reach, yield sustainable and nourishing results.

I couldn't agree more. My entire cooking philosophy is aligned with Annemarie's. It might be summed up like this: Go to the market, grab the best-looking food, hopefully freshest from the farmer's field, make it taste great, and enjoy the repeat business. Today we call this a whole food diet, but Grandma used to just call it "dinner."

Our species nourished itself in this way for millennia. Isn't it telling that only now, after we've gotten so far away from eating thoughtful, well-balanced, whole food meals, so many chronic diseases are flourishing? This epidemic of illness (and epidemic really is the operative word) has finally lit a fire under scientists to investigate how foods heal.

Eventually, science will catch up, and I'll be able to tell you exactly why, for example, roasted butternut squash goes so well with dark leafy greens laced with garlic and walnuts toasted with cumin and coriander, and how those three components synergize to super-charge the absorption of vital nutrients that can extend both our life span and our "health span." (In the meanwhile, you can taste the delicious results if you make the recipe for Swiss Chard and Roasted Butternut Squash Tart, on page 112.) All the pieces of this jigsaw puzzle are slowly coming together, and it thrills me. But does it surprise me? No, not really. I am first and foremost a cook. I've seen the joy and sense of wellness that delicious, health-ful foods bring to those who eat them. So, with no further ado, let's start getting acquainted with some of these foods.

The Culinary Pharmacy

It's fun when something that started out as almost an afterthought takes on a life of its own. In my last book, *The Cancer-Fighting Kitchen*, I thought it would be neat to list many of the ingredients used in the recipes and describe their health benefits based on research published in peer-reviewed scientific journals. I thought it might appeal to some of my research-oriented readers.

It turned out to be some of the most popular text in the book. In retrospect, I realize I shouldn't have been surprised. Readers shared my fascination that something as basic as, say, black pepper has been shown to stimulate digestive enzymes, improve absorption of cancer-fighting nutrients such as beta-carotene, and wipe out dangerous microbes.

Given the response, I've included a culinary pharmacy in this book too, updated with information from about five hundred studies, many of them covering new scientific ground. I especially focused on research into nutrients that fight inflammation, because chronic inflammation is now seen as being linked to impaired immune system function and increased risk of many chronic diseases.

Take your time digesting the tasty tidbits here. I guarantee that, once you've read this section, you'll be hooked on the healing power of delicious foods. To find recipes that include each ingredient, consult the index.

Allspice. *Antimicrobial. Digestive support.* Allspice contains eugenol, a phytochemical that helps with digestive problems such as nausea, bloating, and diarrhea. It has also been shown to protect foods from spoiling. Some studies suggest that eugenol may reduce nerve pain.

Almonds. *Antioxidant. Blood sugar regulation. Heart health.* Almonds have a low glycemic load, which is a fancy way of saying they help prevent blood sugar spikes, which can reduce the risk of type 2 diabetes. This, in combination with their abundant antioxidants, may also reduce the risk of coronary heart disease. Half of the antioxidants in almonds are located in the skin.

Apples. *Anticancer. Anti-inflammatory. Bone health. Cardiovascular health. Digestive support.* Apples are their own little medicine cabinet. They have been shown to reduce levels of C-reactive protein, a marker for inflammation. High levels of C-reactive protein are related to heart disease. Apples contain pectin, which helps soothe the stomach, and a mixture of antioxidants that can protect against the development of certain cancers, including lung cancer. In promising studies, German researchers found an acid in apples inhibited the development of colon cancer tumors, while Italian researchers noted apple extract appeared in animals to protect against stomach damage normally caused by aspirin.

Apricots. *Brain health. Blood pressure reduction.* Researchers have noted the carotenoids in apricots inhibit the formation of beta-amyloid plaques in the brain—one of the defining characteristics of Alzheimer's disease. Apricots are also an excellent source of potassium, a vital player in balancing the body's electrolytes and maintaining healthy blood pressure levels.

Artichokes. *Antioxidant. Digestive support. Liver health.* A study of artichoke extract found it contained tremendous amounts of antioxidants and potentially helps prevent damage to protect liver cells. Artichokes are also an excellent digestive aid, according to a 2011 article in the *International Journal of Food Science Nutrition* that analyzed the results of numerous clinical studies.

Asparagus. *Anti-inflammatory. Antioxidant. Digestive support.* Glutathione is a superstar among antioxidants, and asparagus contains more glutathione than any other vegetable or fruit. In addition, it contains the soluble fiber inulin, which helps bacteria beneficial to digestion flourish in the lower intestine. Asparagus is also particularly rich in the B vitamin folate. High folate levels are thought to reduce blood levels of homocysteine, an amino acid linked to cardiovascular disease and dementia.

Avocados. *Anticancer. Cholesterol reduction.* If you're worried about bad cholesterol (LDL), look to avocados and their high levels of oleic acid for help. One study found that regular consumption of oleic acid lowered LDL cholesterol by nearly 50 percent compared to a control group who ate mostly complex carbohydrates. Those who ate avocados also maintained high levels of good cholesterol (HDL). In addition, avocados have been shown to destroy cancerous and precancerous cells.

Basil. *Antibacterial. Anti-inflammatory. Liver health.* Bacteria have a lot to fear from basil: its volatile oils have been shown to slow the growth of disease-causing bacteria such as staphylococcus, including drug-resistant strains. Eugenol, present in basil and several other herbs and spices, inhibits COX, an enzyme related to inflammation, in a manner similar to the action of nonsteroidal anti-inflammatory drugs. Basil extract has also been shown to protect liver cells.

Bell peppers. *Antioxidant. Eye health.* In terms of vitamin C content, eating a bell pepper is like downing a glass of orange juice: one cup of chopped raw green bell pepper contains nearly 200 percent of the recommended daily intake of vitamin C, and red bell peppers contain over 300 percent. Bell peppers contain numerous other antioxidants, notably vitamin A and folate. In fact, 1 cup of chopped raw red bell pepper provides almost the entire recommended daily intake of vitamin A. Vitamin A is linked to maintaining retinal function and protecting the body's mucosal linings, which form a protective barrier against a variety of pathogens.

Black cod. *Anti-inflammatory.* Black cod, also known as sablefish, is as rich in omega-3 fatty acids as wild salmon. Diets rich in omega-3s lower inflammation, which may offer a host of health benefits, including reducing the risk of heart disease, cancer, and rheumatoid arthritis. Research also indicates that there may be a link between high omega-3 intake and lower levels of nerve and brain disorders, including psychiatric conditions.

Blueberries. *Anti-inflammatory. Antioxidant. Brain health. Heart health.* Next time you forget where you put your car keys, try eating some blueberries. Studies indicate that the anthocyanins responsible for blueberry's deep color are associated with improving memory and possibly lowering depression. These anthocyanins also offer anti-inflammatory benefits that led researchers to suggest that dark berries are "essential" to heart health.

Broccoli. *Anticancer. Bone health. Heart health.* If you're concerned about osteoporosis, consider eating more broccoli. It's rich in vitamin K, which increases the density of bone and lowers the risk of fracture. Broccoli also has anticancer properties, and research has shown that cooking doesn't significantly impact the antioxidants that play a role in this benefit.

Buckwheat. *Heart health.* Buckwheat's effects on heart health have been fairly well studied. A notable study conducted in a region of China known for high buckwheat intake found an association between buckwheat consumption and lower overall levels cholesterol. It was also linked with a better ratio of good cholesterol (HDL) to bad cholesterol (LDL). Buckwheat is also relatively high in magnesium, a mineral that dilates vessels and can potentially help lower blood pressure.

Cabbage. *Anticancer. Liver health.* Eating cabbage may be a great way of keeping cancer at bay. It contains glucosinolates, compounds that the body can convert into an array of cancer-fighting agents. Glucosinolates also help improve the liver's detoxification functions. For women concerned with developing hormone-related breast cancer, studies found that the glucosinolate by-product indole-3-carbinol doubled the effectiveness of the liver in removing estrogen from the body.

Cardamom. *Anti-inflammatory. Breath freshener. Digestive support.* Long a staple of traditional Chinese medicine and ayurvedic medicine, cardamom is legendary for aiding digestion. This may be due to cineole, a phytochemical that helps break down mucus. In the gut, cardamom lessens the gas produced as a result of consuming mucus-producing foods, notably dairy products. Its mucus-fighting capacity may help people struggling with chronic obstructive pulmonary disease (COPD); in one six-month study of more than two hundred patients with COPD, those who took cineole experienced improved lung function. Cardamom also freshens the breath, which is why it is often offered at the end of a meal or at the checkout counter in Indian and Chinese restaurants.

Carrots. *Anticancer. Cardiovascular health. Eye health.* Carrots contain a kaleidoscope of antioxidants. In fact, a 1-cup serving provides more than four times the recommended daily intake of vitamin A. Their superlative antioxidant profile has been shown to protect against damage to the cardiovascular system and may lower the risk of colon cancer. Studies show eating carrots regularly lowered the incidence of glaucoma in women.

Cauliflower. *Anticancer. Anti-inflammatory. Liver health.* Studies have shown that a diet that includes plenty of cauliflower can offer protection against breast, colon, prostate, and ovarian cancer. In addition, cauliflower is rich in sulfur, which plays a role in some of the liver's detoxification pathways. It's also rich in both vitamin K and glucosinolates, which may protect against overreaction of the immune system.

Celery. *Blood pressure reduction. Cholesterol reduction. Immune support.* Celery is full of promise, at least in animal studies. Among its active compounds, phthalides have been shown to aid blood vessel dilation, lower blood pressure, and decrease cholesterol levels by triggering the release of more bile, which binds to cholesterol and sweeps it out of the system. In addition, its coumarins can improve the efficiency of certain white blood cells, enhancing immune system function.

Cherries. *Anti-inflammatory. Antioxidant.* Talk about potential: according to a 2011 study in the journal *Critical Reviews in Food Science and Nutrition,* cherries are rich in nutrients linked to decreased risk of cancer, cardiovascular disease, diabetes, inflammatory disease, and Alzheimer's disease. Other research notes that cherries, notably Bing cherries, contain more antioxidants than almonds or dark chocolate, and that's saying a lot.

Chicken. *Bone health. Muscle health. Thyroid health.* Ounce for ounce, when it comes to getting protein, which plays a vital role in maintaining muscle mass and bone density, chicken rules. A four-ounce serving can provide as much as two-thirds of the recommended daily intake of protein. Chicken is also rich in the mineral selenium, which is important for proper thyroid function. Just be sure to use organic chicken to avoid exposure to antibiotics and a host of other unsavory substances.

Chickpeas (aka garbanzo beans). *Cell metabolism support. Digestive support.* Mitochondria, the little energy factories within cells, are protected from free radicals by the antioxidant mineral manganese, which is found in abundance in chickpeas. A serving of chickpeas also contains a tremendous amount of insoluble fiber, which promotes colon health

Chile peppers. *Anticancer. Appetite regulation.* Cayenne and other hot chile peppers, which are members of the genus *Capsicum,* contain capsaicin, which may help control certain types of pain. Capsaicin can also trick the body into feeling fuller, so chile peppers are a good choice for people who want to avoid overeating. Their spiciness stimulates the brain's satiation receptors, triggering the same appetite suppressing hormones that the stomach normally sends out when it's full.

Chives. *Anticancer. Anti-inflammatory.* Like garlic, leeks, and onions, chives are a member of the genus *Allium* and are rich in sulfur compounds. National Cancer Institute Researchers found that men who ate a just small amount (10 grams) of allium vegetables daily had a far lower risk of prostate cancer. In animal studies, French researchers similarly found that these sulfur compounds help lower the risk of colorectal and stomach cancer, and possibly other cancers, as well.

Chocolate (dark). *Anti-inflammatory. Antioxidant. Blood pressure reduction. Heart health.* Eat chocolate and live longer. This sounds wonderful, and it may well be true. Animal studies suggest that the flavanols in dark chocolate can prevent coronary artery disease and reduce the impact of heart attacks. Spanish researchers who reviewed numerous studies of chocolate noted that these flavanols can also help reduce blood pressure and insulin resistance and protect red blood cells. And here's a factoid that probably won't come as a surprise: studies also show that dark chocolate is an excellent mood enhancer.

Cilantro and coriander. *Anticancer. Antioxidant. Antimicrobial. Cholesterol reduction. Liver health.* Cilantro, aka coriander, could be your liver's best friend. It has been used in the treatment of jaundice, and studies show that it reduces fatty deposits that can collect in the liver and impair its function. Additionally, cilantro appears to inhibit the growth of that nasty bug *E. coli*. In animal studies, eating coriander seeds was associated with a significant drop in triglycerides and total cholesterol levels. In addition, coriander has been shown to lower the risk of colon cancer, and there's also a potential link between high coriander consumption and low rates of cancer among populations in the Eastern Bloc.

Cinnamon. *Anti-inflammatory. Diabetes prevention. Digestive support. Pain relief.* Cinnamon is a mighty powerful spice. It stimulates the production of digestive enzymes and works wonders in the pancreas. One common precursor to diabetes is a growing resistance to insulin, which helps regulate blood sugar levels. In animals, cinnamon has been shown to make the body more receptive to insulin and decrease other risk factors for diabetes, such as high triglycerides. One compound in cinnamon, cinnamaldehyde, reduces inflammation. In addition, cinnamon contains salicylates (also found in aspirin), which can reduce pain and promote heart health by preventing blood clots.

Coconut milk and coconut oil. *Antibacterial. Anti-inflammatory. Antimicrobial. Bone health.* Eating coconut is the equivalent of an internal antiseptic treatment because coconut is an outstanding source of lauric acid, which the body converts into potent antiviral and antibacterial compounds. Coconut is also rich in magnesium, which promotes bone health. So if you're concerned about osteoporosis, reach for the coconut.

Corn. *Anticancer.* Beta-cryptoxanthin, which is responsible for the lovely color of yellow corn kernels, also has the potential to lower the risk of lung cancer. Because of its excellent antioxidant profile, corn may also protect against other cancers, particularly colon cancer, due to its high fiber content.

Cranberries. *Antibacterial. Anti-inflammatory. Cardiovascular health. Oral health.* Most women are well aware of cranberry's curative powers for urinary tract infections, thanks to proanthocyanidins, which prevent bacteria from attaching to the bladder wall. These and other compounds in cranberries also reduce inflammation, notably in the mouth and gums. In addition, cranberries can inhibit the activity of enzymes related to the development of heart disease and stroke.

Cumin. *Anticancer. Appetite stimulator. Digestive support. Pain reduction.* In animals, cumin revs up the production of pancreatic enzymes that enhance appetite and aid digestion. Various compounds in cumin have also been shown to neutralize carcinogens, improve antioxidant efficiency, and decrease cancer-related inflammation. In addition, cumin can relieve pain due to inflammation when consumed or applied topically.

Edamame (immature soy beans). *Anti-inflammatory. Blood sugar regulation.* All soy is not created equal. Research shows that getting soy directly from soybeans, rather than processed soy products, offers the greatest health benefits. Soy consumption has been linked with bone and cardiovascular health, cancer prevention, and relief from the hot flashes associated with menopause. However, these benefits haven't been definitively established, and they may hinge on consuming other foods as well. The ability to digest soy and absorb its nutrients, which differs among individuals depending on genetics, may also be a factor. In animals fed limited polyunsaturated fats, soy intake decreased insulin resistance, which could help stave off type 2 diabetes.

Eggs. *Anti-inflammatory. Eye health.* One way the brain creates and retains memory is through acetylcholine, which is made from choline, and eggs contain abundant choline. High levels of choline in the diet have also been shown to reduce several inflammation markers in the body. In addition, two antioxidants in eggs, lutein and zeaxanthin, appear to be helpful in preventing macular degeneration.

Fennel. *Anti-inflammatory. Digestive support.* Fennel contains the phytochemical limonene, which appears to offer anticancer and anti-inflammatory benefits, at least in animal studies and in vitro. More definitive work indicates that anethole, another phytochemical in fennel, can improve digestion and soothe the tummy. Anethole is also thought to have excellent antibacterial and antifungal properties.

Garlic. *Antibacterial. Anti-inflammatory. Antimicrobial. Cardiovascular health.* The potent smell of garlic has an equally potent effect on numerous body systems. As a member of the genus *Allium*, garlic contains a number of sulfur compounds, including allicin, that help prevent free radical damage to the linings of blood vessels. This limits inflammation, which may ward off heart attacks and stroke. Garlic has also been shown to prevent certain yeast infections and a type of bacterial infection in burn patients.

Ginger. *Anti-inflammatory. Arthritis relief. Digestive support.* Mothers have long turned to ginger to soothe their children's tummy aches, but that just touches the surface of this rhizome's healing properties. To mention just a few, clinical studies show that ginger consumption can decrease pain related to arthritis, and animal studies indicate that it protects against liver damage.

Green tea. *Anticancer. Anti-inflammatory. Antioxidant. Appetite suppressant. Blood pressure reduction. Cholesterol reduction.* If you're fond of acronyms, commit EGCG to memory. It stands for epigallocatechin gallate, an antioxidant that is abundant in green tea and has numerous healing properties. EGCG can be useful in treating breast, lung, and prostate cancer. It can also inhibit the conversion of glucose (blood sugar) into fat and decrease appetite. In addition, evidence suggests that green tea prevents cholesterol plaques from forming on blood vessel walls, and a clinical study found that people who consumed green tea daily decreased their risk of being diagnosed with high blood pressure by up to 65 percent.

Halibut. *Anticancer. Anti-inflammatory. Blood pressure reduction. Cardiovascular health. Stroke prevention. Triglyceride reduction.* Just 4 ounces of halibut provides at least 25 percent of the recommended daily intake of vitamin B_{12}, omega-3s, phosphorus, niacin (40 percent), protein (60 percent), and selenium (75 percent). Regular consumption of omega-3s has been shown to lower rates of colorectal cancer, lymphoma, high blood pressure, and high triglycerides. The link in all of these may be the ability of omega-3 to lessen systemic inflammation. In addition, vitamins B_6, also abundant in halibut, and B_{12} limit production of homocysteine, a metabolic by-product that damages blood vessels.

Hibiscus. *Blood pressure reduction. Cardiovascular health. Diabetes prevention.* Researchers at Tufts University discovered that drinking hibiscus tea benefited people at risk for hypertension, dropping their systolic blood pressure (that's the top number) significantly in just six weeks. Mexican researchers found hibiscus effective against metabolic syndrome, a precursor to diabetes and heart disease marked by insulin resistance, high blood sugar levels, and high cholesterol levels.

Honey. *Antimicrobial. Antiviral. Cholesterol reduction. Triglyceride reduction.* Honey's reputation for fighting infection is so robust that some hospitals use it to combat staph bacteria in their wards. And although it's a sweetener, it's been shown to help reduce levels of cholesterol and triglycerides.

Kale. *Anticancer. Anti-inflammatory. Cholesterol reduction. Eye health.* Like all cruciferous vegetables, kale has numerous health benefits. It goes way off the charts with certain nutrients, providing more than *ten times* the recommended daily intake of vitamin K, a key regulator of inflammation, and three times the recommended daily intake of vitamin A, which is vital to eye health and maintaining moisture in the skin and mucous membranes. Kale's high fiber vacuums cholesterol out of the body, while its isothiocyanates are associated with reducing risk of breast, ovarian, and colon cancer. Animal studies and in vitro research suggests that a compound in kale, glucobrassicin inhibits inflammation in animals with induced arthritis.

Kombu. *Anticancer. Detoxification. Immune support.* Like many sea vegetables, kombu contains fucoidans, molecules with a host of healing properties. Studies show that they bind to carcinogens to help move them out of the body. They seem to have a dual effect on the immune system, either enhancing or limiting immune response as needed. Fucoidans have also shown potential to relieve pain associated with inflammation due to arthritis, to reduce metabolic syndrome (which is associated with diabetes and cardiovascular disease), and to inhibit herpes viruses.

Leeks. *Anti-inflammatory. Cardiovascular health.* The major player in leeks is a photochemical called kaempferol, which is well studied in regard to protecting blood vessels from free radical damage. Leeks are also rich in folate, which reduces levels of homocysteine (linked to cardiovascular disease).

Legumes. *Antioxidant. Blood pressure reduction. Blood sugar regulation. Heart health.* All beans are rich in fiber, which aids in digestion and elimination and slows the release of sugars into the bloodstream. The soluble fiber found in beans is also linked to lower heart attack rates. Generally, beans are extremely high in antioxidants and minerals, particularly manganese, phosphorus, iron, and magnesium. Lentils are also an outstanding source of potassium, and a huge clinical study found a link between high levels of potassium and lower blood pressure.

Lemons. *Antioxidant. Cardiovascular health. Immune suppport.* The abundance of vitamin C content in lemons could have numerous health benefits. As a powerful antioxidant, vitamin C protects immune and cardiovascular system function. In animal and in vitro studies, another compound found in lemons, limonene, offered some resistance to the development of breast, colon, mouth, and lung cancers. Other studies suggest that limonene could lower production of bad cholesterol (LDL).

Lemongrass. *Antibacterial.* The volatile oils in lemongrass, including citral, have been the subject of a fair number of animal and in vitro studies. These oils show promise in controlling the spread of *E. coli* bacteria, responsible for many food-borne ailments. Lemongrass extract killed or impaired the function of animal and human leukemia cells. Other animal studies showed that lemongrass has the potential to lower blood pressure.

Limes. *Anti-inflammatory. Antimicrobial.* It kind of makes sense that limes would contain compounds called "liminoids," and it's a good thing they do. Liminoids actively combat cancers of the colon, mouth, skin, and breast. The high levels of vitamin C in limes also appears to limit the impact of rheumatoid arthritis. And on the international front, limes are perhaps the most inexpensive cure for the world-wide scourge of cholera; notably in West Africa, where consuming lime juice with daily meals helped limit the cholera outbreaks.

Maple syrup (Grade B). *Antioxidant. Heart health. Immune support. Prostate health.* The flavor alone is enough to warrant seeking out maple syrup, but it also has some outstanding health benefits. It's a good source of zinc and an excellent source of manganese. Zinc plays a vital role in the effectiveness of immune cells and cells that line the walls of blood vessels. Manganese helps enzymes protect the cells' mitochondria from damage.

Mint. *Anticancer. Anti-inflammatory. Antimicrobial. Appetite suppressant. Breath freshener. Digestive support.* A little chopped mint goes a long way toward enhancing well-being. Your friends will appreciate the breath-freshening aspects of mint, and you'll be rewarded with both improved digestion and decreased appetite. The most potent member of the mint family may be peppermint, which is a culinary pharmacy in itself. It has antimicrobial qualities that destroy germs in the food it contacts, its abundant limonene and luteolin show promise for cancer prevention, and its rosmarinic acid inhibits the formation of coronary plaques. Peppermint has been shown to soothe the tummy by decreasing gas and relaxing stomach muscles, and it can also help combat *H pylori*, a cause of stomach ulcers.

Miso. *Breast health. Bone health. Cardiovascular health. Immune support. Joint health.* Researchers have long theorized that higher soy consumption is linked to better health and lower rates of breast cancer among certain Japanese populations. A study using mice found that those who were given miso in their diet developed fewer breast malignancies than the control group. Miso is also high in zinc, which plays a key role in supporting the immune system and in healing lacerations. Other minerals found in miso, manganese and copper, help blood vessels and joints remain pliable.

Mustard seeds. *Anticancer. Antimicrobial.* Mustard seeds are produced by plants in the genus *Brassica*, which also includes nutritional superstars such as cabbage, Brussels sprouts, and broccoli, and like their cousins, they help combat cancer-causing enzymes. In vitro studies showed that mustard seeds caused human colon cancer cells to implode and greatly reduced the growth of new colon cancer cells. Mustard seeds also help destroy bacteria in other foods they come in contact with.

Olives and olive oil. *Anticancer. Anti-inflammatory. Heart health. Stroke prevention.* Renowned for its link to longevity, the Mediterranean diet has put the scientific spotlight on two popular ingredients: olives and olive oil. Long known for its monounsaturated (healthier) fat, extra-virgin olive oil contains large amounts of oleocanthal, a compound that helps protect the heart. According to Spanish researchers, olive oil helped reduce inflammation in patients with autoimmune disorders, and a recent study of more than seven thousand people found a 41 percent reduction in strokes among those who consumed olive oil. On top of all of that, research also suggests that olive oil can decrease the risk of cancers in the respiratory system, upper GI tract, colon, and breasts.

Onions. *Antibacterial. Anti-inflammatory. Antimicrobial. Bone health.* Once you realize how good onions are for you, you'll never shed another tear. Studies show that onion consumption increases bone thickness by 15 percent and may limit bone loss. The American Cancer Society noted that quercetin, which is abundant in onions, helped protect against colon cancer in animal studies. Other research indicates that onions help fight many common dangerous microbes, including forms of staph, strep, candida, and *E. coli*.

Oranges. *Anticancer. Anti-inflammatory. Cardiovascular health*. Oranges are the standard-bearer for vitamin C in fruits, with each orange containing more than 100 percent of the recommended daily intake. Vitamin C has been linked to reduction in many cancers, notably colon cancer. Its antioxidant capacity may also lower inflammation and associated arthritic conditions. In addition, the World Health Organization reported that diets rich in citrus had cardiovascular benefits.

Oregano. *Anti-inflammatory. Heart health*. Both oregano and individual compounds within it have gone under the microscope with favorable findings. Two phytochemicals in oregano, oleanolic acid and ursolic acid, reduce cholesterol levels, while other compounds prevent the formation of arterial plaque.

Parsley. *Anticancer. Anti-inflammatory. Cardiovascular health*. Though studies of parsley's impact as a whole food are scarce, the effectiveness of its components is well studied. Parsley's volatile oils help activate glutathione, a vital cancer-fighting antioxidant, and have shown promise in limiting the development of lung cancer in animal studies. It's a good source of folate and an excellent source of vitamin C. Folate impairs production of homocysteine, which can damage blood vessels, and abundant vitamin C in the diet is known to reduce inflammation associated with rheumatoid arthritis. Animal studies have also shown that parsley can help repair the lining of the stomach.

Peas. *Anti-inflammatory. Blood sugar regulation. Cholesterol reduction*. Researchers at Tulane University were curious whether legumes in the American diet (specifically peas) have the same cholesterol-lowering effects as soybeans, which are common in Asian diets. They pored through 140 studies, and the answer was a resounding yes. In addition to helping lower cholesterol, the rich fiber content of peas can help regulate blood sugar. Surprisingly, peas also contain a decent amount of omega-3s, which play a role in controlling inflammation.

Pistachios. *Antioxidant*. In animal studies, pistachios are like a panacea for the cardiovascular system. Greek researchers looking at an extract from pistachio nuts found that it kept the aorta from thickening while also lowering levels of bad cholesterol (LDL) and raising levels of good cholesterol (HDL). Italian investigators sang the praises of the antioxidants in pistachios, particularly in the skins, while Turkish researchers found that pistachios increased antioxidant activity in rats with high cholesterol.

Pomegranate. *Anti-inflammatory. Heart health*. Nitric oxide helps blood vessels relax, making it vital for cardiovascular health, and pomegranates have been shown to pump up levels of nitric oxide in heart cells and also lower systolic blood pressure. In animal studies, pomegranate extract also helped slow the absorption of sugar into the blood, which could be beneficial for those at risk of metabolic syndrome, which is associated with type 2 diabetes and insulin resistance. Pomegranate antioxidant levels are so high that Russian physicians used it to reduce the effects of radiation exposure following the nuclear disaster at Chernobyl.

Potatoes. *Brain health. Nervous system health. Thyroid health.* A recent article in *Prevention* magazine caught my eye. Entitled "The Happiness Diet," it noted that red and blue potatoes are filled with iodine and other nutrients crucial for optimal functioning of the thyroid gland, one of the body's major mood regulators. Most potatoes contain high levels of vitamin B_6, which is a key player in the creation of neurotransmitters critical to communication between brain cells, and some of the affected neurotransmitters are vital for combating depression (serotonin) and sleep disturbances (melatonin). Is it any wonder that potatoes are a universal comfort food?

Quinoa. *Blood sugar regulation. Heart health.* When it comes to quinoa, the magic word is *lignans*, which are also abundant in sesame seeds and flaxseeds. A Finnish study of nearly 1,900 men found that those with high levels of a compound associated with lignan consumption suffered less mortality from heart and cardiovascular disease. Another key study, which looked at more than 40,000 African-American women, found those who regularly consumed magnesium from whole grains such as quinoa had significantly lower rates of type 2 diabetes; the reduction is even greater when calcium is added to the mix.

Raspberries. *Anticancer. Anti-inflammatory.* Raspberries contain ellagic acid, which as been well studied and is associated with potentially inhibiting development of cancers of the skin, lung, liver, esophagus, and also with destroying the human papilloma virus (HPV) responsible for cervical cancer. An emerging area of study involves resveratrol, which is present in raspberries and abundant in red wine, cocoa powder, and, surprisingly, peanuts. In vitro studies have shown that resveratrol may help inhibit Alzheimer's and Parkinson's disease, but this research is in a very early phase. There are also theories, at this point far from proven, that resveratrol could delay normal cell death, perhaps slowing the aging process.

Red meat (grass-fed). *Antioxidant. Heart health.* Red meat can be part of a health-promoting diet, if eaten in moderation. Choose organic, grass-fed beef to reduce your exposure to antibiotics, hormones, pesticides, and other toxins, and to obtain even higher levels of certain nutrients abundant in lean beef, notably vitamin B_{12}, selenium, and, to a lesser extent, omega-3s. Vitamin B_{12} can help lower levels of homocysteine, a metabolic by-product associated with heart disease. Selenium is important for proper functioning of antioxidants that fight cancer, notably glutathione.

Rice (brown). *Anti-inflammatory. Heart health.* While brown rice per se hasn't been well studied, like many other whole grains it is rich in fiber and lignans, which have received plenty of scientific attention. In population-based studies, those who consumed high levels of whole grains had a decreased risk of insulin resistance, a precursor of type 2 diabetes. Lignans are converted into enterolactone in the body, and enterolactone is believed to lower the risk of breast cancer and heart disease. In addition, women who ate larger quantities of the kind of insoluble fiber found in brown rice suffered significantly fewer gallstones, perhaps because fiber decreases the amount of bile, produced by the gallbladder, required for digestion.

Saffron. *Brain health.* Saffron's health benefits are undeniable. There's preliminary evidence that it helps protect the kidneys, eyes, and heart and, perhaps of greatest interest, the brain. Animal and in vitro studies point to a possible connection between saffron extract and cognitive improvement, and a small Iranian study, with fifty-four human subjects, found a small improvement in patients with mild to moderate dementia. Australian researchers reviewing herbal medicine studies found preliminary evidence that saffron has antidepressant properties, as well.

Sage. *Anti-inflammatory. Antioxidant. Brain health.* Herbs in general are packed with healthful antioxidants, and sage contains especially robust amounts. Antioxidants play a key role in neutralizing compounds associated with promoting inflammation in the body. In addition, limited clinical studies indicate that sage extract can improve short-term memory.

Salmon (wild). *Anticancer. Anti-inflammatory. Brain health. Cardiovascular health. Joint health. Skin health.* No fish offers higher concentrations of healthful omega-3 fatty acids than wild salmon. Omega-3s are credited with decreasing inflammation throughout the body and thereby improving brain, cardiovascular, skin, and joint health. Omega-3s may even play a role in reducing the risk of a leading cause of blindness: macular degeneration. Wild salmon is also a top source of vitamin D, which is hard to find in abundance in food sources, and getting sufficient vitamin D is linked to reduced risk of colon, prostate, and breast cancer.

Sardines. *Anticancer. Bone health. Brain health. Heart health.* Like salmon, sardines are a great source of omega-3s. An interesting Dutch study of 1,613 forty-five- to seventy-year-olds analyzed their diet and gave them cognition tests over a five-year period. Those who ate the highest amounts of fish-based omega-3s scored best; those whose diets tilted toward saturated fats and cholesterol consumption fared worse. Sardines are also rich in vitamin D, which helps ward off certain cancers, and vitamin B12, which helps maintain strong bones.

Scallops. *Anti-inflammatory. Brain health. Cardiovascular health.* An interesting area of heart research is electrophysiology, the study of how electric current runs through the heart muscle, keeping it beating properly—or not. It might seem counterintuitive, but having a little variability in the timing between beats can ward off arrhythmias and heart attacks, and consumption of omega-3s, which are abundant in scallops, can accomplish this in just a few weeks. In addition, scallops are rich in vitamin B12, potassium, and magnesium, which also contribute to improved cardiovascular health.

Shiitake mushrooms. *Anticancer. Anti-inflammatory. Cholesterol reduction.* Shiitake mushrooms contain the cholesterol-lowering compound eritadenine. In animal and in vitro studies, shiitake extracts appear to prompt certain cancer cells to self-destruct.

Shrimp. *Anticancer. Antioxidant.* Though diminutive, shrimp are big, bad mommas when it comes to selenium levels, and selenium is like emergency roadside service, traveling throughout the body to seek out and repair cells and DNA that have been damaged by free radicals. Selenium travels well armed, as it has been shown to blast cancer cells out of existence.

Sesame seeds and tahini. *Anti-inflammatory. Bone health. Cholesterol reduction. Joint health. Rheumatoid arthritis relief.* Sesame seeds are extremely rich in copper, a mineral that's often in short supply in the diet. Copper has anti-inflammatory properties that promote bone and joint health and help reduce arthritis pain. Sesame seeds also contain lignans, which are linked to lowering cholesterol. In animal studies, lignans have been shown to improve synthesis of vitamin E.

Spinach. *Anticancer. Anti-inflammatory.* A nutritional powerhouse forever immortalized by a certain cartoon sailor, spinach has been shown to slow the growth of ovarian, stomach, and prostate cancer. It's a rich source of magnesium, which could benefit people who experience headaches because of not getting enough magnesium in their diet. Animal studies also suggest that spinach can prevent or delay the onset of certain dementias.

Squash (winter). *Antibacterial. Anti-inflammatory. Antioxidant.* A superb source of vitamin A, winter squash also has an unusual combination of carotenoid antioxidants and healthful albeit tongue-twisting compounds called cucurbitacins, which have antibacterial and anti-inflammatory properties. The types of omega-3s in winter squash have also been shown to suppress inflammation. In vitro tests also suggest that winter squash could limit cholesterol production in the body.

Strawberries. *Anticancer. Skin health.* Most us don't think of skin as a defense mechanism, but that's exactly what it is: a barrier that keeps damaging intruders from breaking into the body. The rich vitamin C content of strawberries aids in the production of collagen, which helps keep skin supple and protects against microtears. Compounds in strawberries have been shown to kill certain cancer cells while helping normal cells repair themselves. In addition, researchers at Tufts University found that older rats given regular rations of strawberries performed tasks as accurately as younger rats.

Sweet potatoes. *Blood pressure regulation. Cardiovascular health. Immune support.* Sweet potatoes contain compounds that are like police dispatchers, directing the immune system to produce cells that engulf invading bacteria and escort them permanently off the premises. These healthful tubers have an excellent nutrient profile that includes good amounts of vitamin B6 and potassium, the former linked to lowering homocysteine levels and thus reducing the risk of stroke or heart attack, and the latter with helping keep high blood pressure in check. (By the way, the vegetables sold as yams in the United States are, in most cases, actually sweet potatoes.)

Swiss chard. *Anti-inflammatory. Blood sugar regulation. Bone health. Liver health.* Swiss chard is a nutrition superstar, with numerous health benefits. Some of its compounds synergize with the antioxidant glutathione to aid the liver in detoxification. Others slow the breakdown of sugars, keeping blood sugar levels steadier and preventing insulin spikes. Its vitamin K levels are off the charts, with one cup of cooked chard offering more than *seven* times the recommended daily intake, making it a tremendous food for anyone concerned about bone health.

Thyme. *Antibacterial. Antimicrobial.* Like many spices, thyme contains volatile oils that excel at decontaminating foods, notably produce such as lettuce. They have been shown to help neutralize many common pathogens, including strains of *E. coli* and staph that can cause serious illness. Kaempferol, a flavonoid in thyme, has been fairly well studied and may help reduce the risk of cardiovascular disease and certain cancers.

Tomatoes. *Bone health. Cardiovascular health. Cholesterol reduction.* Tomatoes contain abundant lycopene, a phytonutrient that's been linked with lowering both overall cholesterol and bad cholesterol (LDL) and providing antioxidant support for the heart and bones. It may also help prevent obesity. In animal studies, lycopene reduced the growth of brain and breast tumors.

Turkey. *Bone health. Brain health. Muscle health.* An excellent source of protein, which is essential for bone and muscle health, turkey is probably best known nutritionally for its abundance of tryptophan. This essential amino acid ("essential" meaning it has to come from a food source) also helps the body produce serotonin, a neurotransmitter that controls mood. Low serotonin levels have been linked to a variety of issues, including depression and eating disorders.

Turmeric. *Anticancer. Anti-inflammatory.* Researchers are excited about the potential healing properties of turmeric's curcumin, and especially its anti-inflammatory abilities. Curcumin may limit the impact of GI diseases such irritable bowel syndrome. In vitro studies have shown that curcumin fights cancer in several ways, including preventing cancer cells from growing new blood vessels to feed themselves and inducing the death of existing cancer cells. Investigations focused on Alzheimer's disease found that curcumin broke up accumulated amyloid plaque, considered a prime marker or cause of the disease when it occurs in the brain.

Walnuts. *Anti-inflammatory. Bone health. Heart health.* A great source of omega-3s (just ¼ cup provides nearly 100 percent of the recommended daily intake), walnuts offer tremendous heart health benefits. They reduce inflammation, bad cholesterol (LDL), and risk of blood clots and can help prevent bone loss.

Wasabi. *Anticancer. Liver health.* Wasabi, which is actually the root of a cruciferous vegetable, is full of isothiocyanates, compounds that have been linked to reduced risk of cancer. A team at Ohio State noted that isothiocyanates appear to help prevent DNA damage, and researchers at Vanderbilt University who focused on the liver found that these compounds increased levels of enzymes vital to detoxification.

Yogurt. *Digestive support. Immune health.* This may not paint the prettiest picture, but we owe much of our gut health to hundreds of species of bacteria that reside there. Unfortunately, illness and antibiotics can easily wipe them out. On the upside, yogurt with live cultures is excellent for restoring or maintaining their populations. Consuming yogurt cultured with lactic acid bacteria can help prevent or decrease inflammation of the GI tract, which is helpful against conditions such as irritable bowel syndrome, diarrhea, and Crohn's disease.

Eating to Enhance and Enjoy Life: From the Science to the Plate

Knowing the health benefits of various foods is great, but to put that knowledge into action (and for balanced nutrition), you'll need to combine those foods into tasty dishes. In addition to providing more flavor, combining ingredients creates a synergy among ingredients that boosts their health-promoting qualities. While many of my recipes have ingredients that can, say, boost immunity or reduce stress, each of the recipes listed below includes numerous foods known for supporting a particular aspect of health and wellness.

Immune Boosters

Magic Mineral Broth 2.0 (page 55); Chicken Magic Mineral Broth 2.0 (page 56); Vampire Slayer's Soup (page 64); Bento Box Soup (page 66); Chicken Tortilla Soup (page 70); Rustic Lentil Soup (page 72); Peppino's Cowboy Minestrone with Herb Mini Meatballs (page 78); Avocado Lover's Salad (page 83); Carrot Apple Slaw with Cranberries (page 84); Mexican Cabbage Crunch (page 86); Asian Cabbage Crunch (page 87); Roasted Asparagus Salad with Arugula and Hazelnuts (page 88); Strawberry, Fennel, and Arugula Salad (page 91); Latin Kale (page 95); Sweet-and-Sour Asian Cabbage and Kale (page 96); Indian Greens (page 97); Mediterranean Greens (page 98); Maple-Glazed Brussels Sprouts with Caraway (page 99); Broccoli with Red Onion, Feta, and Mint (page 104); Roasted Wild Salmon with Olive and Mint Vinaigrette (page 139); Shrimp via My Ma (page 143); Catherine's Survival Shooters (page 199); Green Tea Cooler with Ginger, Papaya, and Lime (page 202)

Stress Reducers

Magic Mineral Broth 2.0 (page 55); Velvety Mediterranean Gazpacho with Avocado Cream (page 58); Summer's Sweetest Corn Bisque (page 60); Cozy Roasted Vegetable Soup (page 63); Bento Box Soup (page 66); Dahl Fit for a Saint (page 69); Lemon Chive Potatoes (page 102); Roasted Fingerling Potatoes with Pesto (page 103); Sweet Potato and Zucchini Pancakes (page 105); Bella's Moroccan-Spiced Sweet Potato Salad (page 106); Swiss Chard and Roasted Butternut Squash Tart (page 112); Farro with Kale-Basil Pesto (page 121); Brown Rice

Pilaf with Saffron and Ginger (page 123); Hot-and-Sour Sesame Soba Noodles (page 126); Braised Chicken with Artichokes and Olives (page 146); Herby Turkey Sliders (page 153); Sweet Potato Bars (page 160); Gluten-Free Blueberry Mini Muffins (page 164); Thyme Onion Muffins (page 166); Chamomile Lemonade with Green Apple (page 199)

Mind Enhancers

Magic Mineral Broth 2.0 (page 55); Roasted Asparagus Salad with Arugula and Hazelnuts (page 88); Tuscan Beans and Greens (page 100); Golden Roasted Cauliflower (page 111); Layered Frittata with Leeks, Swiss Chard, and Tomatoes (page 132); Good Mood Sardines (page 135); Roasted Halibut with Lime and Papaya and Avocado Salsa (page 137); Black Cod with Miso-Ginger Glaze (page 138); Roasted Wild Salmon with Olive and Mint Vinaigrette (page 139); Smoked Salmon Nori Rolls (page 140); Wild, Wild Salmon Burgers (page 142); Pan-Seared Scallops with Citrus Drizzle (page 144); Greek Chicken Salad (page 145); Moroccan Mint Lamb Chops (page 154); Silk Road Spiced Walnuts (page 167); Curried Deviled Eggs (page 173); Green Tea Cooler with Ginger, Papaya, and Lime (page 202)

Blood Sugar Regulators

Chicken Tortilla Soup (page 70); Peppino's Cowboy Minestrone with Herb Mini Meatballs (page 78); Tuscan Beans and Greens (page 100); Sicilian Green Beans (page 101); Lemony Lentil and Quinoa Salad (page 117); Quinoa with Edamame, Ginger, and Lime (page 118); Layered Frittata with Leeks, Swiss Chard, and Tomatoes (page 132); Smoked Salmon Nori Rolls (page 140); Greek Chicken Salad (page 145); Flat-Out Good Chicken (page 148); Mediterranean Kebabs (page 150); Moroccan Mint Lamb Chops (page 154); Apple Slices with Banana and Almond Butter (page 159); Sweet Potato Bars (page 160); Gluten-Free Blueberry Mini Muffins (page 164); Silk Road Spiced Walnuts (page 167); Curried Deviled Eggs (page 173)

Flexibility Promoters

Chicken Magic Mineral Broth 2.0 (page 56); Curried Butternut Squash Soup (page 65); Golden Roasted Cauliflower (page 111); Layered Frittata with Leek, Swiss Chard, and Tomatoes (page 132); Good Mood Sardines (page 135); Black Cod with Miso-Ginger Glaze (page 138); Roasted Halibut with Lime and Papaya and Avocado Salsa (page 137); Roasted Wild Salmon with Olive and Mint Vinaigrette (page 139); Smoked Salmon Nori Rolls (page 140); Wild, Wild Salmon Burgers (page 142); Pan-Seared Scallops with Citrus Drizzle (page 144); Braised Chicken with Artichokes and Olives (page 146); Flat-Out

Good Chicken (page 148); Herby Turkey Sliders (page 153); Moroccan Mint Lamb Chops (page 154)

Liver Boosters

Roasted Asparagus Salad with Arugula and Hazelnuts (page 88); Many-Herb Gremolata (page 181); Parsley Mint Drizzle (page 189); Catherine's Survival Shooters (page 199); Chamomile Lemonade with Green Apple (page 199); Spa in a Pitcher (page 200); Simon's Most Nourishing Elixir (page 203)

Heart Strengtheners

Rustic Lentil Soup (page 72); Ridiculously Good Split Pea Soup (page 73); Roasted Asparagus Salad with Arugula and Hazelnuts (page 88); Walnut, Date, and Herb Salad (page 92); Tuscan Beans and Greens (page 100); Lemony Lentil and Quinoa Salad (page 117); Not Your Typical Tabouli (page 120); Roasted Wild Salmon with Olive and Mint Vinaigrette (page 139); Pan-Seared Scallops with Citrus Drizzle (page 144); Gluten-Free Blueberry Mini Muffins (page 164); Silk Road Spiced Walnuts (page 167); Edamame Wasabi Spread (page 172)

Skin Enrichers

Avocado Lover's Salad (page 83); Carrot Apple Slaw with Cranberries (page 84); Strawberry, Fennel, and Arugula Salad (page 91); Papaya and Avocado Salsa (page 191); Spa in a Pitcher (page 200); Green Tea Cooler with Ginger, Papaya, and Lime (page 202); Simon's Most Nourishing Elixir (page 203); Hibiscus Pomegranate Cooler (page 205); Mango Lassi (page 208); Roasted Strawberries with Pomegranate Molasses and Basil (page 214); Raspberry Hibiscus Sorbet (page 215)

LDL Cholesterol Reducers

Rustic Lentil Soup (page 72); Carrot Apple Slaw with Cranberries (page 84); Strawberry Arugula Salad (page 91); Walnut, Date, and Herb Salad (page 92); Tuscan Beans and Greens (page 100); Lemony Lentil and Quinoa Salad (page 117); Not Your Typical Tabouli (page 120); Good Mood Sardines (page 135); Roasted Wild Salmon with Olive and Mint Vinaigrette (page 139); Smoked Salmon Nori Rolls (page 140); Silk Road Spiced Walnuts (page 167); Edamame Wasabi Spread (page 172); Gregg's Morning Protein Shake (page 206); Apple-Raspberry Nut Crumble (page 218).

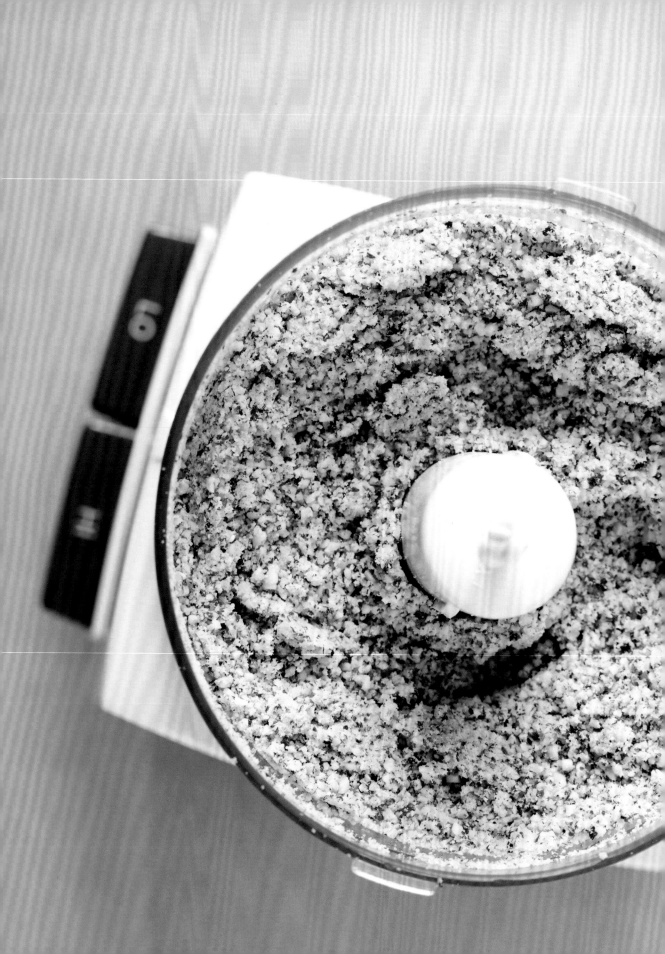

CHAPTER 3

Making the Most of This Book

As you set out to use this book, please be very forgiving of yourself right from the start.

Cooking is a process of trial and error. The fact that you're willing to engage that process, be it one time or a thousand, makes you a success in my eyes. Plus, I have faith in the allure of the kitchen, and promise that, if you're patient, you'll find yourself wanting to cook more and more. In the long run, creating meals that enhance your health and well-being while caressing your taste buds is irresistible. You'll see.

If you haven't done much cooking (or have mostly done it under duress), I encourage you to read this entire chapter closely. In the next section, Getting Started, I'll share the advice I offer when I work with people who want to learn how to cook and are looking for equal parts of inspiration, perspective, and time-tested advice. This will give you a jump start on making the kitchen your favorite room in the house.

Folks with a little more cooking experience might want skip past that section and dive into what I think of as the longevity tool kit: a potpourri of culinary knowledge that will help you turn your kitchen into a lean, mean wellness machine. I offer advice on how to develop your own culinary GPS (page 41) and how to adjust recipes to hone in on your taste preferences. Learning what you like and how to create it can work wonders in overcoming any resistance you may feel toward cooking or eating well. Needless to say, you can also use these approaches to tailor your cooking to others and help them to connect or reconnect with enjoyable nourishment. I'll also help you bring the power of umami, an elusive but important taste sense, into your cooking, and offer guidance on using spices and herbs.

Getting Started

I want to take you by the hand here for a few minutes and welcome you into *our* kitchen. I say "our," because I really want you to feel that cooking for longevity is something we'll do together, and that you'll never be alone in the process. I often work with people who are incredibly enthusiastic about making changes and eating in a way that will improve their health and quality of life in the present and hopefully for decades to come. The problem they run into, and why they end up turning to me for help, is that it's one thing to have the desire to cook, but sometimes quite another to take courageous steps in the kitchen. That's not hyperbole; it takes guts to step across that threshold, especially if you're cooking for other people too. I want to help you stand up to that pesky little judge, the one who sits on your shoulder and says, "Just who do you think you are? You'll never cook as well as (fill in the blank), so who do you think you're kidding?!" I know that voice well. Believe it or not, it still pops up on occasion even for me. When it does, I just laugh (most of the time, anyway) and tell it to go sit in the corner and nibble on a carrot—quietly.

Most people either want to eat well or have been told they need to by someone who means well. The latter usually involves what I call The List: someone—a physician, a friend, a cousin, or anyone with your well-being in mind—hands you a list of healthy foods and expects that, somehow, by some act of prestidigitation, you can turn that two-dimensional printout into living, breathing, delightful, delicious meals.

Receiving that list and being told go do it is like suddenly being told you've been entered in the Olympic 100-meter dash, and, oh, by the way, here are your shoes, and there are the starting blocks. Before you know it, the gun has gone off, the other runners are halfway down the track, and you're still on one knee yelling, "*Wait!* I haven't even tied my laces yet!" At that point, it can be pretty tempting to toss away the shoes and walk off the track barefoot, muttering, "Why did I even bother?" So how do you transition from "I really need to eat well" to "Let's do it!"? That's where a cooking pal comes in.

Everyone who's about to enter the kitchen for the first time or embarking on a new culinary adventure needs a cooking pal, someone with a little more cooking experience to show them the ropes. You've got some nice embers of enthusiasm at the moment; that's why you picked up this book. I want to help fan the flames and turn them into a roaring passion for cooking. How you approach cooking is too important, for your own health and that of your loved ones, to risk having those embers cool to inaction. I'm not gonna let that happen. Eventually, perhaps far sooner than you think, you'll find other kitchen mentors, people you know who can really help you raise your game. But for now, let me be your culinary coach. I've got tips that will help you maximize the time you invest in cooking and can show you how to create flavors that will delight anyone lucky enough to partake of the fruit of your labors, including, most importantly, you.

Believe me, the magic is in simply trying and then experiencing the scrumptious results. Flavor is what brings people back to the table again and again. The knowledge that great flavors and great nutrition can joyfully coexist on the same plate makes it a win-win proposition. Remember, if food doesn't taste good people are unlikely to eat it, no matter how healthful it is.

An interesting thing happens over time. Even people who don't have much interest in nutrition begin to notice how they feel when they regularly eat nutritious, satiating meals—or, in some cases, they notice how they *don't* feel, as in bloated, tired, and so on. Eating more healthful meals just a few times a week can start to turn the tide. Eventually, even people who grew up on Oscar Mayer bologna begin gravitating toward a more healthful diet.

Trust me on this: all it takes to set the wheels of change in motion is one dish that combines sensational flavors and superior nutrition. So take it slow and be kind to yourself. Why? Because these foods will be very kind to you and to those you cherish.

Discovering Your Culinary GPS

Everything you need to know about connecting with healthful, life-enhancing food is already inside you. It may just need a little prompting to bring it out into the open. That's where my culinary GPS questionnaire (see page 43) comes up. It's a fun exercise with an incredible payoff. It will help you pinpoint where you stand in relation to food: the tastes and textures you love, the regional cuisines that most tempt your palate, your attitudes about eating, the times you felt nourished or not nourished, and even the support systems available to help you succeed in the kitchen. There are no right or wrong answers; rather, your response will allow you to discover reference points that can help orient you as you embark on your culinary adventure.

Best off, it really works. I recently met a lovely lady who genuinely believed that eating well was absolutely essential to living a long, happy life, but wasn't sure how to get from point A to point B. She was a network TV producer in her midthirties who worked long hours and had high stress, a poor diet, and a past history of serious illness. Plus, as she stated in the first five seconds of our meeting, "I don't cook!"

Yet that wasn't true. Using the questionnaire, we spent the next 45 minutes exploring her culinary landscape. As it turned out, she went to the farmers' market every week to get the freshest ingredients for her green smoothies. Unfortunately, she didn't like the way they tasted; they were so bitter that it took all of her willpower to drink them. Nevertheless, and despite her statements to the contrary, her efforts did indeed constitute cooking.

As we talked, it became increasingly clear that she didn't need motivation so much as direction. She had absorbed a tremendous amount of information about good nutrition, but instead of freeing her, it had led to culinary paralysis. It had never occurred to her that healthy foods could be delicious, so she focused on just getting them down quickly rather than enjoying food. That never works in the long term.

So I turned the focus to foods that she had loved earlier in life. She told a story about her mother, who was raised on traditional Asian cuisine and made a special stewed chicken and lots of stir-fries with high-quality ingredients. The change in her body language as she transitioned from talking about her bitter green smoothies to her mom's cooking was dramatic. One minute her face was pinched as she sat with her arms pulled in protectively across her chest, and the next she was smiling and gesturing expansively, her eyes sparkling at the recollection of how nourished her body and soul felt at her mother's table.

This was the opening I was looking for—the compass bearing to her culinary future. Keying on her fondness for Asian cuisine, I asked if she would be willing to throw those greens from the farmers' market into a skillet instead of a blender. I asked if she knew what a Microplane grater was. She said she had one and used it for lemon zest, because she had heard about how healthful it is. I explained how she could rub a little garlic and ginger across the Microplane, rip the kale off the stems, chop it into small pieces, add some olive oil and tamari, and suddenly she'd have a sauté reminiscent of her mother's cooking.

You could almost see the proverbial lightbulb go off over her head. From that point on, we were completely in sync. I asked what her favorite protein was, and she said, "Chicken, good-quality chicken, but I don't have always time to cook it." So I suggested that she could pick up a roasted bird to put on top of the sauté, and she said she was happy to do that. As for those green smoothies, she said she needed them because they were quick to make and she could drink them on the way to work. So I suggested that she switch to a protein shake like the one my husband makes (page 206). She liked that idea and figured that if it was good enough for my family, it was good enough for her.

Again and again I went back to the questionnaire, peeling back the layers of what made eating appealing for her: "Do you like eating from a bowl or plate?" "Ooh . . . a pretty bowl." Forks or chopsticks? "Chopsticks!" You could see her mind creating a beautiful picture: a nourishing meal, lovingly made and consumed—in an environment she had created or, to use a more apt phrase, cooked up.

That's the whole point of the questionnaire. It can take anyone from where they are, in terms of diet, to where they want to be. If you want to translate your preferences into life-enhancing meals, it will set you on your course, and the recipes in this book will keep you moving in the right direction. If cooking is really daunting for you, I suggest working with a local cook who's dedicated to healthy fare made with fresh ingredients so you can get more hands-on training. Likewise, if you have specific nutritional concerns or health issues, consider meeting with a nutritionist, who can help you transform a list of foods that enhance longevity into meals you'll find yourself willing and able to make.

Discovering Your Culinary GPS

- What are your favorite foods?

- Why do you like them? What, specifically, do you like about them?

- What are your comfort foods? What foods make you happy?

- If you were stuck on a desert island, what's the one food you would take with you and why?

- What kinds of food do you crave and why?

- What are your favorite flavors? If your taste buds could travel around the world, where would they go? Multiple landings are allowed!

- What are your favorite or least favorite textures? Do you enjoy crispy, crunchy, or smooth textures?

- What foods do you not like or dislike?

- How often to you drink hydrating beverages, such as water or herbal or green teas?

- What kind of relationship do you have with food? Did you grow up with family members who cooked? Was gathering at the dinner table generally a happy or upsetting experience?

- Where are your ancestors from?

- Do you have any specific comforting food memories?

- How many meals do you eat a day? Do you eat small meals more often or one or two big meals a day?

- Do you take your time and savor your food, or do you eat while distracted or on the run?

- How do you feel when you're eating and at the end of a meal? Do you feel nourished and satiated?

- Do you eat to live, or do you live to eat?

- Do you cook, or does someone else in your family cook? How often do you cook?

- Do you want to cook or be a part of the cooking process? Can you identify a friend or family member you could cook with?

- How much time would you be willing to devote to cooking during the week or weekend?

- What are your goals pertaining to food? For example, do you want to become inspired or make a transition to a more healthful and sustainable way of eating?

- Do you have a family history of chronic disease?

- Do you currently have any health challenges?

Balancing Flavor with FASS

Like all good tools, FASS is easy to both grasp and use. FASS is an acronym that stands for fat, acid, salt, and sweet. These are the four tastes that many cooks balance by instinct in each dish. While we do sense other flavors (more on that in a bit), these four are at the forefront, constantly vying with each other for our attention, and if there's an imbalance, boy do we notice! If, on the other hand, you can get them to work in harmony, their synergies are practically orchestral. They build on each other to create a crescendo of flavor far more resonant than each individual taste.

Keeping FASS in mind helps ensure that all the players stay in perfect pitch, and it's almost as simple as using a tuning fork. In my book (literally!), it involves just four pantry staples: olive oil (fat), lemon juice (acid), sea salt (salt), and Grade B organic maple syrup (sweet). Before I show you how they work together, let's take a look what each brings to the party.

Olive Oil

Like all fats, olive oil is a delivery system for flavor. Like me, when you were growing up you may have heard that different parts of the tongue held different taste receptors: bitter in back, sweet up front, and so on. As it turns out, that's not the case. Receptors for all tastes reside in little islands spread across the tongue and even on the roof of your mouth.

In FASS, olive oil is like a Caribbean ferry that goes island-hopping, carrying different ingredients and tastes all across the tongue. It guarantees that flavors reach every possible taste bud destination. This is vital because as we age, our taste buds become less sensitive, so we don't taste food as well. One way to fight that is to incorporate some fat into the food to ensure that all of your taste buds are in play. If you're wondering why I use olive oil for this purpose, it goes right back to the topic of this book: if you study the cuisine of the most long-lived populations, you'll find that many of them make extensive use of olive oil. There's not a healthier oil or fat out there, and if you use the good stuff, its flavor can't be beat. Additionally, healthy fats slow the release of sugars into the bloodstream.

Lemon Juice

I like working with lemon juice because, unlike other acids, such as vinegar, it isn't overpowering. Acids have a brightening effect, energizing the taste buds the way a lightning bolt cuts through a dark sky. I turn to lemon and its close citrus kin, lime and orange, when a dish is a bit flat and needs something to get noticed; adding a squeeze of citrus is the quickest way to get the flavors to pop.

Adding acids also confers a nice a health bonus. Like fats, acids slow the release of sugars into the bloodstream, lowering their glycemic load. That's great for folks concerned with high blood sugar or diabetes. Acids also jump-start the salivary glands, improving digestion.

Sea Salt

Sea salt is my salt of choice, because unlike refined table salt, it retains up to eighty different trace minerals. Salt may be the most misunderstood ingredient. From a cook's viewpoint, its primary purpose is to work its way into other ingredients, where it has an action like little scrubbing bubbles that allows it to break down fiber, particularly in vegetables. This helps the food's inherent tastes come forth. Sea salt also gives the sensation of moving flavors toward the front of the mouth.

From a health viewpoint, salt has often been seen as the enemy, something to be avoided. That awareness is important when dealing with processed foods because salt and sodium are extremely overused by manufacturers and are also hidden in many of their tongue-twisting ingredients such as hydrolyzed yeast and monosodium glutamate. But in this book, almost every ingredient is a whole food, so the only sodium they have is what nature gave them. That's my way of saying that, unless your doctor has restricted your sodium intake, the amounts of sea salt I suggest using will benefit both your health and your taste buds.

Maple Syrup

Grade B organic maple syrup is my go-to sweetener for a few reasons. First off, it's far more healthful than refined sugar. Katie, one of my kitchen assistants, is always amazed at how little syrup is needed. Even when I'm working with a large stockpot of soup, she calls the amount of syrup I use medicinal in quantity. I also prefer maple syrup's taste profile; it has a mellow rather than overwhelming sweetness, and it has a way of rounding out the flavors in a dish. If you wonder why I use Grade B rather than Grade A, Grade B has more minerals and a slightly richer flavor.

FASS in Action

I often demonstrate FASS with soups, because that's the perfect canvas for showing how taste can be adjusted quickly. One of my favorite things to do when teaching is purposely throw off the flavor of a soup while it's cooking. Then I ask students to come up, taste, and offer suggestions. Everyone is shy at first; no matter how it tastes, they usually say, "It's okay." I just look at them and say, "'Okay?' Who wants to settle for 'okay' what you can have 'great!' Now tell me, what do you think it needs?" It doesn't take them long to start offering ideas, and with just a bit of experimentation, they get it.

If the balance of flavors is off, the solution is usually to add a bit of sea salt, lemon juice, or maple syrup. It's a bit like flying an airplane; if you've ever had the wheel in your hands, you probably learned mighty quickly that it only takes a minute turn to send the plane off in another direction. Likewise, course corrections with food generally require just a pinch of salt, a spritz of lemon juice, or a restrained drizzle of maple syrup. If the flavors are in the ballpark but the soup is missing mouthfeel—that satiating feeling when food hits the palate—olive oil or another healthful fat is usually the answer.

It's a blast to see people take a soup to that ideal place incrementally, through trial and error. You can hear excitement in their voices as they taste, squeeze in a bit of lemon juice, taste again, say, "Better, better, but it still needs . . . a pinch of salt," taste again, say "Ooh, it's close, . . . close," add another spritz of lemon juice, taste, and exclaim, "Yes, *yes, yes!!!*"

FASS FOR FLAVOR AND NUTRITION

	EXAMPLES	FUNCTION	HEALTH BENEFITS
Fat	Olive oil, butter, coconut oil, ghee, sesame oil, avocado, nuts	Distributes flavor across the palate.	Can optimize healthy gene expression (antioxidant, anti-inflammatory).
Acid	Lemons, limes, oranges, vinegar	Brightens flavors.	Increases absorption of minerals and stimulates digestion.
Salt	Sea salt, tamari, fish sauce, miso	Brings out the flavor of foods. Moves flavor to the front of the tongue where it's best perceived.	In balances with potassium, facilitates energy production and cellular metabolism.
Sweet	Grade B maple syrup, honey	Tames harsh, sour, or spicy flavors. Rounds out or harmonizes flavors.	Increases sense of pleasure.

FASS FIXES IN THE KITCHEN

PROBLEM	FASS FIX
Too sweet?	Add lemon juice or another acid.
Too sour?	Add maple syrup or another sweetener.
Too bland?	Add salt.
Too salty?	Add lemon juice or another acid, which will erase the taste of salt.
Just needs a spark?	Add lemon juice or another acid, or an aromatic ingredient (discussed shortly, under Spicy Solutions), at the end of cooking.
Too harsh?	Add 1/8 to 1/4 teaspoon Grade B maple syrup.

Source: Rebecca Katz, MS, with Jeanne Wallace, PhD, www.nutritional-solutions.net.

FASS is about building awareness and trusting that you can coax the finest flavors out of anything you choose to make. That's so important when you're embracing new foods, especially vegetables that may, on their own, be a tad bitter. With FASS, challenging flavors become malleable, a mere starting point for what you craft into a phenomenal finished product. In time, you'll look at the ingredients in any dish and, like a painter gazing at the colors on a palette, know how the elements will blend. You'll recognize how varying temperatures can unlock the inherent sweetness of certain ingredients (which is why I love roasting veggies), and how FASS can take those flavors over the top—especially with the help of two other categories of ingredients . . .

Umami

For the past few decades, cooks, scientists, and gourmands have been debating whether umami (pronounced OOH-mommy), a certain something that is as elusive as its name suggests, is a taste or a sensation. The word, borrowed from the Japanese term for savoriness, is often used to describe the weight, gravity, brothiness, or meatiness that certain foods lend to a dish. When you're looking for that quality in a dish, take a gander at the list of umami ingredients below and choose one that suits your fancy. As you look it over, you'll probably be surprised at how diverse these foods are, ranging from beef to green tea to tomatoes:

- Beef
- Carrots
- Chicken
- Eggs
- Green tea
- Kombu

- Miso
- Parmesan cheese
- Pomegranate
- Potatoes
- Red wine
- Scallops

- Shiitake mushrooms
- Shrimp
- Sweet potatoes
- Tamari
- Tomatoes

Spicy Solutions

Another category of ingredients that's an absolute must-use, from the standpoint of both flavor and longevity, is aromatics: spices, herbs, and alliums, such as garlic, onions, shallots, leeks, and chives.

Aromatics serve several important roles. They're incredibly stimulating to the mouth, nose, and eyes, offering a culinary telegram to the brain consisting of three words: time to eat! There's immense pleasure associated with that message. It could be argued that when you crave a certain kind of food—Italian, Indian, and so on—what you really want is the aromatics associated with that cuisine.

Receiving the sensory input that those aromatics are just around the corner creates almost a Pavlovian response, like a little kid hearing the chimes of an ice cream truck coming down the street. Just think of how your nose has sometimes pulled you out of from whatever you may have been doing in another part of the house, offering a simple but irresistible command: "Go the kitchen. Now!" That's aromatics at work.

If you haven't used these ingredients a lot, fear not. The recipes in this book will help you get more familiar with them, and then you can start improvising. When you're ready to put together your own creations, you can use the following global "flavorprints" to help you capture the essence of different cuisines.

GLOBAL FLAVORPRINTS

REGION	INGREDIENTS
Asian	basil, bay leaves, chiles, cilantro, coriander, curry powder, five-spice powder, garlic, ginger, kaffir lime leaves, lemongrass, lime juice and zest, mint, miso, red pepper flakes, turmeric
Indian	cardamom, chiles, cilantro, cinnamon, cloves, coriander, cumin, curry powder, garlic, ginger, mint, mustard seeds, nutmeg, red pepper flakes, saffron, sesame seeds, turmeric
Latin	chiles, cilantro, cinnamon, cumin, garlic, oregano, sesame seeds
Mediterranean	basil, bay leaves, fennel, garlic, marjoram, mint, nutmeg, oregano, parsley, red pepper flakes, rosemary, saffron, sage, thyme
Middle Eastern	allspice, cilantro, cinnamon, coriander, cumin, garlic, marjoram, mint, oregano, sesame seeds, thyme
Moroccan	cilantro, cinnamon, coriander, cumin, garlic, ginger, mint, red pepper flakes, saffron, thyme, turmeric

Source: The American Spice Trade Association.

Gram for gram, no ingredients are more powerful for stimulating the appetite and satisfying the taste buds than herbs and spices. Their power to heal is no less outstanding, as a quick review of the Culinary Pharmacy (page 21) will reveal. Over the past decade or so, numerous aromatic ingredients have gone under the microscope. A major impetus for this may well have been the prolific use of spices in folk medicine; they have been revered by traditional healers from around the globe for centuries.

Now the research from many top-notch medical centers is coming in, and results indicate that those healers may have been on to something. Many aromatics contain compounds capable of modifying gene expression. Genes often have the equivalent of on and off switches, and they typically flip on and off rapidly to meet the changing needs of the body. When this system is operating well, one of its functions is to create molecules and proteins

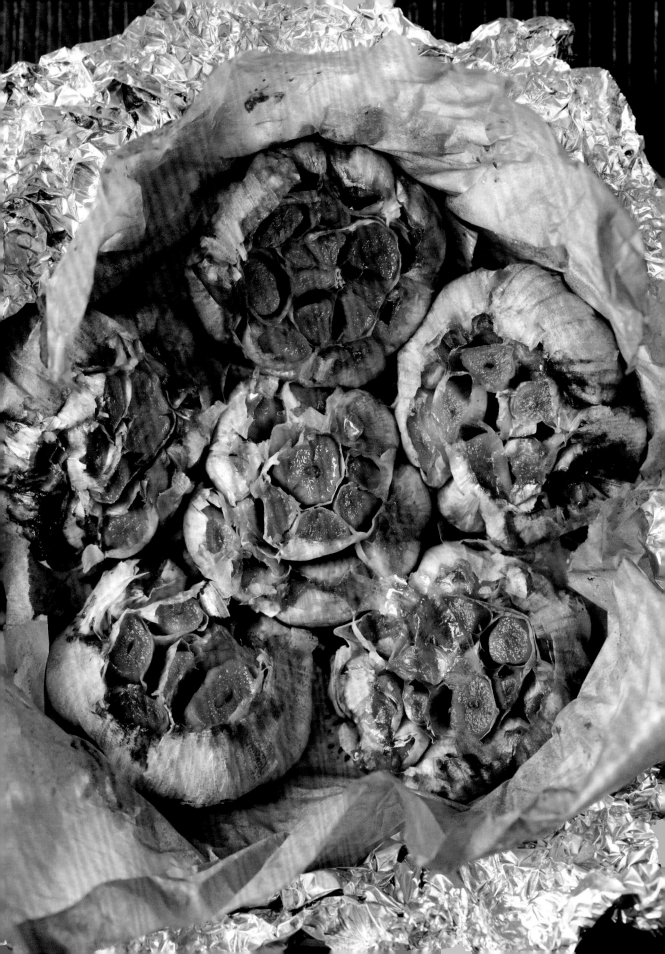

that keep cancer and many other diseases at bay. Spices appear to play a huge role in this process. Similarly, many aromatics contain compounds that provide immune support, control inflammation, and ward off bacteria and viruses.

What more could you ask for? Great taste, copious health benefits, and possibly increased longevity—that's what I'd call literally a pinch in time.

Why Organic Matters

Before you dive into the recipes, I want to be sure we're on the same page about the importance of purchasing organic ingredients wherever possible. Eating for longevity is all about tilting the odds in your favor, and organic food can make a difference. As a cook, I was initially drawn to organic ingredients because of their flavors. To my taste buds, organic ingredients—fruits, veggies, meats, and more—are always superior. But the focus of this book is on how food affects your health, for better and worse, so let's take a quick look at some of the health benefits of organics.

Food raised organically, without pesticides and synthetic fertilizers, is consistently more nutrient dense. One possible explanation is that fruits and vegetables that rely on their own defenses to survive and thrive have a different, richer nutrient profile than their non-organic kin. When it comes to fish, fowl, and other animal products, consider that animals raised conventionally are often given numerous drugs and hormones to enhance their growth, and this can negatively affect their nutritional profile. As an example, farm-raised salmon have far higher levels of omega-6 fatty acids than their wild cousins. While omega-6s do have some health benefits and are present in many healthful foods, the ratio of omega-6s to omega-3s is crucial. Unfortunately, most people consume excessive amounts of omega-6s and too few omega-3s, a dietary pattern that's been linked to inflammation and to a host of other deleterious effects on the body. Steering clear of non-organic animal products is one way to address this problem.

Amazingly, up to this point there hasn't been a great deal of research into how consuming pesticides and hormones affects human health. However, the general consensus among physicians and researchers is that while these substances may or may not be harmful, they certainly aren't beneficial. As someone who always likes to stay a step ahead of the science, I'll go out on a limb and say I think the recommendation to avoid various pesticides, hormones, and such will only increase over time.

The great news about organics is that their growing popularity has made them more available and affordable. Some supermarket chains even have house brands of different organic products, and they wouldn't invest their money in that unless they saw a booming market. Personally, I like getting organics right from the source: local farmers who raise their produce and meats ethically and sustainably. If you don't do so already, check out your local farmers' markets, where you can meet face to face with the people who raise your food. As a bonus, they often enjoy chatting about the foods they've raised.

Still, there are times when organic options are either expensive or unavailable. Depending on where you live and your budget, sometimes you may need to purchase conventional produce. If so, try to be well informed about which produce items typically have more pesticide residues. Fortunately, there are good resources to help you out here. The Environmental Working Group (www.ewg.org), a nonprofit organization that conducts research and publishes information on threats to the environment and human health, produces an annual list of the Dirty Dozen and Clean Fifteen. In 2012, their Dirty Dozen list recommended avoiding the following conventionally raised produce:

- Apples
- Celery
- Sweet bell peppers
- Peaches
- Strawberries

- Grapes
- Nectarines (imported)
- Spinach
- Lettuce

- Cucumbers
- Blueberries (domestic)
- Potatoes

On the upside, the following conventionally raised fruits and vegetables have relatively minimal amounts of pesticide residues:

- Onions
- Sweet corn
- Pineapples
- Avocados
- Cabbage
- Sweet Peas

- Asparagus
- Mangoes
- Eggplant
- Kiwi fruit
- Cantaloupe (domestic)

- Sweet potatoes
- Grapefruit
- Watermelon
- Mushrooms

For a more complete list, ranking many common produce items, visit www.ewg.org/foodnews/list.

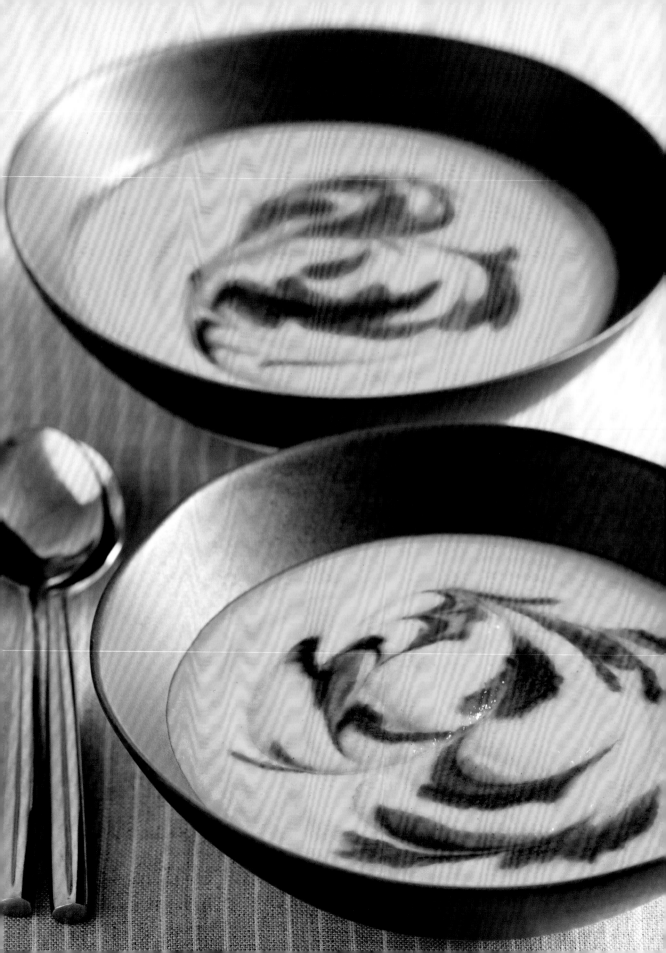

CHAPTER 4

Life-Enhancing Soups and Broths

There's nothing I'd rather do, day in, day out, than make soup.

If aliens dropped in from Mars and, after I fed them, said to me, "We need to bring everything in your kitchen back for our next Ladies Club Auxiliary lunch, but since we appreciate your hospitality, we'll leave you your two favorite kitchen tools," I'd grab my wooden soup spoon and jump in my 24-quart stockpot. Don't laugh; I fit.

To me, soups are pure comfort, so much so that I prefer to call them "cozy bowls." In my book, they're the gift that keeps on giving. They taste great right out of the pot, and in most cases it's simple to make extra, so that you can freeze a few quarts and reheat them on days where you just don't feel like cooking from scratch.

Soups are also an ideal way to get a blast of life-enhancing nutrients. People who normally disdain vegetables willingly embrace them in the aromatic headiness of a soup. The recipes in this chapter are incredibly nutrient-dense, and while they are great as written, they're not set in stone. Soups are literally a melting pot that invites creativity. If you want to swap out one veggie for another, or if you crave a certain spice, go for it! From a cook's viewpoint, soups are the perfect living lab; no other dish allows you to tinker with the flavors throughout the entire cooking process in the same way. (And if you read my tips about FASS on page 44, I'll show you a foolproof way to course-correct any soup while it's on the stove.)

I have to warn you, making soup is addictive. The prep work is meditative; the sound of the knife hitting the cutting board creates a lulling rhythm that's uniquely your own. It's also a great training ground. Chopping a big old root vegetable into smaller and smaller pieces will help you get familiar with handling produce in a hurry. Plus, there's something just plain fun about the chop and toss routine, especially if you stop for a moment to consider the amazing fuel you're creating for your body. It's like the gas that goes into a high-performance automobile: high-test all the way, filled with a king's ransom of antioxidants, minerals, vitamins, phytochemicals . . . you name it, it's in the broth.

And what a broth it is! The base broth for most of these recipes is my Magic Mineral Broth 2.0 (page 55) or Chicken Magic Mineral Broth 2.0 (page 56). Either has enough nutrients to make your grandmother put down her knitting and applaud or, at the very least, to smile and say, "It's about time!"

Magic Mineral Broth 2.0

I'll admit it: I'm a little obsessive. I'll be darned if I'm going to send anything out of my kitchen that I wouldn't eat—and love—myself. Sometimes that means it takes a lot of time and patience to perfect a recipe. Such is the case here. It took 65 gallons, scores of attempts, and a full rotation of the earth around the sun before I came up with what I've come to call Magic Mineral Broth: a delicious, nutrient-dense veggie broth with amazing health properties. Magic Mineral Broth became my go-to broth, and after I published the recipe in my previous cookbooks, it became many other people's go-to broth as well. I've created a new, jazzed-up version for this book—let's call it Magic Mineral Broth 2.0—adding fennel and thyme for their outstanding longevity properties. While you could just use it in recipes, it's also wonderful on its own, as a dazzling and hydrating elixir of life. MAKES 6 QUARTS

1 fennel bulb, with tops
2 unpeeled yellow onions, cut into quarters
6 unpeeled carrots, cut into thirds
1 leek, white and green parts, cut into thirds
1 bunch celery, including the heart, cut into thirds
2 unpeeled sweet potatoes, cut into chunks
1 unpeeled garnet yam, cut into chunks
1 large bunch fresh flat-leaf parsley
6 sprigs fresh thyme
12 large cloves unpeeled garlic, smashed
1 (3-inch) piece of unpeeled fresh ginger, cut in half lengthwise
1 (8-inch) strip of kombu
12 black peppercorns
4 juniper berries or allspice berries
2 bay leaves
8 quarts cold filtered water, plus more if needed
1 teaspoon sea salt

Rinse all the vegetables well, including the kombu. Put the fennel, onions, carrots, leek, celery, sweet potatoes, yam, parsley, thyme, garlic, ginger, kombu, peppercorns, juniper berries, and bay leaves in a 12-quart or larger stockpot. Add the water, cover, and bring to a boil over high heat. Decrease the heat to low and simmer uncovered for 2 to 4 hours. As the broth simmers, some of the water will evaporate; add more if the vegetables begin to peek out. Simmer until the full richness of the vegetables can be tasted.

Strain the broth through a large, coarse-mesh sieve placed over a large heatproof container. Stir in the salt. Let cool to room temperature before refrigerating or freezing.

Variation: For extra immune-boosting action, add 8 whole shiitake mushrooms, 1 (6-inch piece) of burdock root (washed and cut into quarters), or both.

PREP TIME: 10 minutes COOK TIME: 2 to 4 hours
STORAGE: Store in an airtight container in the refrigerator for up to 6 days or in the freezer for up to 4 months.
PER SERVING: Calories: 10; Total Fat: 0.25 g (0 g saturated, 0 g monounsaturated); Carbohydrates: 3 g; Protein: 0.25 g; Fiber: 0.75 g; Sodium: 70 mg

COOK'S NOTES: Like fine wine, this broth gets better with age. The longer you simmer it, the more flavor and nutrient density it will have. If you don't want to have to tend to it for hours on end, you can also cut the recipe in half and make it in a slow cooker. Once the broth is cooked, you may want to add about 1/8 teaspoon each of lemon juice and sea salt to bring the flavors to life.

Chicken Magic Mineral Broth 2.0

Can you make a fantastically tasty and nourishing broth even better? Why not! It all comes down to dem bones—or, more precisely, it comes down to the nutrients Magic Mineral Broth can pull from chicken bones during a good, long simmering. Many of these nutrients help build healthy cartilage, immune cells, blood cells, and, not surprisingly, bone itself. Of course, chicken bones enrich the flavor. MAKES 6 QUARTS

1 fennel bulb, with tops
2 unpeeled yellow onions, cut into quarters
6 unpeeled carrots, cut into thirds
1 leek, white and green parts, cut into thirds
1 bunch celery, including the heart, cut into thirds
2 unpeeled sweet potatoes, cut into chunks
1 unpeeled garnet yam, cut into chunks
1 large bunch fresh flat-leaf parsley
6 sprigs fresh thyme
12 large cloves unpeeled garlic, smashed
1 (3-inch) piece of unpeeled fresh ginger, cut in half lengthwise
1 (8-inch) strip of kombu
12 black peppercorns
4 juniper berries or allspice berries
2 bay leaves
1 tablespoon vinegar or freshly squeezed lemon juice
1 organic chicken carcass, or 2 pounds organic chicken bones
8 quarts cold filtered water, plus more if needed
1 teaspoon sea salt

COOK'S NOTE: Once you've skimmed the fat from the surface of the broth, you can remove even more by dabbing the surface of the broth with paper towels to sop it up.

Rinse all the vegetables well, including the kombu. Put the fennel, onions, carrots, leek, celery, sweet potatoes, yam, parsley, thyme, garlic, ginger, kombu, peppercorns, juniper berries, bay leaves, vinegar, and chicken carcass in a 12-quart or larger stockpot. Add the water, cover, and bring to a boil over high heat. Decrease the heat to low and simmer uncovered for 2 to 4 hours. As the broth simmers, some of the water will evaporate; add more if the vegetables begin to peek out. Simmer until the full richness of the vegetables can be tasted.

Strain the broth through a large, course-mesh sieve placed over a large heatproof container. Stir in the salt. Let cool to room temperature, then refrigerate overnight. Skim off as much fat from the top of the broth as you can, then portion into airtight containers and refrigerate or freeze.

Variation: For extra immune-boosting action, add 8 whole shiitake mushrooms, 1 (6-inch piece) of burdock root (washed and cut into quarters), or both.

PREP TIME: 10 minutes COOK TIME: 2 to 4 hours
STORAGE: Store in an airtight container in the refrigerator for up to 6 days or in the freezer for up to 4 months.
PER SERVING: Calories: 50; Total Fat: 1.5 g (0 g saturated, 0 g mono-unsaturated); Carbohydrates: 11.5 g; Protein: 1.2 g; Fiber: 2 g; Sodium: 144 mg

WHO KNEW? You say "sweet potato"; I say . . . "yam"? There are two main types of sweet potatoes: those that have pale flesh that cooks up with a dry texture, and those that have darker, orange flesh that's more moist. In the US, the term "yams" is often used for orange-fleshed sweet potatoes, creating some confusion because, in most of the world, "yam" refers to a plant from an entirely different family. To further cloud the issue, the USDA requires that any sweet potato labeled as a yam also bear the label "sweet potato." I'm sure they're trying to be helpful, but . . . So, just to set the record straight, the garnet yams called for in this recipe are actually sweet potatoes.

Chilled Curried Cucumber Soup

Yogurt plays an important role the cuisine of many cultures renowned for longevity, and there's probably a link. Yogurt with live cultures is the GI tract's best friend, aiding digestion, fighting off infections, and soothing an upset tummy. Yogurt is also a versatile culinary performer, making a delicious appearance in everything from breads to smoothies to dollops and beyond. My friend Catherine says this soup reminds her of being in an Armenian grandmother's kitchen. It's wonderfully refreshing, with the yogurt serving as a canvas for cucumber, garlic, cumin, ginger, mint, and curry powder. To me, this soup is as summery as long walks at sunset, fireflies, and shimmering pitchers of iced tea. MAKES 4 SERVINGS

2¼ cups organic plain yogurt
1 pound, 4 ounces English cucumbers, peeled, seeded, and chopped
1 teaspoon minced fresh ginger
½ teaspoon chopped garlic
1¼ teaspoons curry powder
½ teaspoon sea salt
½ teaspoon ground cumin
2 teaspoons freshly squeezed lemon
1 teaspoon grated lemon zest
1 tablespoon chopped fresh mint

Put the yogurt, cucumbers, ginger, garlic, curry powder, salt, cumin, lemon juice, and lemon zest in a blender and process until extremely smooth. Taste; you may want to add as much as ¾ teaspoon of salt. Transfer to a glass container, cover, and refrigerate for at least 2 hours. Just before serving, stir in the mint.

PREP TIME: 10 minutes COOK TIME: 2 hours for chilling
STORAGE: Store in an airtight container in the refrigerator for up to 5 days.
PER SERVING: Calories: 105; Total Fat: 5 g (3 g saturated, 1 g mono-unsaturated); Carbohydrates: 10.5 g; Protein: 6 g; Fiber: 1.5 g; Sodium: 267 mg

WHO KNEW? According to nutrition expert Kathie Madonna Swift, MS, RD, LDN, coauthor of *The Inside Tract: Your Good Gut Guide to Great Digestive Health*, the majority of both the human body's immune system (60 percent) and neurotransmitters are located in the gut. The GI tract even has its own command center, called the enteric nervous system. It's no wonder some scientists now refer to the gut as the second brain.

Velvety Mediterranean Gazpacho with Avocado Cream

Some folks like shots of tequila. My coauthor, Mat, sips Grand Marnier, and my husband, Gregg, is happy with a finger of twelve-year-old Scotch. Me? My choice is this Mediterranean gazpacho, which is an orgy of vegetables: cucumbers, red bell peppers, cherry tomatoes, red onions, fennel, garlic, and more. At this point, you may be rebelling at the thought of chopping all those vegetables, and I totally understand that instinct. When I was at culinary school, gazpacho prep was the equivalent of Ninja Knife Skills Boot Camp. Teachers actually walked around the kitchen with rulers to make sure each veggie was uniformly diced. That's nuts and, you'll be glad to know, totally unnecessary. In this recipe, all of the ingredients are simply coarsely chopped, then they're thrown into the blender and—*shazam!*—it's party time. I took this to an Independence Day dinner, poured it into shot glasses, and topped it with a creamy avocado concoction. You know you're doing something right when everyone corners you for the recipe. MAKES 8 SERVINGS

AVOCADO CREAM WITH BASIL
1 avocado, halved and flesh scooped out
2 tablespoons water
2 teaspoons coarsely chopped fresh basil
3/4 teaspoon freshly squeezed lemon juice
1/8 teaspoon sea salt

GAZPACHO
3 cups low-sodium tomato juice
1/4 cup extra-virgin olive oil
1 tablespoon plus 1 teaspoon freshly squeezed lemon juice
1 tablespoon Grade B maple syrup
1 teaspoon sea salt
1/2 teaspoon ground cumin
1/4 teaspoon ground coriander
1/8 teaspoon cayenne
2 cloves garlic, coarsely chopped
1 fennel bulb, cut into quarters and cored
3 celery stalks, coarsely chopped
1 English cucumber, peeled, seeded, and coarsely chopped
1 red bell pepper, seeded and coarsely chopped
2 cups cherry tomatoes
1 small red onion, coarsely chopped
1/4 cup coarsely chopped fresh basil, cilantro, or a combination

To make the avocado cream, put all the ingredients in blender and process until very smooth. Transfer to a small bowl. (No need to rinse the blender before proceeding.)

To make the gazpacho, put all the ingredients in a large bowl and stir to combine. Working in batches, transfer to the blender and process until completely smooth. Taste; you may want to add a pinch of salt or a bit of maple syrup. Pour into small glasses and garnish with the avocado cream.

PREP TIME: 20 minutes
STORAGE: Store the gazpacho in an airtight container in the refrigerator for 5 days or in the freezer for up to 1 month. Store the avocado cream with a spritz of lemon or lime on top in an airtight container in the refrigerator for up to 2 days.
PER SERVING: Calories: 125; Total Fat: 7.5 g (1 g saturated, 5.5 g monounsaturated); Carbohydrates: 13.5 g; Protein: 2 g; Fiber: 3.5 g; Sodium: 314 mg

WHO KNEW? According to nutrigenomics expert Colleen Fogarty Draper, MS, you can increase the body's ability to absorb nutrient supplements by taking them with certain foods. "I suggest eating foods high in that particular nutrient concurrently to ensure maximum absorbability," says Draper. This makes sense, considering that the interplay of different substances within a given food often makes a particular nutrient, say vitamin C, more bioavailable to the body.

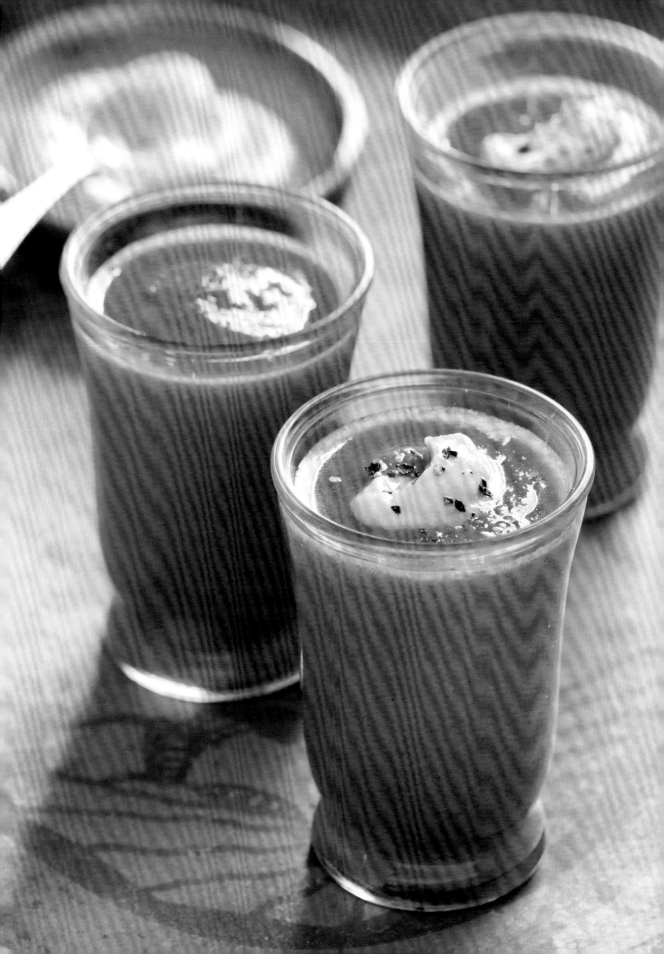

Summer's Sweetest Corn Bisque

Corn has gotten a bad rap lately, and that's a shame. It's true that adulterated versions, from high-fructose corn syrup to corn oil, are downright unhealthy. But freshly shucked corn is amazingly rich in phytonutrients, and in flavor. Believe me, I know good corn. There used to be huge cornfields within walking distance of my childhood home. I vividly remember coming home with a bushel of summer corn, planting myself outside our back door, and ripping away the husks with glee. Flash forward just a wee bit and now I have my Gen Y kitchen angels Jen and Katie out on my back porch, sipping lemonade and giggling over how they're knee-deep in husks. In this soup, shaved corncobs make for an outrageous broth, and the whazzed-up kernels create a richness that lets the honey-like flavor linger on the tongue like a slow sunset. If you could put summer in a pot, this would be it. MAKES 8 SERVINGS

12 ears of corn
10 cups filtered water
Sea salt
2 tablespoons extra-virgin olive oil
2 cups diced yellow onions
Chive Oil (page 178), for garnish

Cut the kernels off the corn and set aside. Put the corncobs, water, and 2$^1/_2$ teaspoons of salt in a large stockpot over medium heat. Cover and cook for 30 minutes.

Meanwhile, heat the olive oil in a large skillet over medium heat. Add the onions and a generous pinch of salt and sauté until golden, about 7 minutes. Add the corn kernels and a generous pinch of salt and sauté until the corn is just tender, about 4 minutes more.

Remove the corncobs from the stockpot and discard. Working in batches, pour some of the broth in a blender. Add some of the corn mixture and process until very smooth. For a velvety texture, after pureeing each batch, strain it through a fine-mesh sieve, pushing with the back of a spoon to extract as much liquid as possible. Return the soup to the stockpot and stir in a pinch of salt. Cook over low heat until just heated through. Serve garnished with a drizzle of Chive Oil.

Variation: To create a chunky chowder, reserve 1 cup of the corn and onion mixture. After blending the soup, stir in the reserved corn and onions, along with $^1/_4$ cup peeled and diced carrot, $^1/_4$ cup diced celery, and $^1/_2$ cup diced red potatoes. Simmer over low heat, stirring occasionally, until the potatoes and carrots are just tender, about 8 minutes.

PREP TIME: 20 minutes COOK TIME: 40 minutes
STORAGE: Store in an airtight container in the refrigerator for up to 5 days or in the freezer for up to 4 months.
PER SERVING: Calories: 220; Total Fat: 6 g (1 g saturated, 3.5 g monounsaturated); Carbohydrates: 42 g; Protein: 6.5 g; Fiber: 5.5 g; Sodium: 860 mg

Julie's "Spring Is Busting Out All Over" Soup

Each of us has a little clock of hope in our head. It starts ticking in the quiet depths of winter and reminds us that, although the scene outside may be still and solemn, the earth will soon awaken with spring's vivacious explosion of color. For me and my "soup sister" Julie, that mental metronome kicks in as soon as we hear rumors that the first stalks of asparagus are soon to arrive at the farmers' market. In this soup, asparagus provides a feast not just for the mouth, but also for the eyes. Asparagus is one of my Super Sixteen longevity foods (see page 2), in large part because it contains copious quantities of the powerful antioxidant glutathione. And since spring is the season when everything comes alive, it's only appropriate that this soup pairs asparagus with four other high-ranking longevity partners: garlic, thyme, mint, and yogurt. MAKES 8 SERVINGS

2 tablespoons extra-virgin olive oil
1 cup finely chopped yellow onion
Sea salt
Freshly ground black pepper
1 cup finely chopped leek, white part only
1 tablespoon finely diced shallot
2 teaspoons minced garlic
1/4 teaspoon dried thyme
2 pounds asparagus, tough ends snapped off and discarded, then cut into 1/2-inch pieces
1/2 cup frozen peas, thawed
6 cups vegetable broth, homemade (page 55) or store-bought
1/4 cup finely chopped fresh flat-leaf parsley
2 teaspoons freshly squeezed lemon juice
Organic plain yogurt, for garnish
1 tablespoon chopped fresh mint, for garnish
Chive Oil (page 178), for garnish

COOK'S NOTE: *Deglazing* refers to adding liquid and scraping up bits of food stuck to the bottom of the skillet. (Those bits, which stick because of the food's natural sugars, are outrageously delicious!) Just add a little liquid (wine, broth, or water) and quickly move the food around with a spoon or spatula to loosen all of those flavorful bits of yum.

Heat the olive oil in a skillet over medium heat. Add the onion, a pinch of salt, and a pinch of pepper and sauté until golden, about 8 minutes. Add the leek and shallot and sauté for 5 minutes. Stir in the garlic and thyme. Add the asparagus, 1/4 teaspoon of salt, and 1/4 teaspoon of pepper and sauté for 3 minutes. Stir in the peas. Pour in 1 cup of the broth to deglaze the skillet, stirring to loosen any bits stuck to the pan. Cook until the asparagus is just tender. Remove from the heat.

Pour 1 1/2 cups of the broth in a blender. Add one-third of the vegetable mixture and blend until smooth. Transfer to a soup pot over low heat and repeat the process two more times, using 3 cups of the remaining broth. Stir in the parsley, lemon juice, 1/4 teaspoon sea salt, and the remaining 1/2 cup broth. Cook just until heated through. Taste; you may want to add a squeeze of lemon juice and a couple of pinches of salt. Serve garnished with a dollop of yogurt, a sprinkling of the mint, and a drizzle of Chive Oil.

Variation: Substitute mint or dill for the parsley.

PREP TIME: 15 minutes COOK TIME: 20 minutes
STORAGE: Store in an airtight container in the refrigerator for up to 4 days.
PER SERVING: Calories: 110; Total Fat: 4.5 g (1 g saturated, 3 g monounsaturated); Carbohydrates: 15 g; Protein: 4.5 g; Fiber: 5 g; Sodium: 246 mg

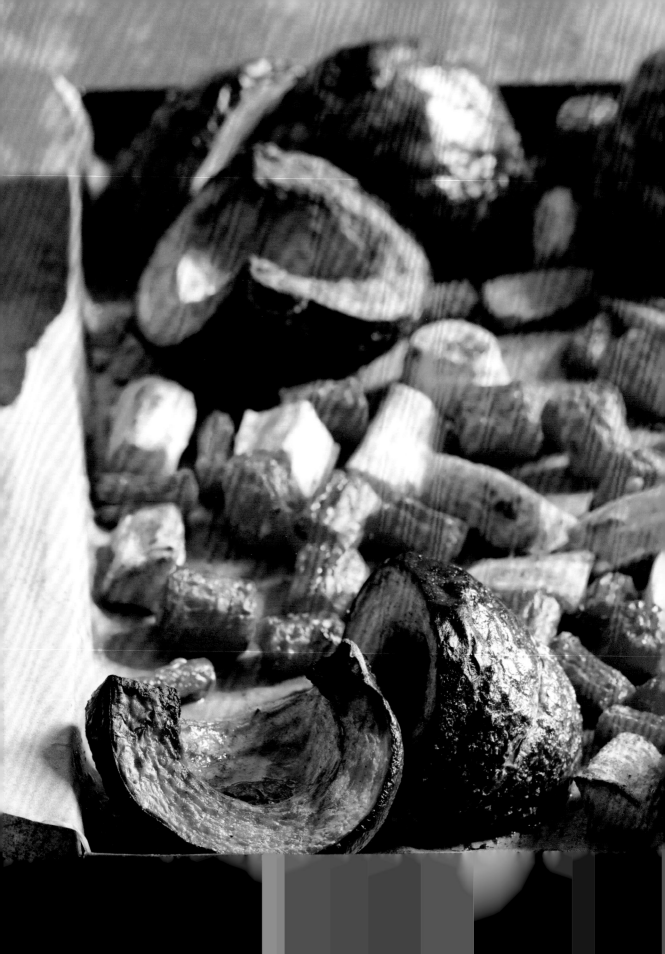

Cozy Roasted Vegetable Soup

Winter squash and root vegetables are a real comfort food, especially when roasted. Here, my favorite hardy veggies are blended into a soup (pictured on page 52) that will revive you after an autumn romp (or a good raking session), thanks to the kabocha squash, which is packed with immune-boosting compounds and beneficial fiber. Soups like this always welcome a spice blast, and I've obliged this one with cinnamon, allspice, cardamom, nutmeg, ginger, and thyme. It's like lighting your internal fireplace to keep autumn's chill at bay. MAKES 8 SERVINGS

5 tablespoons extra-virgin olive oil
Sea salt
$^1/_2$ teaspoon ground ginger
$^1/_4$ teaspoon ground cinnamon
$^1/_4$ teaspoon ground allspice
$^1/_4$ teaspoon red pepper flakes
$^1/_8$ teaspoon ground cardamom
$^1/_8$ teaspoon freshly grated nutmeg
2 cup peeled and cubed carrots
1 cup peeled and cubed parsnips
3 pounds kabocha squash, cut into quarters and seeded
1 yellow onion, diced
1 tablespoon minced garlic
2 teaspoons minced fresh ginger
$^1/_4$ teaspoon dried thyme
8 cups vegetable broth, homemade (page 55) or store-bought, plus more as needed
1 tablespoon freshly squeezed lemon juice
2 tablespoons pomegranate molasses, homemade (page 192) or store-bought, for garnish

COOK'S NOTE: Blenders work most efficiently if you put liquids in first, then add the rest of the ingredients.

Preheat the oven to 400°F. Line a rimmed baking sheet with parchment paper.

Combine 3 tablespoons of the olive oil, $^1/_4$ teaspoon of salt, and the ground ginger, cinnamon, allspice, red pepper flakes, cardamom, and nutmeg in a small bowl and stir.

Put the carrots and parsnips in a bowl. Drizzle with half of the olive oil mixture and toss until evenly coated. Rub the remaining olive oil mixture into the cut sides of the squash using your hands or a pastry brush. Put the squash in the corners of the lined baking sheet and spread the carrots and parsnips in an even layer in the center of the baking sheet. Bake for 40 minutes, until tender. Let cool.

Meanwhile, heat the remaining 2 tablespoons of olive oil in a skillet over medium heat. Add the onion and a pinch of salt and sauté until golden and translucent, about 6 minutes. Add the garlic, fresh ginger, and thyme and sauté until fragrant, about 30 seconds. Remove from the heat.

When the squash is cool enough to handle, scoop the flesh into a large bowl. Add the carrots, parsnips, and onion mixture and stir to combine. Pour one-third of the broth into a blender. Add one-third of the squash mixture and process until smooth, adding more liquid as needed. Transfer to a soup pot over low heat and repeat the process two more times. Cook just until heated through. Stir in the lemon juice and $^1/_4$ teaspoon of salt. Taste; you may want to add a spritz of lemon juice or a pinch of salt. Serve garnished with a drizzle of the pomegranate molasses.

PREP TIME: 15 minutes COOK TIME: 55 minutes
STORAGE: Store in an airtight container in the refrigerator for up to 5 days or in the freezer for up to 2 months.
PER SERVING: Calories: 200; Total Fat: 9 g (1.5 g saturated, 7 g monounsaturated); Carbohydrates: 29 g; Protein: 3 g; Fiber: 6 g; Sodium: 289 mg

Vampire Slayer's Soup

Garlic has a long list of health benefits: antibacterial, antimicrobial, anti-inflammatory, anti-vampiric (okay, I admit it's been hard to find research studies on that last one), and much, much more. Garlic lovers will gravitate toward this soup, but I want to convince those of you who say, "Garlic? *Eww!*" to try it. Those overwhelmed by garlic's natural pungency will delight in how roasting transforms the garlic into a caramelized, sweet-smelling delight. In this recipe, roasted garlic is simmered in the broth, adding to the gentle mellowing. Further fortified with Yukon gold potatoes, thyme, pepper, onion, and a spritz of lemon, this nutritious soup will arm you to the teeth . . . so to speak. MAKES 4 SERVINGS

4 heads garlic
2 tablespoons plus 4 teaspoons
    extra-virgin olive oil
Sea salt
1 cup diced yellow onion
2 teaspoons minced garlic
1 cup peeled and finely diced Yukon
    gold potatoes
1 teaspoon minced fresh thyme,
    or 1/4 teaspoon dried
1/4 teaspoon freshly ground black
    pepper
3 1/4 cups vegetable broth, home-
    made (page 55) or store-bought
Chive Oil (page 178), for garnish

COOK'S NOTE: Roasted garlic is creamy, nutty, and eminently spreadable, so you may want to roast extra garlic or set aside a few cloves for later use. It's great for perking up vegetables and marinades. To speed preparation of the soup, you can roast the garlic in advance. Once it has cooled, store the roasted heads in an airtight container in the refrigerator for up to up to 3 days.

Preheat the oven to 400°F.

Cut the tops off of the heads of garlic and discard. Drizzle each head of garlic with 1 teaspoon of the olive oil, then sprinkle with a pinch of salt. Wrap the garlic in parchment paper in one bundle, and then wrap in aluminum foil. Bake for 45 to 50 minutes; the aroma will tell you when it's ready. The flesh should be soft and golden brown. Remove from the oven to cool.

Heat the remaining 2 tablespoons of olive oil in a skillet over medium heat. Add the onion and a pinch of salt and sauté until translucent, about 4 minutes. Add the minced garlic, potatoes, thyme, pepper, and 1/4 teaspoon of salt and sauté for 5 minutes. Pour in 3/4 cup of the broth to deglaze the skillet, stirring to loosen any bits stuck to the pan. Simmer until potatoes are tender and the liquid has mostly evaporated. Remove from the heat.

When the garlic is cool enough to handle, squeeze the flesh into a bowl and mash with the back of a spoon to form a paste.

Pour the remaining 2 1/2 cups of broth into the blender. Add the roasted garlic and the onion mixture and blend until smooth. Transfer to a soup pot over low heat and stir in 1/4 teaspoon salt. Cook just until heated through. Do a FASS check (see page 44); you may want to add a spritz of lemon juice and a pinch of salt. Serve garnished with Chive Oil.

PREP TIME: 20 minutes COOK TIME: 1 hour
STORAGE: Store in an airtight container in the refrigerator for up to 3 days or in the freezer for up to 3 months.
PER SERVING: Calories: 210; Total Fat: 11 g (1.5 g saturated, 8 g mono-unsaturated); Carbohydrates: 27 g; Protein: 4 g; Fiber: 3.5 g; Sodium: 343 mg

Curried Butternut Squash Soup

Butternut squash is the utility infielder of vegetables; wherever you place it on the culinary diamond, it does a great job. Stuffed in ravioli, as part of a risotto, roasted with herbs—it's far more versatile than its tubby exterior suggests. In this soup, it's blended with coconut milk to create a sensual, buttery texture that carries a phenomenal spice blend that delights the tastes and delivers superior nutrition. The cinnamon and turmeric help regulate blood sugar, have anti-inflammatory properties, and help fight cancer, while cumin boosts immunity and energy. MAKES 8 SERVINGS

2 tablespoons extra-virgin olive oil
1½ cups diced yellow onion
1 tablespoon minced fresh ginger
2 teaspoons turmeric
2 teaspoons ground cumin
Sea salt
1½ pounds butternut squash, cut into 1-inch cubes (about 5 cups)
4½ cups vegetable broth, homemade (page 55) or store-bought, plus more if needed
1 cinnamon stick
1 (15-ounce) can coconut milk
2 teaspoons freshly squeezed lime juice
¼ teaspoon Grade B maple syrup
4 teaspoons Parsley Mint Drizzle (page 189) or pomegranate molasses, homemade (page 192) or store-bought, for garnish

COOK'S NOTE: Here's an important physics safety note: Blending hot liquids causes pressure to rise in the container, which can blow the lid right off. To help prevent this, leave at least one-third of the container empty. To be safe and avoid burns, put a kitchen towel over the loosely placed lid and hold the lid in place before you hit the power button. This will also keep the blender from creating unwanted spin art on your kitchen walls.

Heat the olive oil in a soup pot over medium heat. Add the onion, ginger, turmeric, cumin, and a pinch of salt and sauté for about 3 minutes. Add the squash and ¼ teaspoon of salt and sauté for 30 seconds. Pour in ½ cup of the broth to deglaze the pot, stirring to loosen any bits stuck to the pot. Cook until the liquid is reduced by half. Add the remaining 4 cups broth and the cinnamon stick. Increase the heat to high and bring to a boil. Decrease the heat to low and stir in the coconut milk. Cover and simmer until the squash is tender, about 15 minutes.

Remove the cinnamon stick. Stir in the lime juice, maple syrup, and ¼ teaspoon of salt. Remove from the heat.

Working in batches, transfer the soup to a blender (see note) and process until very smooth, adding additional broth or water for a thinner consistency if you like. Return the soup to the pot and cook over low heat just until heated through. Serve garnished with the Parsley Mint Drizzle.

Variation: Pumpkin and kabocha squash also work well in this recipe.

PREP TIME: 15 minutes COOK TIME: 30 minutes
STORAGE: Store in an airtight container in the refrigerator for up to 5 days or in the freezer for up to 3 months.
PER SERVING: Calories: 100; Total Fat: 4 g (0.5 g saturated, 3 g monounsaturated); Carbohydrates: 17.5 g; Protein: 2 g; Fiber: 3.5 g; Sodium: 105 mg

Bento Box Soup

The Japanese are renowned for their longevity. As of 2011, their average life expectancy was 82.3 years. (The United States came in fiftieth, at 78.4 years.) Researchers often credit their diet, and this soup is my way of cramming as much of their healthy cuisine into a bowl as possible. It's called Bento Box Soup because of the traditional Japanese take-out bento box lunch, which is full of compartments, each containing a tasty treat: fish or meat, rice, pickled or cooked veggies, and other goodies. The base is a miso broth; if you're not in the know about miso, it's a salty fermented soy product that aids digestion and improves immune function. In case white miso isn't available, use any mellow (light) miso. I kicked those healing properties up a notch by infusing green tea into the broth for an extra immune boost, then added shiitakes, spinach, kombu, scallions, and tamari. MAKES 6 SERVINGS

4 ounces soba noodles

4 cups organic vegetable or chicken broth, homemade (page 55 or 56) or store-bought

$^1/_2$ teaspoon toasted sesame oil or hot pepper sesame oil

1 (6-inch) strip of kombu

3 green tea bags

1 carrot, peeled and grated

$^1/_2$ cup stemmed and sliced shiitake mushrooms

4 ounces firm tofu, cut into $^1/_2$-inch cubes

2 tablespoons tamari

$^1/_4$ cup white miso

2 scallions, white and green parts, sliced diagonally

1 tablespoon freshly squeezed lemon juice

$1^1/_2$ cups loosely packed baby spinach

COOK'S NOTE: If you're sensitive to gluten, be sure to purchase 100 percent buckwheat soba noodles. Also, be aware that prolonged cooking or high heat will kill the beneficial nutrients in miso, so add it at the end of recipes and heat it gently.

Fill a soup pot halfway with water and bring to a boil over high heat. Add a pinch of salt and the soba noodles and decrease the heat to medium. Cook, stirring gently on occasion, until just tender, about 5 minutes. Drain and rinse well under cold water to remove the starch. Immediately transfer to a bowl, drizzle with $^1/_4$ teaspoon of the sesame oil and toss gently to coat.

Put the broth in the same pot and bring to a boil over high heat. Decrease the heat to low, add the kombu and tea bags, and simmer for 4 minutes. Remove the kombu and tea bags with a slotted spoon. Add the carrot, mushrooms, tofu, tamari, cover, and simmer for 5 minutes.

Put $^1/_4$ cup of the hot broth in a small bowl, add the miso, and stir with a fork until the miso is dissolved. Stir the mixture back into the broth, then stir in the scallions, lemon juice, and remaining sesame oil.

Distribute the soba noodles and spinach among six bowls and ladle in the soup.

Variations: You can substitute udon noodles for the soba. Another option is to omit the soba and instead put add $^1/_4$ cup of cooked brown rice in each bowl, and then ladle the soup over the rice.

PREP TIME: 20 minutes COOK TIME: 15 minutes
STORAGE: Store the soba and soup separately so the soba doesn't fall apart. Store the soup in an airtight container in the refrigerator for up to 4 days, and the soba in an airtight container in the refrigerator for no more than 1 day.
PER SERVING: Calories: 140; Total Fat: 1.5 g (0 g saturated, 0.5 g monounsaturated); Carbohydrates: 27 g; Protein: 7 g; Fiber: 5.5 g; Sodium: 834 mg

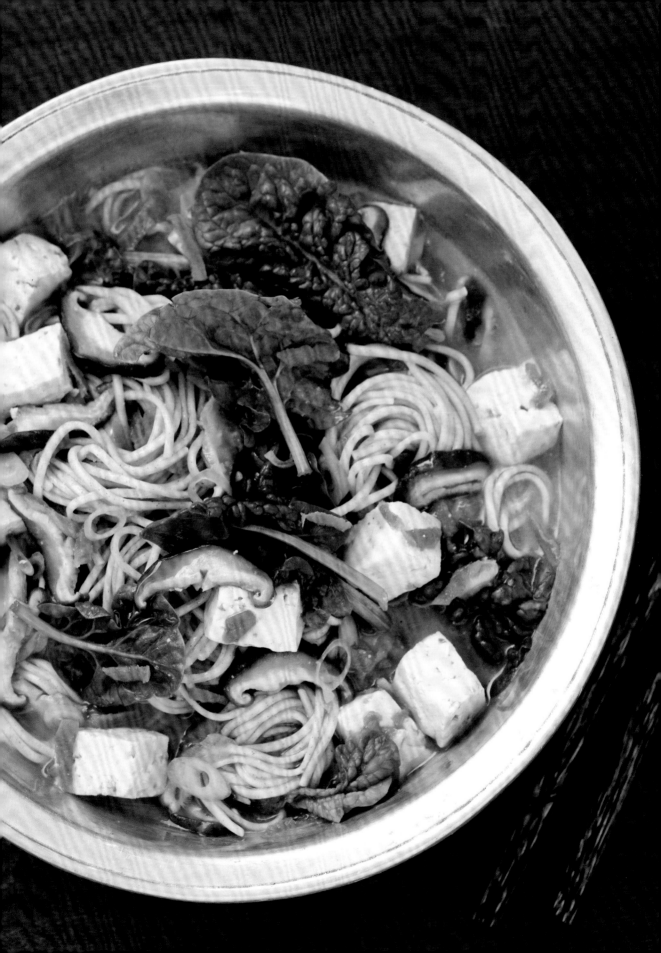

Costa Rican Black Bean Soup with Sweet Potato

Costa Rica is renowned for longevity; if you're born and raised there, you're four times more likely than a US citizen to reach age ninety. Ask Costa Ricans what they're likely to eat often, and from a young age, and the answer is likely to be "beans, beans, *beans!*" A particular favorite is black beans, which have a deep color indicating their rich phytochemical content and plenty of fiber to help control blood sugar levels. The sweet potato provides beautiful color and sweetness, with cayenne, cinnamon, cumin, and garlic providing the flavorprint associated with this Central American paradise.

Prepare ahead: Soak the beans in cool water for 8 hours or overnight before cooking; this will make them more digestible and decrease the cooking time. MAKES 8 SERVINGS

2 tablespoons extra-virgin olive oil
2 cups diced yellow onions
Sea salt
1 1/2 teaspoons seeded and finely diced jalapeño chile
1 tablespoon minced garlic
1 1/2 teaspoons dried oregano
1/2 teaspoon ground cumin
1/4 teaspoon ground cinnamon
Pinch of cayenne
8 cups vegetable broth, homemade (page 55) or store-bought
2 cups dried black beans, soaked, rinsed, and drained
1 (6-inch) strip of kombu
1 cinnamon stick
1 bay leaf
2 cups finely diced orange-fleshed sweet potato, such as garnet yams
2 teaspoons freshly squeezed lime juice
1/4 cup chopped fresh cilantro, for garnish
Ancho Chile Relish (page 180), for garnish

COOK'S NOTE: You can use 2 (14.5-ounce) cans of cooked black beans. Rinse, spritz with lemon juice, and sprinkle with salt. Add them just before deglazing the pot and simmer the soup for just 15 minutes before adding the sweet potato.

Heat the olive oil in a soup pot over medium heat. Add the onions and a pinch of salt and sauté until translucent, about 4 minutes. Add the jalapeño, garlic, oregano, cumin, cinnamon, cayenne, and 1/4 teaspoon of salt and sauté for 1 minute. Pour in 1/2 cup of the broth to deglaze the pot, stirring to loosen any bits stuck to the pot. Cook until the liquid is reduced by half. Add the remaining 7 1/2 cups broth, along with the black beans, kombu, cinnamon stick, and bay leaf. Increase the heat to high and bring to a boil. Decrease the heat to medium-low, partially cover, and simmer briskly (bubbles should break the surface regularly), until the beans are tender, about 1 hour and 15 minutes.

Stir in the sweet potato and 1/4 teaspoon salt. Cover and simmer until the sweet potato is just tender, about 7 minutes. With a slotted spoon, remove and discard the kombu, cinnamon stick, and bay leaf. Ladle 2 cups of the beans and sweet potatoes into a blender and process until velvety smooth. Stir the blended mixture back into the soup and cook just until heated through. Stir in the lime juice, then do a FASS check (see page 44); you may want to add 1/4 teaspoon of salt and a spritz of lime juice. Serve garnished with the cilantro and a dollop of the Ancho Chile Relish.

PREP TIME: 20 minutes (after soaking the beans)
COOK TIME: 1 hour 30 minutes
STORAGE: Store in an airtight container in the refrigerator for up to 5 days or in the freezer for up to 2 months.
PER SERVING: Calories: 170; Total Fat: 4 g (0.5 g saturated, 3 g monounsaturated); Carbohydrates: 29 g; Protein: 5.5 g; Fiber: 8 g; Sodium: 218 mg

Dahl Fit for a Saint

My first internship when I got out of culinary school was in the kitchen at the Chopra Center for Wellbeing, where they had an entire wall filled with dozens and dozens of spices. I swear that wall looked like a piece of art—in the form of a jigsaw puzzle that I had to figure out. The way you knew you had earned your stripes in the kitchen was when the executive chef finally let you make their famous dahl. Wouldn't you know, the very first time I made it, an honest-to-goodness Indian saint had come to visit. There are rules regarding saints, and at mealtime, the first and foremost is that no one can try the dahl before she does. I must have done something right, because she tasted, smiled, and kissed me gently on the forehead. I treasure that memory, and also appreciate the experience of making that dahl because it taught me that spices—which have phenomenal healing properties—can be the heart of a dish, rather than an add-on to enhance flavor. Here, the blending of spices is what really gives this dish its power, both nutritionally and on the palate. MAKES 6 SERVINGS

2 tablespoons organic ghee or
  extra-virgin olive oil
1 1/2 teaspoons cumin seeds
1 1/2 teaspoons black or brown
  mustard seeds
1 yellow onion, diced small
1 tablespoon minced fresh ginger
2 teaspoons turmeric
2 teaspoons ground cumin
Sea salt
2 cups chopped tomatoes, or
  1 (14.5-ounce) can diced tomatoes, drained and juices reserved
8 cups vegetable broth, homemade
  (page 55) or store-bought
2 cups dried red lentils, rinsed well
  (see note, page 72)
1 cinnamon stick
3 cups loosely packed baby spinach
1 teaspoon freshly squeezed
  lime juice
1/2 teaspoon Grade B maple syrup
1/4 cup finely chopped fresh cilantro
  or mint, for garnish

Heat the ghee in a soup pot over medium heat. Add the cumin seeds and mustard seeds and sauté until they begin to pop. Immediately add the onion, ginger, turmeric, ground cumin, and a pinch of salt and sauté for about 3 minutes. Add the drained tomatoes and 1/4 teaspoon of salt and sauté for 2 minutes. Pour in 1/2 cup of the broth and the reserved juice from the tomatoes to deglaze the pot, stirring to loosen any bits stuck to the pot. Cook until the liquid is reduced by half. Add the lentils and stir well, then add the remaining 7 1/2 cups broth and the cinnamon stick. Increase the heat to high and bring to a boil. Decrease the heat to low, cover, and simmer until the lentils are tender, about 30 minutes.

Stir in another 1/4 teaspoon of salt and simmer for 5 minutes. Remove the cinnamon stick and stir in the spinach, lime juice, and maple syrup. Serve garnished with cilantro.

PREP TIME: 15 minutes COOK TIME: 45 minutes
STORAGE: Store in an airtight container in the refrigerator for up to 5 days or in the freezer for up to 2 months.
PER SERVING: Calories: 365; Total Fat: 7 g (4.1 g saturated, 0.6 g mono-unsaturated); Carbohydrates: 58 g; Protein: 20 g; Fiber: 14 g; Sodium: 300 mg

Chicken Tortilla Soup

If I'd been cast in *The Wizard of Oz*, I'd have been Toto, that tiny troublemaker who can't resist pulling back the curtain to see what's behind it. Maybe it's an occupational hazard of being a cook, but I can't take any meal I eat in a restaurant at face value. I try to figure out the flavors, commit them to culinary memory, and re-create them in my kitchen. When I eat out, I often chance upon dishes that almost work but need a little help to achieve scrumptiousness. Such is the case here. I think both taste and texture are vital for the perfect meal, and too often tortilla soups have good flavor but mushy tortillas. Since I like some crunch, that's an instant turnoff. The solution? In this recipe, fresh, crispy strips of tortilla go on top of the soup at the last second, providing an ideal counterpoint to the soup, which is swirling with delicious, healing ingredients, including cilantro, cumin, oregano, avocado, garlic, onion, and celery. MAKES 6 SERVINGS

---

2 tablespoons extra-virgin olive oil
1 cup finely chopped yellow onion
$^1/_2$ cup peeled and diced carrot
$^1/_2$ cup diced celery
2 teaspoons seeded and diced
    jalapeño chile
$^1/_2$ teaspoon sea salt
2 cloves garlic, chopped
$^1/_4$ teaspoon ground cumin
$^1/_4$ teaspoon dried oregano
1 (14.5-ounce) can diced tomatoes
6 cups organic chicken broth,
    homemade (page 56) or
    store-bought
6 corn tortillas
1 cup thinly sliced cooked organic
    chicken
2 tablespoons plus $^1/_2$ teaspoon
    freshly squeezed lime juice
$^1/_2$ avocado, diced,
2 tablespoons chopped fresh
    cilantro

COOK'S NOTE: This is a good soup to make when you have leftover Flat-Out Good Chicken (page 148) or roasted chicken in the fridge.

Preheat the oven or toaster oven to 350°F.

Heat the olive oil in a soup pot over medium-high heat. Add the onion, carrot, celery, jalapeño, and $^1/_4$ teaspoon of the salt and sauté until the vegetables begin to soften, 3 to 5 minutes. Stir in the garlic, cumin, and oregano. Stir in the tomatoes with their juice and cook 1 minute. Add the broth and bring to a boil. Decrease the heat to low, cover, and simmer for 15 minutes.

Put the tortillas in a stack and cut into $^1/_4$- to $^1/_2$-inch-wide strips. Spread the strips on a baking sheet and bake just until crisp, 7 to 8 minutes.

Add the chicken, 2 tablespoons of the lime juice, and the remaining $^1/_4$ teaspoon of salt to the soup and stir to combine. Simmer uncovered for 5 minutes. Remove from the heat and stir in the remaining $^1/_2$ teaspoon of lime juice. Taste; you may want to add a squeeze of lime juice or a pinch of salt.

To serve, ladle the soup into bowls. Crumble the tortilla strips, then scatter them over the soup. Top with the avocado, and cilantro and serve immediately.

Variations: For added pizzazz, serve with a dollop of Ancho Chile Relish (page 180). You could turn this into a Latin *albóndigas* (meatball) soup by substituting the chicken meatballs from Peppino's Cowboy Minestrone (page 78).

PREP TIME: 15 minutes COOK TIME: 25 minutes
STORAGE: Store in an airtight container in the refrigerator for up to 2 days.
PER SERVING: Calories: 300; Total Fat: 12 g (2 g saturated, 6 g mono-unsaturated); Carbohydrates: 31.5 g; Protein: 15 g; Fiber: 3 g; Sodium: 537 mg

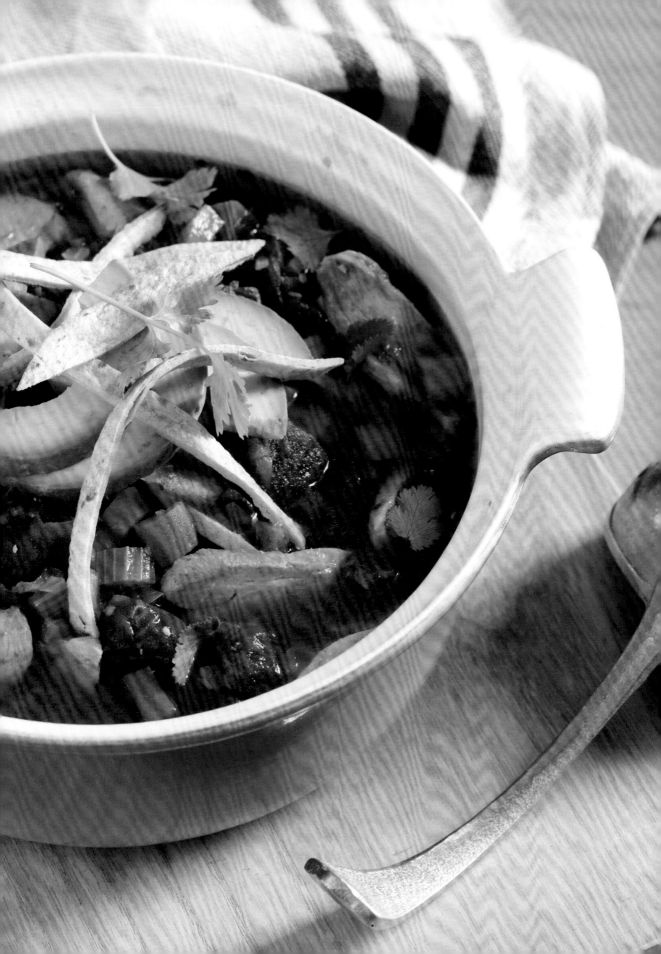

Rustic Lentil Soup

At restaurants, my dad didn't see a set line where the salad bar ended and the soup bar began. He'd stride up, bowl in hand, and ladle away to his heart's content. Other folks may have looked on aghast, but my dad was a real culinary alchemist; he knew which ingredients played well together. This soup pays homage to his wizardry. It has a hybrid quality, probably because it started out as a lentil dish braised in red wine, which I loved, but then realized it was just a few tweaks away from being a hearty lentil soup. Like Dad, I experimented to find the right combination of taste and heft, because to me watery soup is like finding a bill in the mailbox instead of a check. Lentils are so good for helping regulate blood sugar levels that everyone should consume them often; in an effort to lure those who aren't especially fond of lentils, I've made them enticing by surrounding them with mushrooms, red wine, Swiss chard, garlic, and a host of herbs and spices. MAKES 6 SERVINGS

2 tablespoons extra-virgin olive oil
1 yellow onion, diced small
Sea salt
2 carrots, peeled and diced small
2 celery stalks, diced small
1 cup finely diced parsnips
8 ounces cremini mushrooms, sliced
1 tablespoon minced garlic
1/2 teaspoon dried thyme
1/2 teaspoon dried oregano
1/4 teaspoon freshly ground black pepper
1 cup red wine
2 tablespoons tomato paste
1 (14.5-ounce) can diced tomatoes
1 cup dried green lentils, rinsed well (see note)
7 cups vegetable broth, homemade (page 55) or store-bought
1 bay leaf
2 1/2 cups stemmed and chopped Swiss chard, in bite-size pieces (see note, page 97)

COOK'S NOTE: You don't have to presoak lentils, but rinse them well in a bowl of cold water and use your hands to swish them around. Drain and repeat until the water is clear. Don't boil lentils for an extended period of time, which makes them mushy and tends to cause them to fall apart. Let the lentils simmer for a nice, tender texture.

Heat the olive oil in a large skillet over medium heat. Add the onion and a pinch of salt and sauté until translucent, about 4 minutes. Add the carrot, celery, parsnips, mushrooms, and another pinch of salt and sauté until all of the vegetables are tender and becoming deep golden brown, about 12 minutes.

Add the garlic and sauté for about 30 seconds, then stir in the thyme, oregano, pepper, and 1/4 teaspoon of salt. Pour in the wine to deglaze the skillet, stirring to loosen any bits stuck to the pan. Cook until the liquid is reduced by half. Stir in the tomato paste, tomatoes, and lentils. Add the broth and the bay leaf. Increase the heat to high and bring just to a boil. Decrease the heat to low, cover, and simmer until the lentils are tender, about 20 minutes. Taste; you may want to add a spritz of lemon juice or a pinch of salt. Stir in the Swiss chard and cook until it's tender, about 3 minutes.

Variations: Substitute fennel, which is a good digestive aid, for the celery to add more depth to the flavor. If you aren't a fan of mushrooms, just leave them out. You can substitute 1 cup of broth for the wine.

PREP TIME: 20 minutes COOK TIME: 40 minutes
STORAGE: Store in an airtight container in the refrigerator for up to 5 days or in the freezer for up to 3 months.
PER SERVING: Calories: 265; Total Fat: 6 g (1 g saturated, 4 g monounsaturated); Carbohydrates: 39 g; Protein: 10 g; Fiber: 9.5 g; Sodium: 251 mg

Ridiculously Good Split Pea Soup

Working with the youth of America in the kitchen keeps me both in stitches and on my toes. A sassy Jersey girl named Katie Bealer is one of my trusted assistants. Hanging around Katie is like learning a new language, one I think of as Text-o-Talk. She took one taste of this soup and exclaimed, "OMG!" I LOL'd in response. (See, I'm learning.) I was actually thinking of calling this recipe RGSPS in her honor; anyone who comes up with the descriptor "ridiculously good" deserves to be honored. In any case, her unbridled enthusiasm for this soup made it a keeper for the book. If you enjoy traditional split pea soup with ham and want that smoky flavor here, just add smoked paprika or ground chipotle chiles. However, it's the blending of the split peas that drives the taste in this recipe, creating a velvety mouthfeel that's perfect for transporting the flavors of the garlic, carrot, onions, and thyme that round out the soup. As a bonus, especially for those concerned about diabetes, split peas are great for you, being rich in fiber, which fights cholesterol and helps regulate blood sugar levels. As for Katie and me, all I can say is we're BFFs. MAKES 8 SERVINGS

2 tablespoons extra-virgin olive oil
1 cup finely diced yellow onion
Sea salt
1 cup peeled and finely diced carrot
1/2 cup finely diced celery
1/4 teaspoon dried thyme
Freshly ground black pepper
2 cloves garlic, minced
2 cups dried green split peas, rinsed
    well (see note, page 72)
8 cups vegetable broth, homemade
    (page 55) or store-bought
2 teaspoons freshly squeezed
    lemon juice
1 tablespoon finely chopped fresh
    flat-leaf parsley, for garnish
Chive Oil (page 178), for garnish

Heat the olive oil in a soup pot over medium heat. Add the onion and a pinch of salt and sauté until golden, about 8 minutes. Add the carrot, celery, thyme, 1/4 teaspoon of salt, and 1/8 teaspoon of pepper and sauté for about 8 minutes. Stir in the garlic and split peas, then pour in 1/2 cup of the broth to deglaze the pot, stirring to loosen any bits stuck to the pot. Cook until the liquid is reduced by half. Add the remaining 7 1/2 cups of broth. Increase the heat to high and bring just to a boil. Decrease the heat to low and simmer until the split peas are tender, about 40 minutes.

Ladle 2 cups of the soup into a blender and process until velvety smooth. Stir the blended mixture back into to the soup and cook just until heated through. Stir in the lemon juice, 1/4 teaspoon of salt, and a few grinds of pepper. Do a FASS check (see page 44); you may want to add a spritz of lemon juice and a pinch of salt. Served garnished with the parsley and Chive Oil.

Variation: For a smoky flavor, add 1/4 teaspoon of smoked paprika or 2 dried chipotle chiles, rehydrated and minced, when sautéing the onion.

PREP TIME: 15 minutes COOK TIME: 1 hour
STORAGE: Store in an airtight container in the refrigerator for up to 3 days.
PER SERVING: Calories: 245; Total Fat: 4 g (1 g saturated, 3 g monounsaturated); Carbohydrates: 40 g; Protein: 13 g; Fiber: 15 g; Sodium: 289 mg

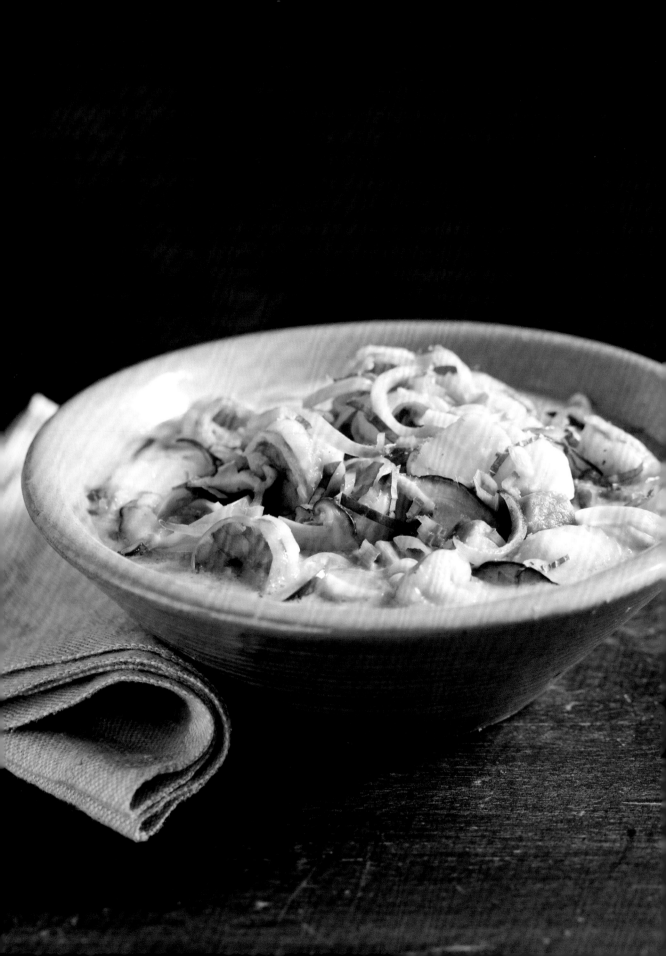

Southeast Asian Seafood Stew

Annemarie Colbin, PhD, my mentor and founder of New York City's Natural Gourmet Institute for Health and Culinary Arts, has spent her career investigating links between nutrition and longevity. She's noted that being breast-fed in infancy confers numerous long-term health benefits. This stew uses luscious coconut milk, which contains lauric acid, also found in mother's milk, to strengthen the immune system. All of the accompanying Thai flavors I delight in make an appearance as well: cilantro, chili paste, lemongrass, kaffir lime leaves ... all doing the backstroke around delicious and omega-3-rich fish. MAKES 6 SERVINGS

1 tablespoon coconut oil or extra-virgin olive oil

1 cup thinly sliced shallots or red onion

Sea salt

1 tablespoon finely chopped fresh ginger

2 teaspoon finely chopped garlic

1 (6-inch) piece of lemongrass, thinly sliced (see note, page 76)

2 kaffir lime leaves, or 1 teaspoon grated lime zest

4 cups vegetable broth, homemade (page 55) or store-bought

1 teaspoon Thai red chili paste

1 (15-ounce) can coconut milk

1 tablespoon fish sauce

3 1/2 ounces wide rice noodles, broken into 2-inch pieces

1 cup finely diced orange-fleshed sweet potato

10 shiitake mushrooms, stemmed and thinly sliced

1 pound black cod or halibut, cut into 2-inch pieces

1 pound shrimp, peeled and deveined

2 tablespoons freshly squeezed lime juice

1/4 cup chopped fresh cilantro, for garnish

2 tablespoons sliced scallion, white and green parts, cut thinly on the diagonal, for garnish

2 tablespoons chopped fresh basil, preferably Thai basil, for garnish

2 tablespoons chopped fresh mint, for garnish

1 small jalapeño chile, seeded and thinly sliced, for garnish

Heat the oil in a soup pot over medium heat. Add the shallot and a pinch of salt and sauté until translucent, about 3 minutes. Add the ginger, garlic, lemongrass, and kaffir lime leaves. Pour in 1/2 cup of broth to deglaze the pot, stirring to remove any bits stuck to the pot. Cook until the liquid is reduced by half.

Put the chili paste and 1 tablespoon of the coconut milk in a small bowl and stir until well combined. Add to the pot, along with the remaining 3 1/2 cups of broth, the remaining coconut milk, and the fish sauce. Decrease the heat to medium-low and simmer for 15 minutes.

Meanwhile, put the rice noodles in a bowl of hot water and soak until tender, about 8 minutes. Drain well.

Stir the sweet potato and mushrooms into the soup and simmer for 6 minutes. Gently stir in the fish and shrimp and simmer until the seafood is tender and cooked through, about 4 minutes, until just opaque. Stir in the noodles, lime juice, and 1/4 teaspoon of salt. Do a FASS check (see page 44); you may want to add a bit of salt and a squeeze of lime juice. Serve garnished with the scallion, basil, mint, and jalapeño.

Variation: For a vegetarian and low-sodium take on this dish, add 5 more shiitake mushrooms and replace the fish and shrimp with 1 pound of extra-firm tofu cut into 1-inch pieces or 1 cup of fresh or frozen shelled edamame, mixed with a spritz of lime juice and a pinch of salt.

PREP TIME: 15 minutes COOK TIME: 35 minutes
STORAGE: Store in an airtight container in the refrigerator for up to 3 days.
PER SERVING: Calories: 390; Total Fat: 19 g (16 g saturated, 1 g mono-unsaturated); Carbohydrates: 33.5 g; Protein: 23 g; Fiber: 4 g; Sodium: 715 mg

White Bean and Chicken Chili

They say identical twins share a kind of telepathy. I think the same holds true for certain cooks who work closely together. I've spent countless hours canoodling in the kitchen with Jersey girl Katie. One day, out of nowhere, I told her, "Be prepared to make a white bean chili tomorrow." Her mouth dropped in shock. "I've been craving that . . . and I've never even had it before!" I told Katie that her homework assignment was to think about what ingredients she'd like to see in the chili, and that I'd do the same and then we'd compare notes. The next day we whipped out our scribbled lists. They were virtually identical: white creamy beans, red bell pepper, garlic, coriander, oregano, cilantro . . . a whole host of tasty longevity delights. I also had one special, secret ingredient: cinnamon. The result was a savory chili with just enough heat from cayenne to kick-start the metabolism without setting off a three-alarm fire. MAKES 6 SERVINGS

---

6 organic chicken thighs, bone in, skin removed
Sea salt
2 1/4 teaspoons ground cumin
1/2 teaspoon cayenne
2 tablespoons plus 2 teaspoons extra-virgin olive oil
2 cups diced yellow onions
1 cup finely diced red bell pepper
1/2 cup finely diced celery
1/2 cup peeled and finely diced carrot
1 tablespoon seeded and finely diced jalapeño chile
1 tablespoon minced garlic
2 teaspoons ground coriander
1 teaspoon dried oregano
1/4 teaspoon ground cinnamon
3 cups organic chicken broth, homemade (page 56) or store-bought
1 tablespoon tomato paste
4 cups cooked cannellini or great northern beans, or 2 (15-ounce) cans, drained, rinsed, and mixed with a spritz of lemon juice and a pinch of salt
1 avocado, sliced, for garnish
1/4 cup chopped fresh cilantro, for garnish
1/4 cup sliced scallion, white and green parts, for garnish
6 lime wedges, for garnish
Ancho Chile Relish (page 180), for garnish

Season the chicken with 1/2 teaspoon of sea salt, 1/4 teaspoon of the cumin, and 1/4 teaspoon of the cayenne.

Heat the 2 tablespoons of olive oil in a heavy soup pot or Dutch oven over medium heat. Add the chicken, working in batches if necessary, and cook until brown on each side, about 3 minutes per side. Transfer to a plate.

Heat the 2 teaspoons of olive oil in the same pot. Add the onions and a pinch of salt and sauté until translucent, about 4 minutes, scraping up the bits from the bottom of the pan. Add the bell pepper, celery, carrot, jalapeño, garlic, coriander, oregano, cinnamon, remaining 2 teaspoons of cumin, remaining 1/4 teaspoon of cayenne, and 1/4 teaspoon of salt and sauté until aromatic, about 5 minutes. Pour in 1/4 cup of the broth to deglaze the pot, stirring to loosen any bits stuck to the pot. Cook until very little liquid remains in the pot. Stir in 1 3/4 cups of the broth and the tomato paste, then add the chicken and any accumulated juices. Decrease the heat to low, cover, and simmer until the chicken is cooked through, about 15 minutes, or until an instant-read thermometer reads 160°F.

Using a slotted spoon, transfer the chicken to a plate and let cool. Add the beans to the pot and cook uncovered until the liquid is reduced by one-quarter, about 20 minutes.

COOK'S NOTE: As a shortcut, you can use 2 cups of shredded leftover cooked chicken rather than chicken thighs. Begin the recipe by sautéing the vegetables in 2 tablespoons of olive oil, then proceed as directed and add the cooked chicken at the end.

Using a slotted spoon, transfer 2 cups of the beans and vegetable mixture to a blender or food processor. Add the remaining 1 cup of broth and process until smooth. Add the mixture back to the pot and stir until well combined. Shred the chicken meat and add it to the pot. Cook just until the chili is heated through. Taste; you may want to add a pinch of salt and a squeeze of lime juice. Serve garnished with the avocado, cilantro, scallions, and lime wedges, and top with a dollop of Ancho Chile Relish.

Variations: For a vegetarian white bean chili, substitute vegetable broth or bean cooking liquid for the chicken broth and omit the chicken. If you want to ring up the alarms, add another 1/4 teaspoon cayenne, or include a minced serrano chile when sautéing the vegetables. Or, for smokier heat, add ground chipotle chiles or a dried chipotle chile, hydrated and then minced.

PREP TIME: 20 minutes COOK TIME: 1 hour
STORAGE: Store in an airtight container in the refrigerator for up to 5 days or in the freezer for up to 2 months.
PER SERVING: Calories: 360; Total Fat: 13 g (2.5 g saturated, 7 g monounsaturated); Carbohydrates: 38 g; Protein: 25 g; Fiber: 11 g; Sodium: 302 mg

Peppino's Cowboy Minestrone with Herb Mini Meatballs

Ever felt like you were in exactly the right place at exactly the right time, and there was nowhere on earth you'd rather be at that moment? That happened not long ago when my friend Paul invited Peppino D'Agostino to play acoustic guitar in our home. His performance was absolutely, utterly mesmerizing. I made this minestrone for Peppino, and given his Italian upbringing, I was a tad nervous about serving it. Not only did Peppino learn cooking at his *nonna*'s knee, but her specialty was—you guessed it—minestrone. I was vibrating like a high E string as he took the first slurp. He looked up, my heart stopped, and he said, "This is so light and flavorful! How did you make these meatballs so light?" I told him, of course (no breadcrumbs). A little while later he announced that he was going to play one of his compositions. "I call this song 'Cowboy Minestrone,'" he said. My jaw dropped. Let's just call this serendipity at its finest. If you think this minestrone is half as good as Peppino's playing, you and I will both be thrilled. MAKES 6 SERVINGS

MEATBALLS

1 organic egg, beaten
1/3 cup cooked brown basmati or jasmine rice
1/4 cup finely chopped fresh parsley or basil
1 tablespoon chopped fresh thyme, or 1 teaspoon dried
1 tablespoon chopped fresh oregano, or 1 teaspoon dried
2 teaspoons minced garlic
1 teaspoon crushed fennel seeds
1/2 teaspoon sea salt
1/4 teaspoon red pepper flakes
1 pound organic ground dark-meat chicken

To make the meatballs, put the egg, rice, parsley, thyme, oregano, garlic, fennel seeds, salt, and red pepper flakes in a bowl and stir to combine. Add the chicken, and mix with your hands or a spatula until just combined (see note, page 79).

To make the soup, heat the olive oil in a soup pot over medium heat. Add the onion and a pinch of salt and sauté until translucent, about 4 minutes. Add the carrots, celery, garlic, thyme, oregano, fennel seeds, and 1/4 teaspoon of salt and sauté for about 3 minutes. Stir in the tomato paste and the juice from the tomatoes to deglaze the pot, stirring to loosen any bits stuck to the pot. Cook until the liquid is reduced by half. Add the tomatoes, broth, and another 1/4 teaspoon of salt. Increase the heat to high and bring to a boil. Decrease the heat to medium-low to maintain a vigorous simmer.

Use a melon baller or tablespoon to scoop out balls of the chicken mixture and gently lower them into the broth. Cover and simmer for 10 minutes, or until the meatballs are cooked all the way through. Add the lemon zest, lemon juice, and another pinch of salt. Put 1/2 cup of spinach in each soup bowl. Ladle the soup over the spinach and garnish with a generous sprinkling of Parmesan cheese and a dollop of pesto.

SOUP

2 tablespoons extra-virgin olive oil

1 yellow onion, diced small

Sea salt

Freshly ground black pepper

2 large carrots, peeled and diced
small

2 large celery stalks, diced small

4 cloves garlic, minced

¼ teaspoon dried thyme

¼ teaspoon dried oregano

¼ teaspoon crushed fennel seeds

1 (14.5 ounce can) diced tomatoes,
with juice

2 teaspoons tomato paste

8 cups organic chicken broth,
homemade (page 56) or
store-bought

1 teaspoon grated lemon zest

2 teaspoons freshly squeezed
lemon juice

3 cups loosely packed baby spinach

Freshly grated organic Parmesan
cheese, for garnish

Basil Pistachio Pesto (page 179), for
garnish

Variations: Substitute ground dark-meat turkey or ground grass-fed beef for the chicken. For a vegetarian dish, substitute 2 cups of cooked cannellini beans for the meatballs. You can use a 15-ounce can of cannellini beans, but be sure to give them the spa treatment: drain, rinse well, and then mix with a spritz of lemon juice and a pinch of sea salt.

PREP TIME: 25 minutes COOK TIME: 30 minutes

STORAGE: Store in an airtight container in the refrigerator for up to 5 days or in the freezer for up to 2 months.

PER SERVING: Calories: 335; Total Fat: 15.5 g (3.5 g saturated, 8 g mono-unsaturated); Carbohydrates: 24 g; Protein: 27 g; Fiber: 3 g; Sodium: 683 mg

COOK'S NOTE: I always get a little nervous when I see instructions like "Don't overwork" or "Don't overmix," so I didn't include anything like that for the meatballs. Instead, I'll just suggest that when it comes to making meatballs, it's best to use a gentle touch. In this recipe, all the other ingredients are first mixed together in a bowl. That way, all you have to do is lightly work in the meat and—*voilà!*—you'll have meatballs that cook up light and fluffy.

WHO KNEW? Can seven words lengthen your life? They just might, if you listen to the advice of Annemarie Colbin, PhD. A preeminent wellness author and founder of the Natural Gourmet Institute for Health and Culinary Arts, Colbin has a wonderful way of getting right to the point no matter what the subject. Here's what she has to say on the topic of foods for optimum health: "My seven criteria are foods that are whole, fresh, real, natural, seasonal, harmonious (with cultural traditions), and delicious." Stick those seven words on the fridge or, better yet, make them an integral part of your grocery shopping routine, and you'll never go wrong. But Colbin, ever the realist, knows we're all likely to stray from time to time. She says that if you do purchase packaged foods, you should read the list of ingredients: "They have to sound like food. If an ingredient doesn't sound like food, it isn't. Don't choose it. You don't need to know why or whether it will hurt you, because it simply isn't real food."

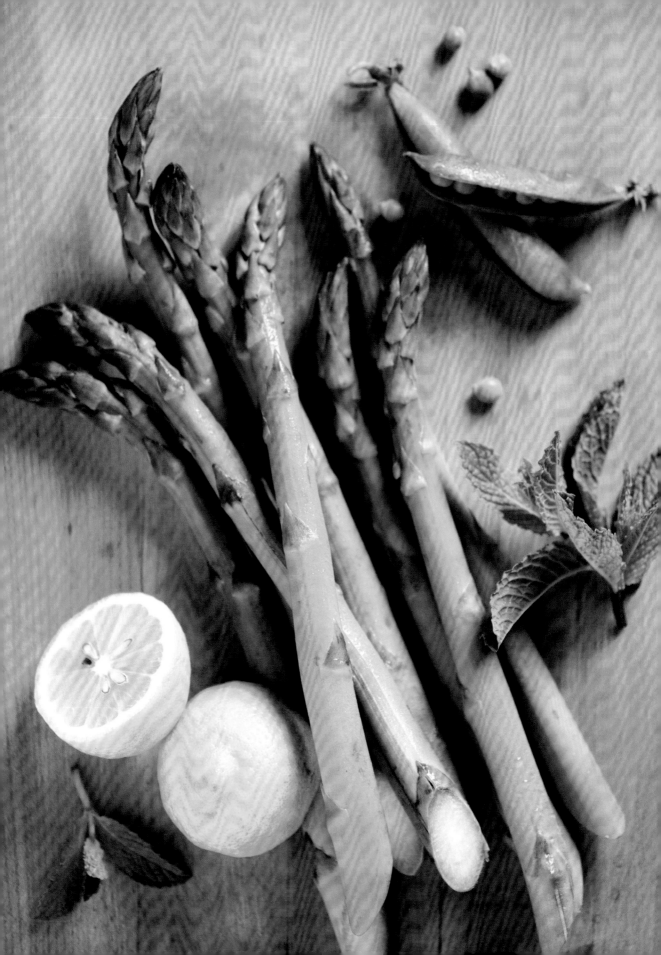

Vital Vegetables

I can (and will) give you a million reasons why you should eat vegetables, but here's the only one that really matters: they taste great.

I know that's hard, maybe impossible, for many people to believe. I get it; half of my generation grew up eating vegetables that were boiled nearly to oblivion. It's not that anybody wanted to destroy both the flavor and the amazing nutrients in those veggies; the average American simply didn't know better back then.

But now? No excuses, my friends. The veggies in this chapter—steamed, roasted, baked, or raw and unadulterated, and infused with luscious herbs, spices, and oils—will make you sigh with pleasure. This explosion of flavor is more than a luxury; it's a necessity if you're intent on eating for maximum health. There's no way to stay at your peak, brimming with vitality and energy, unless veggies are a huge component of your diet. So many of the antioxidants and phytochemicals critical to both short-term and long-term well-being come from vegetables, and it's crucial to stay connected to that source. The only way to do that and not get bored is to bring a kaleidoscope of palate-pleasing veggies into your universe.

That's what this chapter is all about. You can let the flavors seduce you (and believe me, that's easy), knowing that I've done the heavy lifting, pairing complementary ingredients into nutrient-dense dishes and capitalizing on their synergistic properties. The whole really is greater than the sum of its parts in these recipes. As one example, sautéing vegetables in olive oil enhances the body's ability to absorb their nutrients.

Similarly, many herbs and spices influence gene expression. That's a fancy way of saying that they help give your DNA the go-ahead or a stop signal. When paired with vegetables, which deliver phytochemicals with a host of health benefits, herbs and spices act like the station manager at a train terminal, telling the DNA in the switching station which nutrients coming down the track should be sent where and when, and which should be held in the station until further notice.

Veggies also help ward off some of the known effects of the aging process. Take glutathione, a key antioxidant that controls many metabolic functions. Blood levels of glutathione decline as we get older, possibly making us more vulnerable to cancer and other health issues. Fortunately, glutathione is abundant in vegetables such as asparagus, avocados, broccoli, garlic, spinach—all of which, not coincidentally, you'll find in these recipes. As a friend of mine says with love, if not grammar, "Hey, I want you should feel good!"

Avocado Lover's Salad

When my brother Jeff moved to California, he fell in love with avocados. In fact, he became so enamored with this luscious fruit that he began pestering me to create "avotatoes"—an avocado mashed potato recipe—for this book. I'd do almost anything for him, but there are some places a sister just can't go. Still, I wanted to feature avocado because I love them too—for their flavor and texture, and for their incredible antiaging properties. While they do contain a fair amount of fat, it's monosaturated—the kind the body thrives on (in moderation, of course), and they're a great source of the antioxidant glutathione. MAKES 6 SERVINGS

1 head romaine lettuce, torn into bite-size pieces (about 8 cups)
1 English cucumber, peeled, seeded, and diced
1 red bell pepper, diced
Greener Than Green Goddess Dressing (page 186)
1 large avocado, diced
¼ cup pumpkin seeds, toasted (see note)
2 tablespoons chopped fresh mint
2 teaspoons chopped fresh cilantro

Put the lettuce, cucumber, and bell pepper in a large bowl and toss to combine. Drizzle with the dressing and toss again. Add the avocado, pumpkin seeds, mint, and cilantro and toss once more.

PREP TIME: 5 minutes COOK TIME: Not applicable
STORAGE: Store in an airtight container in the refrigerator for up to 5 days.
PER SERVING: Calories: 170; Total Fat: 13 g (2 g saturated, 6 g mono-unsaturated); Carbohydrates: 12 g; Protein: 5 g; Fiber: 6.5 g; Sodium: 122 mg

---

TOASTING SEEDS AND NUTS

Toasting seeds and nuts releases their aromatic oils and makes them more flavorful. To toast a small quantity of seeds or nuts, put them in a small skillet over medium heat. Cook, stirring or shaking the pan often, until they are aromatic and slightly golden. Immediately transfer to a plate or bowl to stop the cooking. For pumpkin seeds (which will puff up a bit as they cook) and most nuts, toasting time is about 4 minutes. For smaller seeds, such as sesame, fennel, or cumin, and for sliced or slivered almonds, toasting time is shorter—just a minute or two. Watch them closely, as they can burn easily.

To toast a larger quantity of seeds or nuts, preheat the oven or a toaster oven to 350°F. Spread the seeds in an even layer on the rimmed baking sheet and toast until aromatic and slightly browned: just a few minutes for small seeds and sliced or slivered almonds; 5 to 7 minutes for pumpkin seeds; 7 to 8 minutes for pecans; 8 to 10 minutes for pistachios; and 10 to 15 minutes for almonds and walnuts. Check them frequently, as they can burn easily. To store any you aren't using right away, let them cool completely, then store in a resealable plastic bag in the freezer for up to 3 months.

Carrot Apple Slaw with Cranberries

Classic slaws usually aren't much to get excited about. Between their homely appearance and goopy consistency, they tend to resemble Spackle. But that's not the case here. This slaw is a feast for the eyes and palate. If Pixar ever created a recipe, this just might be it. Between the carrots, cranberries, apples, and mint, there's enough visual zing to get Peter Max excited. The taste is equally heady, and it offers a host of delightful contrasts for all of the senses: crispy and chewy, tart and sweet, fruits and veggies—all vying for attention in one beautiful package. Plus, apples have a load of health-promoting properties, aiding brain and stomach function. MAKES 4 SERVINGS

1/4 cup unsweetened dried cranberries
1/4 cup very thinly sliced red onion
3 tablespoons freshly squeezed orange juice
1 tablespoon freshly squeezed lemon juice
8 ounces carrots, peeled and thinly sliced into 1/4-inch strips
1 Granny Smith apple, thinly sliced into 1/4-inch strips
1 tablespoon chopped fresh mint
1/4 teaspoon sea salt
2 tablespoons extra-virgin olive oil
1 tablespoon slivered almonds, toasted (see note, page 83)

COOK'S NOTE: The perfect gadget to have around for recipes like this is a julienne peeler. It looks a lot like a regular vegetable peeler, but, like magic, it can cut firm vegetables into thin strips. Julienne peelers are inexpensive and can be found at your favorite kitchen store or online.

Put the cranberries, onion, 1 tablespoon of the orange juice, and the lemon juice in a small bowl and stir to combine. Let sit for a few minutes to allow the juices to penetrate the cranberries and onion.

Put the carrots, apple, mint, salt, cranberry mixture, and remaining 2 tablespoons of orange juice, and salt in a large bowl and toss gently to combine. Drizzle with the olive oil and toss again. Scatter the almonds over the top.

Variations: Add 1/3 cup fresh or frozen shelled edamame, spritzed with lemon juice and a pinch of sea salt, or add 1 cup of finely shredded cabbage. Substitute scallion for the red onion.

PREP TIME: 15 minutes
STORAGE: Store in an airtight container in the refrigerator for up to 3 days.
PER SERVING: Calories: 130; Total Fat: 8 g (1 g saturated, 6 g monounsaturated); Carbohydrates: 14.5 g; Protein: 1.5 g; Fiber: 4 g; Sodium: 142 mg

WHO KNEW? The color of foods can be a key to their health benefits. Generally, the richer the color of a food, the more phytochemicals and antioxidants it contains. One study took the color wheel a step further. Dutch researchers discovered that people who ate the deepest yellow and orange fruits and vegetables (notably carrots) had the lowest risk of developing cardiovascular disease. (In case you wonder, the other colors studied were green, white, and red or purple).

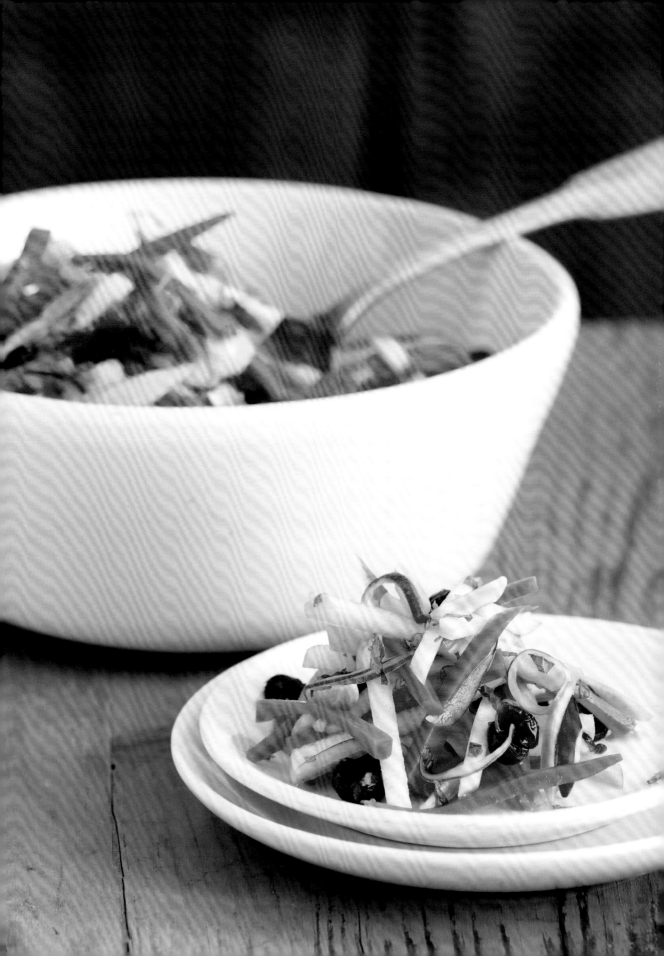

Mexican Cabbage Crunch

Cabbage is a wonderful, healthy alternative for people who like crunchy foods but too often get that mouthfeel from less-than-ideal sources. (There's a reason why snack food is a $28 billion industry.) Here, jicama adds to the crunch factor, and cilantro, diced jalapeños, pumpkin seeds, and a vinaigrette with lime juice and toasted cumin seeds combine to create an irresistible flavor. Bet you can't eat just one bowlful! MAKES 6 SERVINGS

6 cups shredded red cabbage
(see note)
4 cups julienned jicama
1/2 cup finely chopped fresh cilantro
1 tablespoon seeded and diced
jalapeño chile (optional)
1/2 cup of Lime Vinaigrette with
Toasted Cumin Seeds (page 184)
1/2 cup pumpkin seeds, toasted
(see note, page 83)

Put the cabbage, jicama, cilantro, and jalapeño in a large bowl and toss gently to combine. Drizzle with the dressing and toss again. Let sit for a few minutes to allow the dressing to penetrate the cabbage. Sprinkle the pumpkin seeds over the top just before serving.

PREP TIME: 20 minutes
STORAGE: Store in an airtight container in the refrigerator for up to 5 days.
PER SERVING: Calories: 110; Total Fat: 4 g (0.5 g saturated, 0.5 g monounsaturated); Carbohydrates: 14 g; Protein: 6.5 g; Fiber: 4.5 g; Sodium: 368 mg

COOK'S NOTE: To shred cabbage without resorting to a food processor, put the cabbage on a cutting board with the stem side down. Using a sharp chef's knife, cut it in half from top to bottom, then use the tip of the knife to remove the core. Put the halves on the cutting board flat side down and cut in half again. Now you have manageable pieces that you can cut into very thin slices.

Asian Cabbage Crunch

Red cabbage reminds me of that saying "always a bridesmaid, never a bride." It's almost always used as a garnish, a barely glimpsed-then-gone adornment soon discarded in favor of the main course. Well, it's about time for red cabbage to get its moment in the sun. It's a longevity overachiever with anti-inflammatory and antibacterial nutrients. And women concerned about breast cancer, take note; indole-3-carbinol, a compound found in abundance in cabbage, supercharges the liver's ability to break down excess estrogen. MAKES 6 SERVINGS

3 cups shredded red cabbage
  (see note, page 86)
3 cups shredded Napa cabbage
1 cup thinly sliced red bell pepper
3 scallions, white and green parts,
  thinly sliced
1/4 cup finely chopped fresh cilantro
  or basil
2 tablespoons finely chopped
  fresh mint
1/2 cup Sesame Miso Dressing
  (page 187)
1 tablespoon black sesame seeds

Put the cabbages, bell pepper, scallions, cilantro, and mint in a large bowl and toss to combine. Drizzle with the dressing and toss until evenly coated. Sprinkle with the sesame seeds and let sit for a few minutes to allow the dressing to penetrate the cabbage.

Variation: Add 1 cup of fresh or frozen shelled edamame, mixed with a spritz of lime juice and a pinch of salt.

PREP TIME: 20 minutes
STORAGE: Store in an airtight container in the refrigerator for up to 2 days.
PER SERVING: Calories: 75; Total Fat: 2.5 g (0.5 g saturated, 0 g mono-unsaturated); Carbohydrates: 11.5 g; Protein: 3.5 g; Fiber: 3 g; Sodium: 358 mg

Roasted Asparagus Salad with Arugula and Hazelnuts

You can learn a lot sitting on the tailgate of a pickup truck. That's where my buddy Chris, from Zuckerman's Farm, used to sit me down and teach me about all things asparagus. Chris worked hard—awfully hard—as a farmer. He was true salt of the earth, and as generous as they come. Normally, there's an invisible line: farmers behind their wares and buyers on the other side, but Chris always insisted I "step into his parlor." Both of us were always so excited when the first asparagus of the season showed up. He'd put aside a bunch for me, and then we'd both hop up on that tailgate and talk—about recipes, how amazingly nutritious asparagus is, and, a lot of the time, about life and family. Chris passed away not long ago, and I felt the best way I could honor him was to create a recipe featuring his favorite veggie. I think he would have enjoyed this, and I hope you will too. MAKES 4 SERVINGS

1/3 cup hazelnuts

2 bunches asparagus (about 2 pounds), tough ends snapped off and discarded, then peeled (see note)

2 tablespoons plus 2 teaspoons extra-virgin olive oil

Sea salt

2 tablespoons freshly squeezed lemon juice

Freshly ground pepper

4 cups loosely packed arugula

COOK'S NOTE: Peeling the asparagus gets rid of the stringy, sometimes tough outer layer and exposes the sweet flesh underneath. To peel it, use a regular vegetable peeler with a light touch to shave off just the skin. This technique is not necessary with thin asparagus spears.

Preheat the oven to 400°F.

Put the hazelnuts on a rimmed baking sheet. Put them in the oven for 5 to 7 minutes as it preheats, until aromatic and browned. Transfer to a plate or, if you'd like to remove the skins for a more refined texture and appearance, wrap them in a towel and give them a good rub. The majority of the skins will come right off. Coarsely chop the hazelnuts.

Put the asparagus on the same baking sheet in a single layer. Drizzle with the 2 teaspoons of olive oil and generously sprinkle with salt. Toss gently to evenly coat the asparagus. Bake for 8 minutes, until just barely tender.

Put the lemon juice, the 2 tablespoons of olive oil, 1/4 teaspoon of salt, and a few grinds of pepper in a small bowl and mix well with a small whisk.

Put the arugula in a large bowl. Drizzle with half of the dressing and toss until evenly coated. Mound the arugula on individual plates or a platter and arrange the asparagus on top. Drizzle with the remaining dressing and sprinkle the hazelnuts on top.

Variation: Substitute toasted pistachios or walnuts for the hazelnuts.

PREP TIME: 15 minutes COOK TIME: 10 minutes
STORAGE: Store in an airtight container in the refrigerator for up to 5 days.
PER SERVING: Calories: 190; Total Fat: 15.5 g (2 g saturated, 12 g mono-unsaturated); Carbohydrates: 12 g; Protein: 7 g; Fiber: 6 g; Sodium: 210 mg

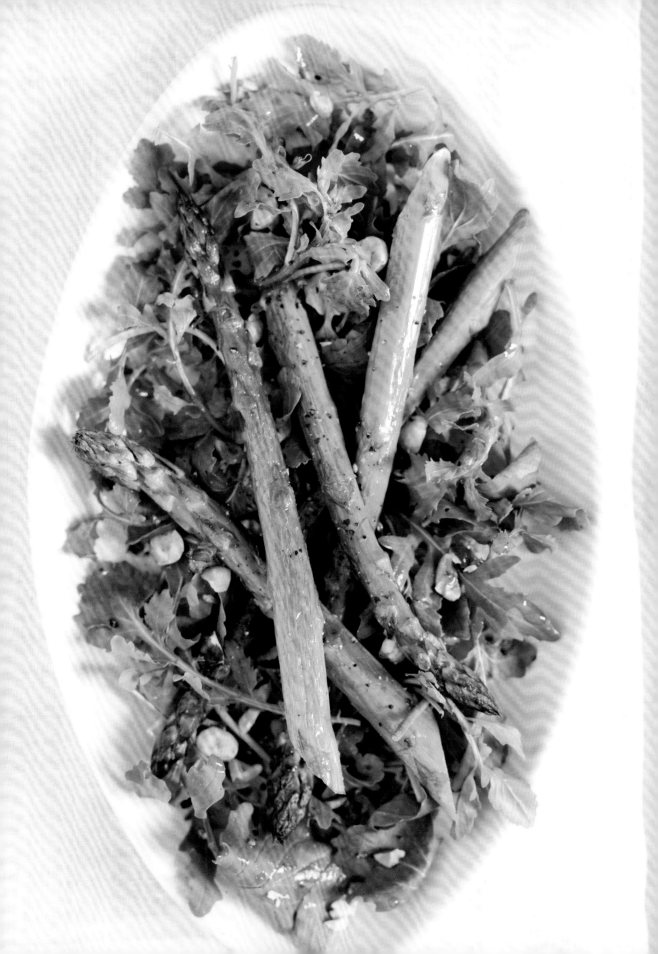

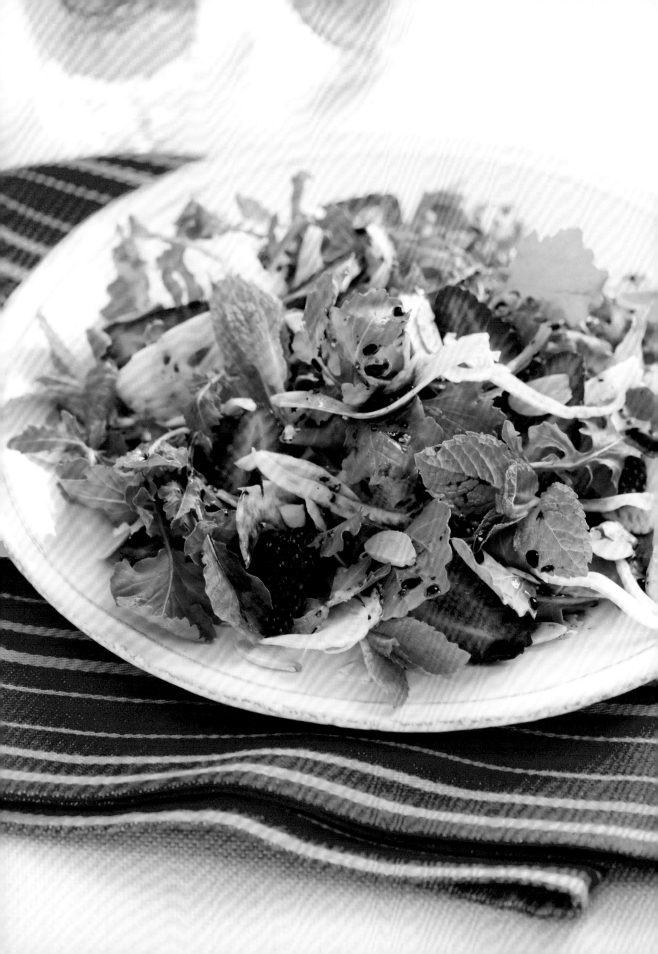

Strawberry, Fennel, and Arugula Salad

Variety isn't just the spice of life; it will also keep you from falling into a food rut. People often tell me that they love salad but get bored with the same old version they always make. This disenchantment can lead folks away from the greens their bodies really need. If that sounds like you, let this salad serve as a springboard for endless seasonal variations. Eating with the seasons isn't just a catch phrase. Each season brings new foods just hitting their peak; in this case, strawberries and arugula, some of the welcome early harbingers of spring. In addition to having an incredibly sweet taste, strawberries have anticancer and anti–inflammatory properties. Plus, when combined with mint and a lemony balsamic vinaigrette, they make for a salad that feels like Pop Rocks going off in your mouth. MAKES 4 SERVINGS

4 cups tightly packed baby arugula
1 cup thinly sliced fennel
12 strawberries, sliced
2 tablespoons chopped fresh mint
6 tablespoons Lemony Balsamic
    Vinaigrette (page 185)
¼ cup sliced almonds, toasted
    (see note, page 83)

COOK'S NOTE: A mandoline (no, you can't strum it) is a handy kitchen tool that allows you to slice vegetables to a uniformed thickness—and perfect for the fennel in this recipe. There are many inexpensive handheld models available at kitchen stores and online.

Put the arugula, fennel, strawberries, and mint in a large bowl and toss gently to combine. Drizzle the vinaigrette over the top and toss again. Scatter the almonds over the top.

Variations: Substitute toasted walnuts for the almonds. Feel free to add a bit of crumbled organic goat cheese.

PREP TIME: 15 minutes
STORAGE: If you must store the salad, don't add the dressing. After combining the greens, fennel, strawberries, and mint, store them in an airtight container in the refrigerator for 1 day at most.
PER SERVING: Calories: 65; Total Fat: 3 g (0.5 g saturated, 2 g monounsaturated); Carbohydrates: 8 g; Protein: 2.5 g; Fiber: 3 g; Sodium: 18 mg

Walnut, Date, and Herb Salad

If you're familiar with that famous scene from *I Love Lucy*, where Lucille Ball freaks out on the chocolate assembly line, that's the way I feel about making finger food. I get overwhelmed, I grow two left thumbs, and I want to cry. (It's really pitiful how cooking calamities can make me feel like a three-year-old.) This salad started off as an appetizer for company, but as their arrival approached, I had made only a few. So I said (and this is the mild form of what I really said), "*Screw it!*" and threw everything into a bowl. Honestly, the format doesn't matter in the least because the flavors work so well together, with sweet dates, peppery arugula, creamy goat cheese, toasty walnuts, and sprightly mint do a lovely dance together. One of the longevity stars here is dates, which first made their earliest culinary appearance (as date honey) in the Old Testament. Who knows, maybe I've stumbled upon Methuselah's secret for a long, long, *long* life. MAKES 4 SERVINGS

4 cups tightly packed baby arugula

$1/2$ cup loosely packed fresh parsley leaves

$1/4$ cup loosely packed fresh mint leaves

$1/2$ cup walnuts, toasted (see note, page 83)

$1/4$ cup chopped dates

4 ounces organic chèvre or other soft goat cheese, crumbled

$1/2$ cup Lemony Balsamic Vinaigrette (page 185)

Put the arugula, parsley, and mint in a bowl and toss to combine. Add the walnuts dates, and chèvre, drizzle with the vinaigrette, and toss again.

PREP TIME: 5 minutes
STORAGE: Not applicable.
PER SERVING: Calories: 365; Total Fat: 32 g (9 g saturated, 14 g mono-unsaturated); Carbohydrates: 15 g; Protein: 9.5 g; Fiber: 3.5 g; Sodium: 372 mg

COOK'S NOTE: You know the old saying "opposites attract"? Dates and arugula are a perfect example. The sweetness of the dates and the peppery flavor of arugula make the perfect couple. If you're an herb lover don't hold back: basil, chives, chervil, dill, tarragon—all are beautiful additions to this salad.

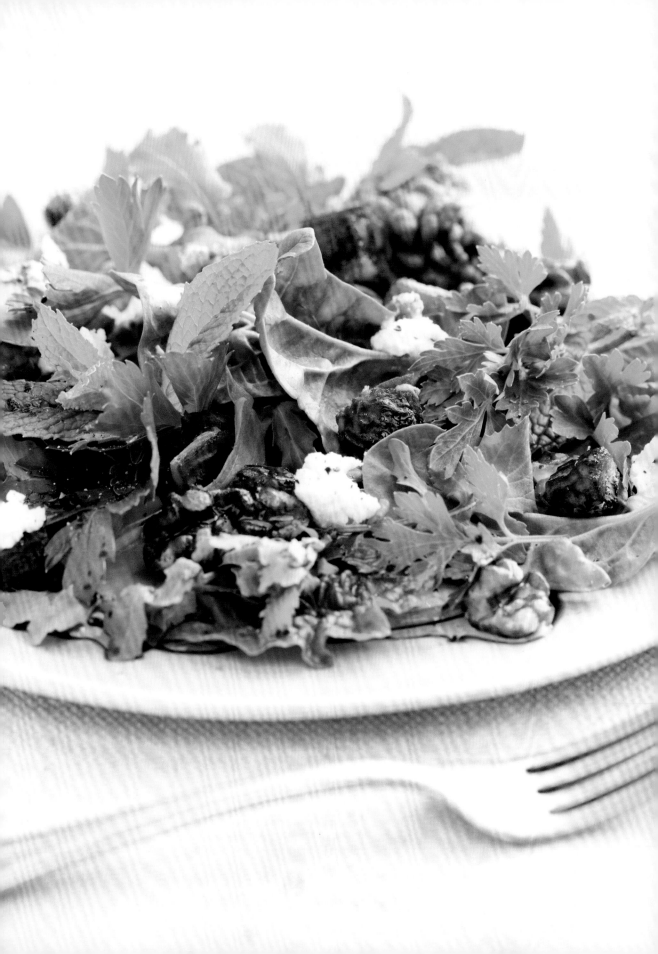

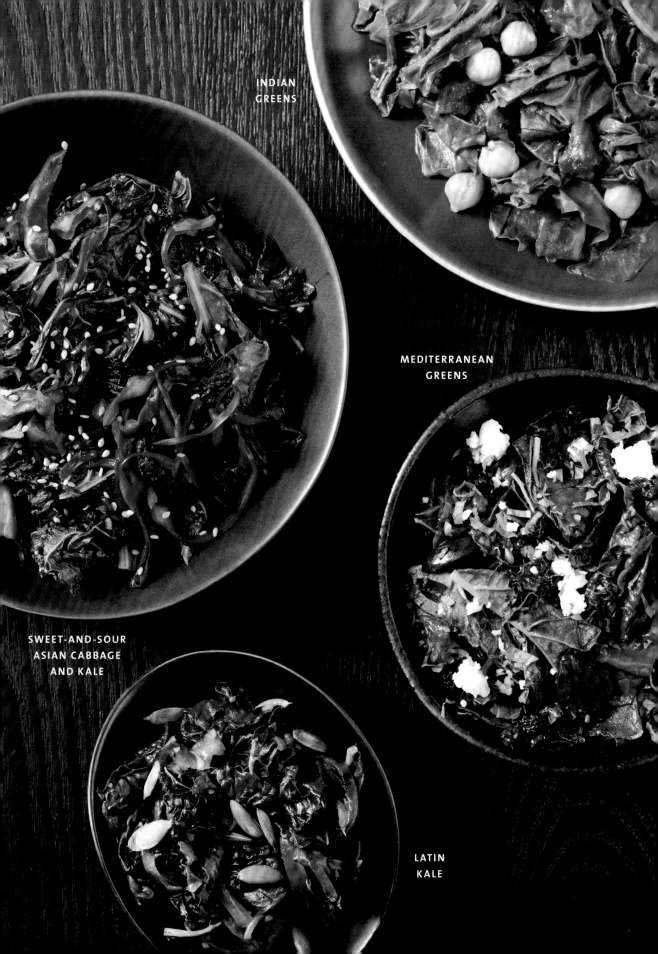

INDIAN
GREENS

MEDITERRANEAN
GREENS

SWEET-AND-SOUR
ASIAN CABBAGE
AND KALE

LATIN
KALE

Latin Kale

With Latin American greens, it's all in the seeds. In this case, toasted cumin and pumpkin seeds (aka pepitas) along with a hit of lime juice give this kale a breezy, fresh Latin feel.

MAKES 4 SERVINGS

8 cups stemmed and chopped lacinato kale, in bite-size pieces
2 tablespoons extra-virgin olive oil
2$\frac{1}{2}$ cups sliced red onions, in half-moons
Sea salt
3 cloves garlic, minced
$\frac{1}{4}$ teaspoon cumin seeds, toasted (see note, page 83)
Pinch of cayenne
1$\frac{1}{2}$ teaspoons freshly squeezed lime juice
1$\frac{1}{2}$ teaspoons freshly squeezed lemon juice
1 teaspoon grated lemon zest
$\frac{1}{2}$ teaspoon Grade B maple syrup
2 tablespoons pumpkin seeds, toasted (see note, page 83), for garnish

COOK'S NOTE: Prepping greens means having to do the rip and strip: Tearing off the tough stems makes greens easier to eat and digest.

Put the kale in a large bowl, add cold water to cover, and set aside.

Heat the olive oil in a large, deep skillet over medium-high heat. Add the onions and a pinch of salt and sauté for 3 minutes. Decrease the heat to medium-low and cook, stirring occasionally, until the onions are slightly golden, about 5 minutes.

Increase the heat to medium. Add the garlic, cumin, cayenne, and a pinch of salt and sauté for 3 to 4 minutes. Drain the kale, add it to the skillet, and sauté until bright green and wilted, about 4 minutes. Cover and cook until just tender, about 4 minutes.

Put the lime juice, lemon juice, lemon zest, and maple syrup in a small bowl and stir to combine. Drizzle over the kale, remove from the heat, and stir to combine. Scatter the pumpkin seeds over the top.

PREP TIME: 10 minutes COOK TIME: 45 minutes
STORAGE: Store in an airtight container in the refrigerator for up to 4 days.
PER SERVING: Calories: 195; Total Fat: 11 g (1.5 g saturated, 6 g monounsaturated); Carbohydrates: 22.5 g; Protein: 7 g; Fiber: 4 g; Sodium: 80 mg

Sweet-and-Sour Asian Cabbage and Kale

Here's a classic sweet-and-sour taste with a mouth-watering, eye-catching twist. Tamari, ginger, and toasted sesame oil combine with lime juice to bring the Great Wall to your great room. And cabbage? That's another super food that's a must-have on the plate.

MAKES 4 SERVINGS

1 tablespoon plus 2 teaspoons
   tamari
1 tablespoon freshly squeezed
   lime juice
1 tablespoon Grade B maple syrup
1 teaspoon toasted sesame oil
1 teaspoon grated fresh ginger
2 tablespoons extra-virgin olive oil
4 cups stemmed and chopped
   lacinato kale, in bite-size pieces
Sea salt
2 cups shredded red cabbage
   (see note, page 86)
1 tablespoon sesame seeds, toasted
   (see note, page 83)

WHO KNEW? Sautéing cabbage helps its fiber bind with the bile that attaches itself to cholesterol, increasing its efficiency in sweeping cholesterol out of the body.

Put the tamari, lime juice, maple syrup, toasted sesame oil, and ginger in a small bowl and stir to combine.

Heat the olive oil in a large, deep skillet over medium-high heat. Add the kale and a pinch of salt and sauté for 4 minutes. Add the cabbage and another pinch of salt and sauté for 2 minutes. Add the tamari mixture and cook until tender, about for 2 minutes. Sprinkle with the sesame seeds and serve immediately.

PREP TIME: 12 minutes COOK TIME: 8 minutes
STORAGE: Store in an airtight container in the refrigerator for up to 4 days.
PER SERVING: Calories: 195; Total Fat: 15.5 g (2 g saturated, 8.5 g mono-unsaturated); Carbohydrates: 14 g; Protein: 4 g; Fiber: 2.5 g; Sodium: 287 mg

Indian Greens

This meal in bowl is filled with fiber and protein from chickpeas and packs flavor that simply has to be experienced to be believed. Coconut milk, curry, turmeric…it's all a taste-bud blast with outrageous anti-inflammatory ingredients. MAKES 4 SERVINGS

8 cups stemmed and chopped Swiss chard, in bite-size pieces (see note)

2 tablespoons extra-virgin olive oil

$1/4$ teaspoon cumin seeds

$1/4$ teaspoon black or brown mustard seeds

1 teaspoon grated fresh ginger

$1/2$ teaspoon turmeric

$1/4$ teaspoon curry powder

$1/8$ teaspoon freshly ground black pepper

Sea salt

1 cup canned diced tomatoes, juices reserved

1 cup canned chickpeas, drained, rinsed, and mixed with a spritz of lemon juice and a pinch of sea salt

$1/4$ cup coconut milk

$1/4$ teaspoon Grade B maple syrup

COOK'S NOTE: Although the recipe calls for removing the chard stems, they're easier to digest than the stems of most greens, and nutritious too. If you'd like to use them, chop them into small pieces and cook them for a few minutes before adding the chopped leaves; that way they'll cook a bit longer and become more tender.

Put the chard in a large bowl, add cold water to cover, and set aside.

Heat the olive oil in a large, deep skillet over medium-high heat. Add the cumin seeds and mustard seeds and sauté until they begin to pop. Immediately stir in the ginger. Add the chard, turmeric, curry powder, pepper, a pinch of salt, and 2 tablespoons of the juice from the tomatoes. Sauté for 2 minutes. Add the chickpeas and tomatoes and sauté for 3 minutes. Stir in the coconut milk and maple syrup and serve immediately.

Variation: If you don't have cumin, mustard seeds, or turmeric handy, omit all three. Sauté the chard with the ginger and increase the amount of curry powder to $2 1/4$ teaspoons.

PREP TIME: 10 minutes COOK TIME: 8 minutes
STORAGE: Store in an airtight container in the refrigerator for up to 4 days.
PER SERVING: Calories: 185; Total Fat: 11 g (4 g saturated, 6 g mono-unsaturated); Carbohydrates: 18 g; Protein: 6 g; Fiber: 4 g; Sodium: 191 mg

WHO KNEW? Want to preserve your memory? Try lowering your homocysteine levels. Dr. Dale Bredesen, a University of California at San Francisco–trained neurologist and founding president of the Buck Institute for Age Research, cites a UK study that found high homocysteine levels were linked with deteriorations in the brain's hippocampus. This damage "is associated with losing your memory," says Bredesen. Fortunately, Bredesen says homocysteine levels, which can be measured by blood tests, can be brought down easily by getting more B12, B6, and folate in your diet. Our suggestion? Eat your dark leafy greens, which have abundant amounts of those key nutrients.

Mediterranean Greens

This is like a taking a two-week cruise around the isles: we go Greek with olives and feta, Sicilian with—surprise—currants, and we'll give the Cypriots credit for the garlic and the mint. Plus a double dose of citrus in the form of lemon and orange zest. MAKES 4 SERVINGS

6 cups stemmed and chopped lacinato kale, in bite-size pieces
2 teaspoons freshly squeezed lemon juice
1 teaspoon freshly squeezed orange juice
2 teaspoons grated lemon zest
1 teaspoon grated orange zest
$\frac{1}{2}$ teaspoon Grade B maple syrup
$\frac{1}{8}$ teaspoon freshly grated nutmeg
1 tablespoon currants
2 tablespoons extra-virgin olive oil
2 cloves garlic, minced
Pinch of red pepper flakes
Scant $\frac{1}{4}$ teaspoon salt
1 tablespoon water
$\frac{1}{4}$ cup kalamata olives, sliced
$\frac{1}{4}$ cup crumbled organic goat's milk or sheep's milk feta cheese
2 teaspoons chopped fresh mint, for garnish

Put the kale in a large bowl, add cold water to cover, and set aside.

Put the lemon juice, orange juice, lemon zest, orange zest, maple syrup, and nutmeg in a small bowl and stir to combine. Stir in the currants.

Heat the olive oil in a large, deep skillet over medium heat. Add the garlic and red pepper flakes and sauté until the garlic is lightly golden, about 20 seconds. Add the kale to the pan, along with the salt and 1 tablespoon of water. Sauté until the kale is bright green and wilted, about 4 minutes. Add the olives and the currants and their soaking liquid and sauté until the kale is just tender, about 4 minutes. Remove from the heat, sprinkle with the feta cheese and mint, and serve immediately.

PREP TIME: 10 minutes COOK TIME: 8 minutes
STORAGE: Store in an airtight container in the refrigerator for up to 4 days.
PER SERVING: Calories: 175; Total Fat: 12 g (2 g saturated, 8 g monounsaturated); Carbohydrates: 15 g; Protein: 5 g; Fiber: 3 g; Sodium: 307 mg

Maple-Glazed Brussels Sprouts with Caraway

Conquering this recipe reminded me of Charlie Brown's travails with Lucy and that football. There would be Lucy, pleading with Charlie to take one more shot at kicking the football and promising she wasn't going to mess with him anymore—and always pulling away the ball at the last moment. The Brussels sprouts in this recipe played Lucy to my Charlie. They teased me with their offerings of wellness—especially a compound shown to keep DNA from fragmenting during cell reproduction—but they kept refusing to play nice with every taste companion I threw their way. I was about to walk away for good when an email arrived from a friend who knew about my frustrations. She sent along a picture of a beautiful Brussels sprout stalk in her garden, with the small sprouts dotting the stalk, along with a caption that said, "Please give us another chance! We'll be good!' So I said, "Okay. One. Last. Chance." And whaddya know? I finally achieved success. Roasting was the key, creating a golden-brown, sweet-tasting, crunchy treat. MAKES 4 SERVINGS

2 tablespoons extra-virgin olive oil
1 tablespoon Grade B maple syrup
1 tablespoon Dijon mustard
1 teaspoon caraway seeds
Pinch of red pepper flakes
1 pound Brussels sprouts, trimmed, cut in half, rinsed, and patted dry
¼ teaspoon sea salt

WHO KNEW? Caraway contains salicylates, the same inflammation-fighting compounds found in aspirin. Studies also show that it lowers elevated blood sugar but, fortunately, doesn't decrease normal blood sugar levels. Caraway also contains phytochemicals shown to dramatically decrease the amounts of certain enzymes that create carcinogens in the body—by as much as 90 percent. In addition, women dealing with low hormone levels associated with menopause may benefit from caraway, as it is a natural, plant-based source of estrogen.

Preheat the oven to 400°F. Line a rimmed baking sheet with parchment paper.

Put the olive oil, maple syrup, mustard, caraway seeds, and red pepper flakes in a large bowl and whisk to combine. Add the Brussels sprouts and toss until evenly coated. Transfer to the lined baking sheet and spread in an even layer. Sprinkle with the salt. Bake for 20 to 25 minutes, until the outer leaves are crispy and the Brussels sprouts are tender all the way through. Transfer to a bowl and serve immediately.

Variation: Get a little nutty. Sprinkle ¼ cup of coarsely chopped toasted pecans over this dish before serving.

PREP TIME: 15 minutes COOK TIME: 25 minutes
STORAGE: Store in an airtight container in the refrigerator for up to 2 days.
PER SERVING: Calories: 125; Total Fat: 7.5 g (1 g saturated, 5.5 g monounsaturated); Carbohydrates: 14 g; Protein: 4 g; Fiber: 5 g; Sodium: 178 mg

COOK'S NOTE: A wonderful thing happens to Brussels sprouts while they're in the oven. Their outer leaves become crispy and positively addictive. You may want to trim off some of the outer leaves and include them on the baking sheet so you'll have plenty of extra-crispy yum.

Tuscan Beans and Greens

This dish has proven to be my daily revitalizer while working on this book. After a morning in the kitchen, I start to flag. It's not a good idea to get woozy from lack of fuel, especially when you're playing with sharp implements. Lunch is really a make-or-break meal. If you choose the wrong food—and especially if you hit the overload button on carbs and fats, you probably won't get much done in the afternoon. That's where this recipe comes in. The warm, creamy white beans and deliciously sautéed greens will definitely recharge your batteries. One of the longevity players here is kombu, a sea vegetable that has tremendous amounts of iodine, along with phenomenal anti-inflammatory and anticoagulant characteristics. As a bonus, it also makes beans more digestible. Because the beans are high in fiber, they help regulate blood sugar, so you'll be able to chug through the rest of your day with contentment in your belly and no crankiness on your countenance.

Prepare ahead: Soak the beans in cool water for 8 hours or overnight before cooking; this will make them more digestible and decrease the cooking time. MAKES 4 SERVINGS

BEANS
2 sprigs fresh rosemary
6 leaves fresh sage
6 sprigs fresh thyme
1 cup dried white beans, such as great northern beans or cannellini beans, soaked, rinsed, and drained
8 cloves garlic, peeled
1 (6-inch) strip of kombu
1 teaspoon extra-virgin olive oil
1 bay leaf
1 teaspoon sea salt

GREENS
2 tablespoons extra-virgin olive oil
3 large cloves garlic, slivered
Pinch of red pepper flakes
8 cups stemmed and chopped dark leafy greens, such as rainbow chard, lacinato kale, collard greens, or escarole, in bite-size pieces
1/4 teaspoon sea salt
1/2 cup water, bean cooking liquid, or vegetable broth, homemade (page 55) or store-bought
2 tablespoons tomato paste
Juice of 1/2 lemon

Freshly grated organic Parmesan cheese (optional), for serving
Extra-virgin olive oil, for drizzling

To make the beans, put the rosemary, sage, and thyme in a small piece of cheesecloth, gather the corners, and tie with kitchen twine to make a bouquet garni. Put the beans in a saucepan and add water to cover by 3 inches. Add the bouquet garni, garlic, kombu, olive oil, and bay leaf. Bring to a boil over high heat. Decrease the heat to low and skim any foam from the surface. Cover and simmer for 1 hour, stirring occasionally, until tender. Start testing the beans after 45 minutes; when they are tender but still a bit firm, stir in the salt. Check the beans occasionally to see if more water is needed. During the last 15 minutes the beans will soften quickly; test them often to ensure they don't overcook. (If you plan to store and reheat the beans, leave them ever so slightly undercooked.) With a slotted spoon, remove and discard the garlic, kombu, bay leaf, and bouquet garni.

Meanwhile, make the greens. Heat the olive oil in a large, deep skillet over medium heat. Add the garlic and red pepper flakes and sauté until the garlic is lightly golden, about 20 seconds. Add the greens to the pan, along with a pinch of salt. Sauté until the greens are wilted, about 4 minutes. You may need to add the greens in two or three batches, waiting until one batch wilts down before adding the next. Stir in the water and tomato paste, cover, and simmer until the greens are tender but still green, about 3 minutes. Remove from heat and stir in the lemon juice. Taste; you may want to add a bit of salt.

To assemble the dish, stir 2 cups of the beans into the greens. (Store any leftover beans for another use.) Serve topped with Parmesan cheese and a generous drizzle of extra-virgin olive oil.

Variation: Crunched for time? Instead of cooking dried beans, use 1 (15-ounce) can of great northern or cannellini beans, drained, rinsed, and mixed with a spritz of lemon juice and a pinch of salt.

PREP TIME: 10 minutes COOK TIME: 1 hour
STORAGE: To store the cooked beans separately, don't drain them completely. Reserve about 2 cups of the cooking liquid and store the beans in the liquid in an airtight container in the refrigerator for up to 4 days. Store the assembled dish in an airtight container in the refrigerator for up to 3 days.
PER SERVING: Calories: 205; Total Fat: 2 g (0.5 g saturated, 1 g monounsaturated); Carbohydrates: 35.5 g; Protein: 13 g; Fiber: 9 g; Sodium: 448 mg

Sicilian Green Beans

Green beans are in dire need of a culinary makeover. Here, my all-purpose Basil Pistachio Pesto partners with carrots to bring out the wonderful flavor and texture. That's a good thing, as green beans have the power to take on LOX and COX, two enzymes that promote inflammation, and it appears that compounds in green beans may help keep them in their place. Green beans also offer up a nice helping of silicon, which is crucial for bone and connective tissue health. MAKES 4 SERVINGS

1 pound green beans, trimmed
3 carrots, peeled and cut into thin 4-inch long strips
¼ teaspoon sea salt
3 tablespoons Basil Pistachio Pesto (page 179)
2 teaspoons chopped fresh mint, for garnish

Put 2 inches of water in a large saucepan. Put a steamer basket in the pan and bring to a boil over high heat. Add the green beans, cover, and steam for 4 minutes. Add the carrots, cover, and steam just until tender, about for 4 more minutes. Transfer the vegetables to a bowl. Add the pesto and stir gently to combine. Serve warm or chilled, garnished with the mint.

Variation: Substitute ¼ cup of Olive and Mint Vinaigrette (page 181) for the pesto.

PREP TIME: 15 minutes COOK TIME: 10 minutes
STORAGE: Store in an airtight container in the refrigerator for up to 5 days.
PER SERVING: Calories: 120; Total Fat: 7.5 g (1 g saturated, 5 g monounsaturated); Carbohydrates: 14 g; Protein: 3.5 g; Fiber: 5 g; Sodium: 166 mg

Lemon Chive Potatoes

You'd be surprised at the kind of tidbits you pick up at the farmers' market. For years, I've been getting my potatoes from Farmer Little. They were always absolutely delish, and I wanted him to let me in on his secret. "Dry farmed," he drawled. Come again? It turns out that dry farming isn't an oxymoron; it's a technique that utilizes only the moisture in the soil and rainfall, rather than irrigation. The result is potatoes that are outrageously nutrient-dense, and, not coincidentally, tasty to the max. Potatoes have gotten a bad rap here lately, but I'm totally committed to them. Contrary to myth, they can be served with something besides a slathering of sour cream and butter and still be delicious. And depending upon the variety of potato you use and how you prepare them, they need not be a carb fest. That's good news, because potatoes are so great for both mind and body that they're a truly holistic comfort food. They're rich in magnesium and vitamin B_6, which nourish the brain, and potassium and a load of antioxidants to revitalize your cells. I go for colorful potatoes, such as those with purple or red flesh. Rich colors are always an indicator of high antioxidant content, not to mention a feast for the eyes. This simple recipe is a wonderful way to enjoy these benefits: just potatoes, chives, and a lemony vinaigrette. MAKES 4 SERVINGS

1 pound purple Peruvian potatoes, peeled and cut into 1-inch cubes
1/4 cup Lemon Dijon Vinaigrette (page 185)
2 tablespoons chopped fresh chives
Generous pinch of sea salt

Put 4 inches of water in a large saucepan. Put a steamer basket in the pan and bring the water to a boil over high heat. Put the potatoes into the steamer basket, cover, and steam until just tender, 9 to 10 minutes. Remove the steamer basket and pour out the water. Put the potatoes in the pan. Add the dressing, chives, and salt and stir gently to combine. Serve hot or at room temperature.

Variation: Replace the purple Peruvian potatoes with Red Bliss potatoes. There's no need to peel them; just scrub them well.

PREP TIME: 10 minutes COOK TIME: 10 minutes
STORAGE: Store in an airtight container in the refrigerator for up to 3 days.
PER SERVING: Calories: 155; Total Fat: 7 g (1 g saturated, 5.5 g monounsaturated); Carbohydrates: 20.5 g; Protein: 3 g; Fiber: 1.5 g; Sodium: 165 mg

Roasted Fingerling Potatoes with Pesto

If you're wondering how I ever came up with the idea to put pesto on potatoes, it's like those old ads for you-know-what, where a guy walking the street eating a chocolate bar bumps into a girl with an open jar of peanut butter: a complete accident, but what an outcome! I was staring into the refrigerator as fingerling potatoes were coming out of the oven, and what should my eyes chance upon but a container of the pesto. Normally, I'd use the pesto with pasta, but as I discovered that night, it's also wonderful with potatoes. MAKES 6 SERVINGS

2 pounds fingerling potatoes,
    scrubbed and cut into quarters
1 tablespoon extra-virgin olive oil
1/4 teaspoon sea salt
Freshly ground black pepper
3 tablespoons Basil Pistachio Pesto
    (page 179)

Preheat the oven to 450°F.

Put the potatoes, olive oil, salt, and a few grinds of pepper in a large bowl and toss until the potatoes are evenly coated. Transfer to a rimmed baking sheet, spreading the potatoes in a single layer. Bake, turning occasionally, for 30 to 35 minutes, until the potatoes begin to turn golden brown.

Transfer to a serving bowl, add the pesto, and toss until the potatoes are evenly coated. Serve immediately.

PREP TIME: 2 minutes COOK TIME: 15 minutes
STORAGE: Store in an airtight container in the refrigerator for up to 5 days.
PER SERVING: Calories: 180; Total Fat: 7 g (1 g saturated, 5 g monounsaturated); Carbohydrates: 27 g; Protein: 4 g; Fiber: 4 g; Sodium: 36 mg

Broccoli with Red Onion, Feta, and Mint

You don't get to my age without learning something about making changes, especially if you're the cook. Take broccoli: it has major anti–inflammatory and anticancer properties and you should eat it often, but how many times can you serve it with an overly orange cheese sauce? Here I've kept the cheese but with a bit of a curve, using goat's milk or sheep's milk feta, which is lower in casein than cheese made from cow's milk and easier for most folks to digest, especially those who are lactose intolerant. The cheese provides a familiar note for the unsuspecting: "Well, it's broccoli and it has cheese, so it must be good." That allows you to go to town, adding in the sweetness of sautéed onions, the pep of lemon zest, and the pop of cherry tomatoes, which take this dish to a whole new level, in terms of both flavor and healthfulness. MAKES 4 SERVINGS

1 bunch of broccoli
2 tablespoons extra-virgin olive oil
1 tablespoon finely chopped garlic
Pinch of red pepper flakes
$1/_2$ cup thinly sliced red onion, in half-moons
Sea salt
$1/_2$ cup halved cherry tomatoes
3 tablespoons crumbled organic goat's milk or sheep's milk feta cheese
2 teaspoons grated lemon zest
1 tablespoon chopped fresh mint, for garnish

WHO KNEW? Sometimes the nose knows. If you're in the mood for a good detox (like the day after Thanksgiving, for example), Cynthia Geyer, MD, medical director of Canyon Ranch health spa in Lenox, Massachusetts, recommends pointing yourself in the direction of some odiferous fare: "Smelly foods are really power foods: The crucifers and the garlic and onion family are key for detoxification," says Geyer, who adds that antioxidant-rich red and black beans, with their high fiber content, are also good for moving foods through your system.

Put 4 inches of water in a large saucepan. Put a steamer basket in the pan and bring the water to a boil over high heat. Cut the broccoli florets off the stalks, then peel the stems and cut them into bite-size pieces. Put the broccoli florets and stems in the steamer basket, cover, and steam until a lush shade of green, 2 to 3 minutes. Remove the steamer basket, pour out the water, and dry the pot well.

Heat the olive oil in the same pot over medium heat. Add the garlic and red pepper flakes and sauté just until aromatic, about 30 seconds. Add the onion and a pinch of salt and sauté until golden, 4 to 5 minutes. Stir in the broccoli florets and $1/4$ teaspoon of salt and sauté for 2 minutes; the broccoli should still be firm. Gently stir in the tomatoes, cheese, and lemon zest. Garnish with the mint and serve immediately.

Variations: Top with chopped toasted almonds or walnuts if you like. You can substitute freshly grated organic Parmesan cheese for the feta. For extra omega-3s, add 2 chopped white anchovies and 1 teaspoon of rinsed capers just before adding the broccoli.

PREP TIME: 15 minutes COOK TIME: 15 minutes
STORAGE: Store in an airtight container in the refrigerator for up to 2 days.
PER SERVING: Calories: 145; Total Fat: 9 g (2 g saturated, 6 g mono-unsaturated); Carbohydrates: 14 g; Protein: 6 g; Fiber: 5 g; Sodium: 143 mg

COOK'S NOTE: No steamer basket? No problem. Bring a large pot of water to a boil over high heat. Add a generous pinch of salt, broccoli, and broccoli stalks and blanch for 30 seconds. Drain well, then run the broccoli under cold water to stop the cooking.

Sweet Potato and Zucchini Pancakes

Those of us of the Jewish persuasion delight in potato pancakes (we call them latkes) on Hanukah, the Festival of Lights. But my friend Wendy proved they could be enjoyable anytime. Unlike the typical oil-drenched holiday fare, these puppies need no blotting, as just a bit of olive oil is used for frying. MAKES 18 SMALL PANCAKES

8 ounces orange-fleshed sweet potato, such as garnet yam, grated
1 small zucchini, finely grated
$1/2$ small onion, grated
2 organic eggs, beaten
$1/2$ teaspoon sea salt
$1/4$ teaspoon freshly ground black pepper
$1/8$ teaspoon freshly grated nutmeg
$1/2$ cup loosely packed fresh basil leaves, shredded (see note)
4 teaspoons extra-virgin olive oil
1 tablespoon brown rice flour
Organic plain Greek yogurt, for serving

COOK'S NOTE: Shred the basil just before adding it to retain its bright green color. Here's a convenient way to shred it: Stack the basil leaves, roll them into a cigar shape, and snip it with scissors or cut thin slices with a sharp chef knife.

Put the grated sweet potato, zucchini, and onion in a colander and press gently to squeeze out excess moisture.

Put the eggs, salt, pepper, and nutmeg in a large bowl and whisk to combine. Add the vegetables, basil, and flour and stir with a spatula to combine.

Carefully drain the excess moisture from the vegetable mixture. Heat the olive oil in a large skillet over medium heat. Spoon the mixture into the skillet by the heaping tablespoonful, then flatten with the back of spoon. Cook until golden brown on both sides, about 2 minutes per side. Transfer to a platter, keeping the pancakes in a single layer. Serve hot or warm with a dollop of Greek yogurt.

Variation: Top the pancakes with a small slice of smoked salmon, or with arugula and a slice of tomato.

PREP TIME: 25 minutes COOK TIME: 25 minutes
STORAGE: Store leftover batter in an airtight container in the refrigerator for up to 2 days. Wrap leftover pancakes tightly and store in the refrigerator for up to 3 days or in the freezer for 1 month. Reheat refrigerated pancakes in a preheated dry skillet over medium heat, or in a toaster oven. Reheat frozen pancakes in a 350 degree oven for 15 minutes.
PER SERVING: (4 small pancakes) Calories: 295; Total Fat: 5 g (1 g saturated, 2 g monounsaturated); Carbohydrates: 56 g; Protein: 7 g; Fiber: 4 g; Sodium: 123 mg

Bella's Moroccan-Spiced Sweet Potato Salad

And who, pray tell, is this exotic culinary adventuress named Bella? My eight-year-old Portuguese water dog. For a long time now, she's loved carrots. She literally comes running every time she hears the carrot peeler come out of the drawer. My husband and I thought, "Hmm, that's different for a dog," and played the approving parents. Recently, she's expanded her palate to sweet potatoes. No sooner do they hit the counter than she's singing and dancing around my feet. I quarter and square off the potatoes and fling the ends at her, and she's been known to get some serious hang time as she leaps for them. Seriously, Air Bud's got nothing on Bella. Maybe she heard about how healthful sweet potatoes are: their natural sweetness is perfectly balanced with high fiber content, slowing the rush of sugar into the bloodstream, which is great for the vascular system, and for mood. My experience says that's true; whenever I make this salad, Bella's awfully happy. MAKES 6 SERVINGS

2 tablespoons extra-virgin olive oil
1 cup finely diced yellow onion
Sea salt
1 teaspoon grated fresh ginger, or
   $1/2$ teaspoon ground ginger
1 teaspoon ground cumin
$1/2$ teaspoon paprika
1 pound orange-fleshed sweet
   potatoes, such as garnet yams,
   cut into $1/2$-inch cubes
$1/2$ cup water
$1/4$ cup freshly squeezed orange
   juice, preferably blood orange
   juice
1 teaspoon grated orange zest
1 teaspoon grated lemon zest
2 tablespoons freshly squeezed
   lemon juice
2 teaspoons Grade B maple syrup
12 kalamata olives, cut in half
$1/4$ cup finely chopped fresh flat-leaf
   parsley
$1/4$ cup almonds or shelled pistachios, toasted (see note, page 83)
   and coarsely chopped

Heat the olive oil in a deep skillet over medium heat. Add the onion and a generous pinch of salt and sauté until slightly golden, about 5 minutes. Add the ginger, cumin, and paprika and sauté for 1 minute. Add the sweet potatoes, water, orange juice, orange zest, lemon zest, and $1/2$ teaspoon salt and stir to combine. Decrease the heat to medium-low, cover, and cook for 15 minutes.

Uncover and cook, stirring occasionally, until the sweet potatoes are tender and the liquid is reduced to almost a glaze, about 5 minutes. Add the lemon juice, maple syrup, and olives and stir gently to combine. Taste; you may want to add a pinch of salt or squeeze of lemon juice. Transfer to a bowl and sprinkle with the parsley and almonds. Serve at room temperature.

PREP TIME: 20 minutes COOK TIME: 25 minutes
STORAGE: Store in an airtight container in the refrigerator for up to 5 days.
PER SERVING: Calories: 180; Total Fat: 9 g (1 g saturated, 6.5 g monounsaturated); Carbohydrates: 23 g; Protein: 3 g; Fiber: 3.5 g; Sodium: 300 mg

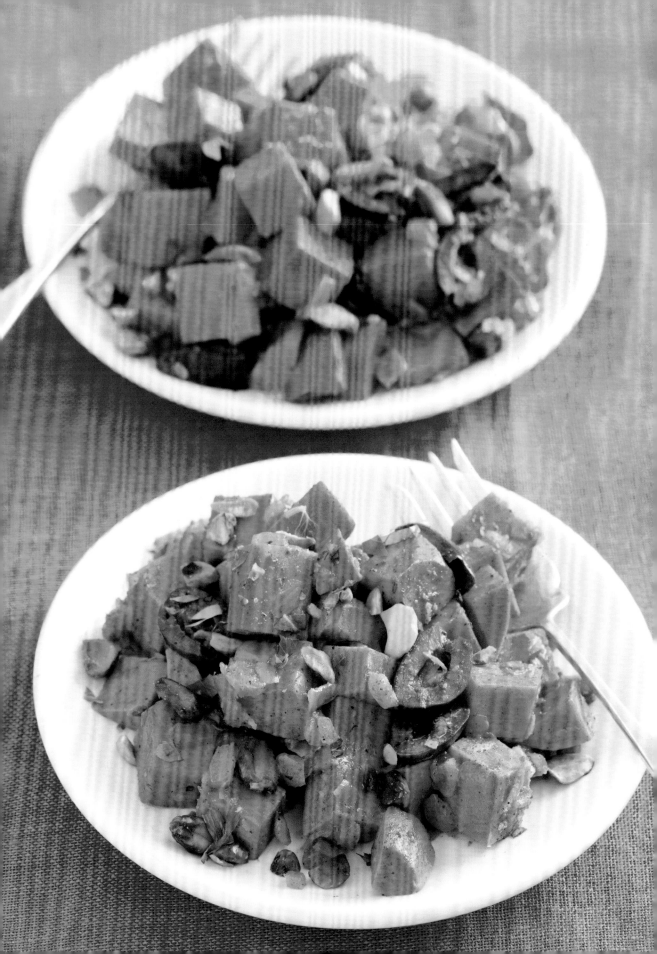

Cauliflower Puree with Cumin and Lime

Maybe the song "The Great Pretender" was written about cauliflower. Here it masquerades as one of my favorite foods: mashed potatoes. It's amazing what steam and a food processor can accomplish. Steaming the cauliflower in broth infused with seasonings takes care of the sulfuric smell it produces as it cooks. Then it gets whazzed in the food processor until the texture is as creamy as Ma's Thanksgiving 'taters. The cilantro and lime juice provide an unconventional but extremely tasty high note. As for health benefits, compounds in cauliflower support several aspects of liver detoxification, help control inflammation, and fight free radical damage. MAKES 4 SERVINGS

3 tablespoons extra-virgin olive oil

2 pounds cauliflower, chopped into florets

2 teaspoons minced garlic

1/4 teaspoon ground cumin

1/2 teaspoon sea salt

3/4 to 1 cup vegetable broth, homemade (page 55) or store-bought

2 teaspoons freshly squeezed lime juice

2 teaspoons finely chopped fresh cilantro or parsley

COOK'S NOTE: You can also mash the cauliflower with a potato masher or fork, but the texture won't be as smooth.

Heat 2 tablespoons of the olive oil in a large skillet over medium heat. Add the garlic and sauté until fragrant, about 20 seconds. Add the cauliflower, cumin, and a 1/4 teaspoon of the salt and sauté for 30 seconds. Decrease the heat to medium-low, pour in 1/2 cup of the broth, cover, and cook until the cauliflower is very tender and most of the liquid has evaporated, about 12 minutes.

Transfer to a food processor, add the remaining 1 tablespoon of olive oil, and process until smooth, adding more of the broth for a thinner consistency if you like. Transfer to a bowl and stir in the lime juice, cilantro, and remaining 1/4 teaspoon of salt.

PREP TIME: 10 minutes COOK TIME: 15 minutes
STORAGE: Store in an airtight container in the refrigerator for up to 3 days.
PER SERVING: Calories: 115; Total Fat: 7.5 g (1 g saturated, 5.5 g monounsaturated); Carbohydrates: 11 g; Protein: 4 g; Fiber: 4 g; Sodium: 220 mg

WHO KNEW? A clean system is a happy system, and food plays an absolutely essential role in detoxification. Jeanne Wallace, PhD, says that clients in her clinical nutrition practice often announce that they're going to go on a detox diet for a while. In her book, that doesn't cut it: "Your liver is busy detoxifying 24/7. You can't decide to detox every year, you need to do it every day, and components of the detox process depend on constituents in the diet." Wallace says cruciferous veggies are great for detoxifying, including broccoli, cabbage, cauliflower, turnips, radishes, Brussels sprouts, arugula, and—ta-da!—wasabi.

Roasted Delicata Squash with Orange and Thyme

As a cook, you never stop learning. I was doing a cooking demo one day in a tiny town in West Marin across from Toby's Feed Barn. As I was prepping and peeling the squash, an extremely seasoned farmer with a weathered face came up to me. He was the kind of guy who normally wouldn't talk even if he were on fire. But what I was doing truly had him flummoxed. He looked at my peeler, smacked his lips in thought, and said, "Y'know, you don't have to peel 'em." He might as well have said it's okay to drive naked. I told him I'd been peeling them forever. "*Nooooo*," he moaned, at what was obviously food blasphemy in his book. "The skin is good—tender. Stop peeling!" It turns out he was right: the skin does indeed taste fine, and once it's cooked, it isn't tough. Squash has excellent anti-inflammatory and immune-boosting nutrients, along with a huge kick of vitamin A. In this incarnation, it also has wonderful sweetness, thanks to the roasting and the addition of a splash of orange juice. MAKES 4 SERVINGS

1 delicata squash
2 tablespoons freshly squeezed orange juice
$^1/_2$ teaspoon grated orange zest
1 tablespoon extra-virgin olive oil
2 teaspoons Grade B maple syrup
1 teaspoon chopped fresh thyme
$^1/_4$ teaspoon sea salt
Freshly ground black pepper

COOK'S NOTE: If you have a melon ball scooper, now is the time to take it out of hibernation; it's the perfect instrument for scooping out squash seeds.

WHO KNEW? Here's another reason to get more fiber and complex carbs into your diet. Simple carbohydrates like refined white sugar promote insulin resistance. According to Jeanne Wallace, PhD, CNC, not only can this lead to type 2 diabetes, it also "creates the damage in the brain that you find in Alzheimer's disease. So much of what we thought of in Alzheimer's as normal brain aging, we now understand that the underpinning of that is insulin resistance."

Preheat the oven to 425°F. Line a rimmed baking sheet with parchment paper.

Cut the stem end off the squash, use a melon baller to scoop out the seeds, and cut the squash into in $^1/_4$-inch-thick rounds; alternatively, cut the squash in half lengthwise, scoop out the seeds, and cut the squash into $^1/_4$-inch-thick semicircles. Put the squash, orange juice, orange zest, olive oil, maple syrup, thyme, salt, and a few grinds of pepper in a large bowl and toss until the squash is evenly coated.

Use a slotted spoon to transfer the squash to the lined baking sheet, spreading it in a single layer. Reserve the liquid in the bowl. Bake for 10 minutes, then flip the squash over and baste with the reserved liquid. Bake for 10 more minutes, until the squash is tender.

PREP TIME: 10 minutes COOK TIME: 20 minutes
STORAGE: Store in an airtight container in the refrigerator for up to 3 days.
PER SERVING: Calories: 85; Total Fat: 3.5 g (0.5 g saturated, 3 g monounsaturated); Carbohydrates: 12.5 g; Protein: 1.5 g; Fiber: 1.5 g; Sodium: 100 mg

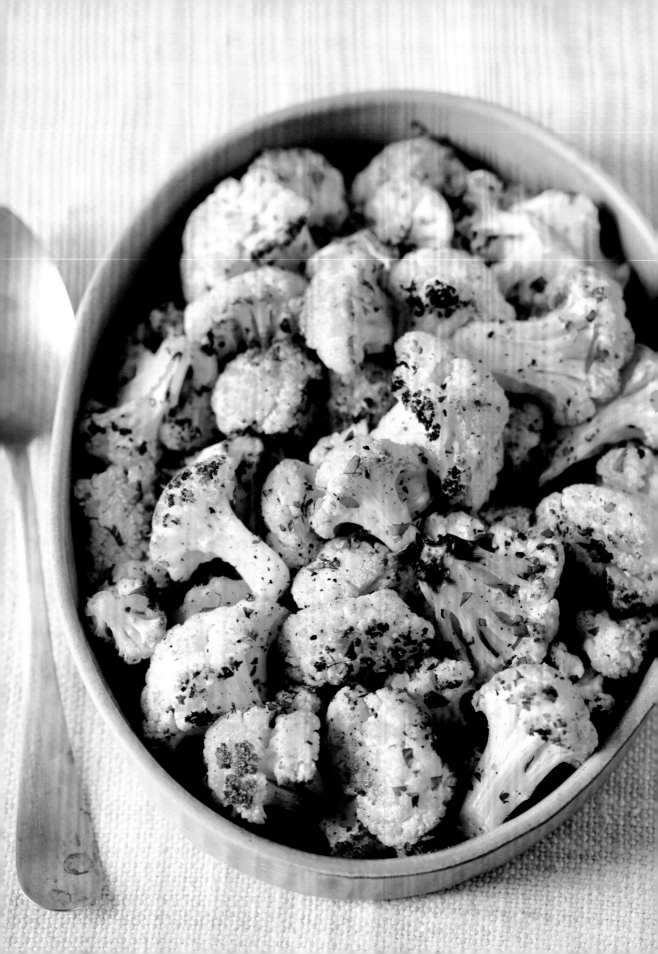

Golden Roasted Cauliflower

My dad was in the salad dressing business, and that meant we never knew what kind of science experiment might show up on the dinner table. One day it might be a new Roquefort dressing, the next day a zesty ranch concoction. There were always plenty of raw veggies available for dipping, and dad's favorite was raw cauliflower with Thousand Island dressing. In fact, for years I just assumed the only way anyone ate cauliflower was raw. I'm glad I know better now. Roasting cauliflower completely transforms it into a candy-like delight that yields to a gentle fork. The spices in this recipe—cumin, coriander, and turmeric—really make it sing. All have health benefits, but turmeric is a superstar: it has anticancer and anti-inflammatory properties and holds great promise for maintaining, and possibly even improving, brain health. MAKES 4 SERVINGS

2 1/2 to 3 pounds cauliflower, cut into 1 1/2-inch florets
2 tablespoons extra-virgin olive oil
1 tablespoon minced garlic
1/2 teaspoon sea salt
1/2 teaspoon turmeric
1/2 teaspoon ground cumin
1/4 teaspoon ground coriander
1/4 teaspoon freshly ground black pepper
1 teaspoon freshly squeezed lemon juice
1 tablespoon finely chopped fresh parsley or cilantro

COOK'S NOTE: Chopping cauliflower releases enzymes that increase the bioavailability of its nutrients. Delaying cooking for 5 to 10 minutes after cutting helps ensure the heat won't destroy the effectiveness of these enzymes. The enzymes need vitamin C to activate, which can be accomplished with a hit of lemon juice.

Position a rack in the middle of the oven and preheat the oven to 425°F. Line a rimmed baking sheet with parchment paper.

Put the cauliflower, olive oil, garlic, salt, turmeric, cumin, coriander, and pepper in a large bowl and toss until the cauliflower is evenly coated. Transfer to the lined baking sheet and spread in an even layer. Bake for 25 to 35 minutes, until the cauliflower is golden and tender. Transfer to a bowl, add the lemon juice and parsley, and toss to combine.

Variation: If you're not in a mood for spices, simply toss the cauliflower with the olive oil, salt, and pepper. You'll love how sweet the cauliflower tastes with this simple seasoning.

PREP TIME: 10 minutes COOK TIME: 35 minutes
STORAGE: Store in an airtight container in the refrigerator for up to 2 days.
PER SERVING: Calories: 120; Total Fat: 8 g (1 g saturated, 5.5 g monounsaturated); Carbohydrates: 12 g; Protein: 4.5 g; Fiber: 4.5 g; Sodium: 265 mg

LIVE LONG AND PROSPER: Reverence for this spice is abundant in Indian ayurvedic traditions, in which turmeric is an important element in healing cuisine. Turmeric's reputation was built on its ability to soothe the stomach, including healing medieval hangovers, and studies confirm that it can be helpful with illnesses of the gastrointestinal system, such as irritable bowel syndrome. A key compound in turmeric, curcumin, is particularly powerful, with some studies indicating that it may help slow the progression of Alzheimer's disease by impairing the growth of the amyloid plaques associated with the disease. Curcumin also has anti-inflammatory properties that hold promise for those seeking relief from pain, particularly joint and arthritis-related discomfort.

Swiss Chard and Roasted Butternut Squash Tart

Like Penn and Teller, opposites often attract—and create magic. So it is here. At first glance, Swiss chard and butternut squash appear to be poles apart, yet they melt into each others arms in a way that enraptures the senses. The sweetness of roasted butternut squash is the perfect foil for chard's tartness, and cranberries and orange zest do a similar tango to heighten the appeal. Visually, the tart is a stunner; topped with walnuts and studded with cranberries and feta, it looks like a still life waiting for the right artiste to saunter by. Chard is also a longevity superstar, full of antioxidants and boasting phytonutrients linked to blood sugar regulation, heart health, and improved detoxification. Note that you'll need a 9-inch tart pan with a removable bottom for this recipe. MAKES 6 SERVINGS

CRUST
1/3 cup corn flour
1 cup plus 2 tablespoons whole wheat pastry flour
1/2 teaspoon sea salt
1 organic egg yolk
1/3 cup extra-virgin olive oil
2 tablespoons ice water
2 teaspoons Grade B maple syrup

FILLING
1 pound butternut squash, cut into 1/2-inch cubes (about 3 cups)
3 tablespoons extra-virgin olive oil
Sea salt
1/2 teaspoon dried thyme
1/2 teaspoon dried sage
1/4 teaspoon freshly ground black pepper
1 cup finely diced yellow onion
1/4 teaspoon red pepper flakes
8 cups stemmed and chopped Swiss chard, in bite-size pieces (see note, page 97)
1/4 cup unsweetened dried cranberries
1 teaspoon grated orange zest
Pinch of freshly grated nutmeg
2 organic eggs, lightly beaten
1/4 cup crumbled organic goat's milk or sheep's milk feta cheese
1/4 cup coarsely chopped walnuts, lightly toasted (see note, page 83)

To make the crust, preheat the oven to 350°F.

Put the corn flour, whole wheat flour, and salt in food processor bowl and pulse until well combined. Put the egg yolk, olive oil, water, and maple syrup in a small bowl and whisk until creamy looking. Pour into the food processor and process until the mixture comes together and just begins to form a ball on the side of the work bowl.

Put a large piece of waxed paper on the countertop and transfer the dough to the waxed paper. Cover with another piece of waxed paper and roll the dough out to an 11-inch circle, so the crust will extend up the sides of the pan. Carefully transfer the dough from the waxed paper to the pan and press it into the bottom and sides of the pan. Prick the bottom of the dough with a fork. Bake for 12 to 15 minutes, until the crust is light golden brown. (It will be baked again once filled, so don't over-bake at this point.)

To make the filling, turn the oven up to 400°F. Line a rimmed baking sheet with parchment paper.

Put the squash, 1 tablespoon of the olive oil, 1/4 teaspoon of salt, and the thyme, sage, and pepper in a bowl and toss until the squash is evenly coated. Transfer to the lined baking sheet and spread in a single layer. Bake for 20 minutes, until tender. Turn the oven down to 350°F.

WHO KNEW? Most people associate fiber with keeping the gut healthy, and it does excel at that, but it's also necessary for getting toxic metals out of the body. When the liver metabolizes heavy metals, the toxins bind with bile. That bile needs a transport mechanism to carry it out of the body, otherwise it—and its dangerous cargo—gets reabsorbed. Fiber fills the bill, escorting bile and company out of the body, but these days most people consume far too little fiber to do the job. "When we existed as hunter-gatherers, we used to eat some 100 to 150 grams of fiber daily, but now it's usually closer to 10 grams," notes nutrition expert Joseph Pizzorno, ND. To up your fiber intake, eat more foods like lentils and dark leafy greens. Pizzorno adds that eating foods rich in vitamin C is also vital for removing heavy metals from the system.

Meanwhile, heat the remaining 2 tablespoons of olive oil in a large skillet over medium heat. Add the onion, red pepper flakes, and a pinch of salt and sauté until the onion is golden, about 5 minutes. Add the chard and $1/4$ teaspoon of salt and sauté until tender, about 5 minutes. Stir in the cranberries, orange zest, and nutmeg. Remove from the heat and let cool briefly.

Transfer to a fine-mesh sieve and press to remove excess moisture. Transfer to a large bowl and fold in the eggs, cheese, and squash.

To assemble and bake the tart, spoon the filling into the crust and sprinkle with the walnuts. Bake for 15 minutes, until the filling is firm and set. Serve immediately.

PREP TIME: 20 minutes COOK TIME: 1 hour 10 minutes
STORAGE: Store in an airtight container in the refrigerator for up to 3 days or in the freezer for up to 1 month.
PER SERVING: Calories: 200; Total Fat: 13.5 g (3 g saturated, 7 g mono-unsaturated); Carbohydrates: 18 g; Protein: 6 g; Fiber: 3.5 g; Sodium: 338 mg

COOK'S NOTE: If you don't feel like making a tart crust, go crust free! Just pour the filling into a pie plate and bake at 350°F oven for 20 minutes, or until firm and set.

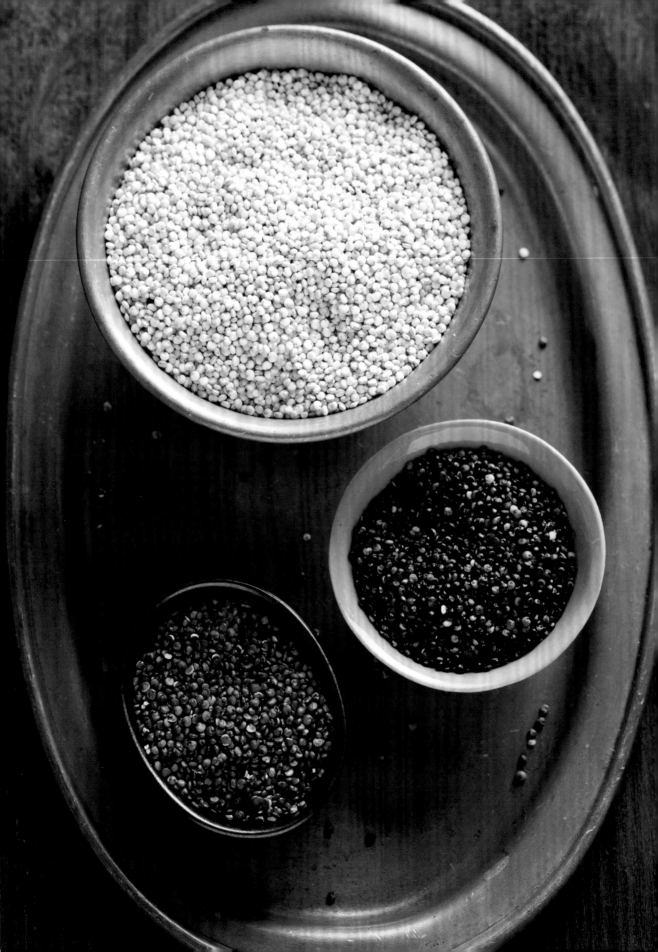

CHAPTER 6

Generous Grains

Talk about time-tested sustenance!

Whole grains have been nourishing our species for millennia—about twenty thousand years, according to anthropologists. Research into the health benefits of whole grains is on the rise, and the findings indicate that consistent consumption of whole grains is linked with promoting health in nearly every body system. They provide protection against heart disease, diabetes, and numerous cancers, especially pancreatic and colorectal cancer and cancer of the small intestine. One large study, which followed over thirty-four thousand people, even suggested that eating whole grains can lower the risk of gum disease. Of course, these benefits are associated with whole, unprocessed grains, which contain numerous nutrients that our bodies crave, particularly iron, vitamin E, B vitamins, fiber (lots of it!), and magnesium, which has calming properties.

As with vegetables, grains come in all sizes and shapes and have diverse, distinct flavors. Most people are familiar with brown rice and turn to it regularly for healthful whole grains. But making that your only whole grain is like listening to a chorus solely made up of tenors. It's hard to get excited about it day after day, and whole grains are too important to fall into the "nah, not today" category. That's while the pages that follow introduce you to several other scrumptious, if less familiar, grains that you might not have cozied up to before: quinoa, buckwheat, and farro. If you're looking to avoid gluten, you'll also appreciate the fact that quinoa and buckwheat are gluten-free, which makes sense when you consider that, botanically, neither is a grain at all. Quinoa is more closely related to beets, and buckwheat is related to rhubarb. Farro, on the other hand, is an ancient form of wheat.

Lemony Lentil and Quinoa Salad

Visual appeal is a vital though often ignored aspect of good digestion, as a mouthwatering response to the food on your plate prompts greater production of saliva, which helps break down food from the moment it hits your tongue. When I'm teaching, I like to use quinoa to underscore the importance of appearances. After an unenthusiastic glance at a bowl of cooked plain quinoa, the response is usually "Doesn't look like much. Kinda tan." Then we go to work on it, studding the quinoa with tiny green lentils and a blast of color from cucumbers, tomatoes, parsley, and mint that gets people excited about this dish. It looks like an edible painting by the time we're done. Now that's *my* idea of art. MAKES 6 SERVINGS

½ cup dried lentils, preferably Le Puy green lentils, rinsed well (see note, page 72)
2 cloves garlic, peeled and smashed
1 bay leaf
Pinch of ground cinnamon
Sea salt
1 ¾ cups water
1 cup white quinoa, rinsed well in cold water and drained (see note)
1 teaspoon ground cumin
½ teaspoon ground coriander
¼ cup freshly squeezed lemon juice
¼ cup extra-virgin olive oil
1 teaspoon grated lemon zest
¼ cup finely chopped fresh mint
½ cup finely chopped fresh flat-leaf parsley
1 small English cucumber, peeled, seeded, and diced
1 cup diced tomato or halved cherry tomatoes
2 tablespoons crumbled organic goat's milk or sheep's milk feta cheese (optional)

COOK'S NOTE: When it comes to quinoa, rinse, rinse, and rinse again! Quinoa is naturally coated with saponins, bitter-tasting resins that protect the seeds from insects. This coating is typically removed during process, but to be sure, put the quinoa in a bowl of cool water, swish it around with your hand, then drain it in a fine-mesh sieve.

Put the lentils, 1 clove of the garlic, the bay leaf, cinnamon, and ¼ teaspoon of salt in a saucepan and add water to cover by 2 inches. Bring to a boil over high heat, then decrease the heat to low, cover, and simmer until the lentils are tender, 20 to 25 minutes. Remove from the heat, drain well, and discard the garlic and bay leaf. Spritz with a bit of the lemon juice and let cool to room temperature.

Meanwhile, put the water, the remaining clove of the garlic, and ¼ teaspoon of the salt in a separate saucepan and bring just to a boil over high heat. Stir in the quinoa. Decrease the heat to low, cover, and simmer for 15 to 20 minutes, until the water is absorbed. Remove from the heat, transfer to a large bowl, and discard the garlic. Add the cumin and coriander and fluff with a fork until well combined. Let cool to room temperature.

Put the lemon juice, olive oil, lemon zest, and salt in a small bowl and whisk to combine. Add to the quinoa, along with the lentils, mint, and parsley, and fluff with a fork until well combined. Chill for at least 2 hours.

Add the cucumbers and tomatoes and fluff with a fork to combine. Do a FASS check (see page 44); you may want to add a squeeze of lemon juice or a pinch of salt. Sprinkle with the feta before serving.

Variation: For a nutritional boost from cruciferous vegetables, add 1 cup of arugula when you add the cucumbers.

PREP TIME: 10 minutes COOK TIME: 25 minutes
STORAGE: Store in an airtight container in the refrigerator for up to 4 days.
PER SERVING: Calories: 280; Total Fat: 13 g (2 g saturated, 7.5 g monounsaturated); Carbohydrates: 33 g; Protein: 10 g; Fiber: 10 g; Sodium: 182 mg

Quinoa with Edamame, Ginger, and Lime

I always think it's wise to carry a small patch and repair kit when you're out bike riding. It comes in very handy if your bike gets a flat tire. Quinoa (say it with me: KEEN-wah) is the food equivalent, an amazing little grain that rebuilds the body when it needs repair, like after a workout. It can do that because it contains all of the essential amino acids (those we must get from dietary sources), allowing the body to build protein. It's also full of magnesium, which is great for relaxing muscles and preventing cramps. From a culinary standpoint, it's wonderful because it doesn't get mushy when combined with other foods; instead, you get a nutty fluff-fest. Here I've paired it with edamame in a salad seasoned with ginger, lemon, and lime. By the way, this dish benefits from being made ahead of time because the flavor deepens as it sits. If you want to take the flavor over the top, try it with a bit of Indonesian Drizzle (page 183). MAKES 6 SERVINGS

2½ cups vegetable broth, home-made (page 55) or store-bought, or water
½ teaspoon sea salt
1½ cups red or white quinoa, rinsed well in cold water and drained (see note, page 117)
1 teaspoon grated fresh ginger
Pinch of cayenne
1 cup fresh or frozen edamame, mixed with a spritz of lime juice and a pinch of salt
½ cup finely diced red bell pepper
2 scallions, white and green parts, finely chopped
2 tablespoons chopped fresh mint
2 tablespoons chopped fresh cilantro, basil, or parsley
2 tablespoons extra-virgin olive oil
2 tablespoons freshly squeezed lemon juice
2 tablespoons freshly squeezed lime juice
1 tablespoon grated lemon zest
1 teaspoon grated lime zest

Put the broth and ¼ teaspoon of the salt in a large saucepan and bring to a boil over high heat. Stir in the quinoa. Decrease the heat to low, cover, and cook for 15 to 20 minutes, until the water is absorbed.

Remove from the heat. Add the ginger, cayenne, and remaining ¼ teaspoon of salt and fluff with a fork until well combined. Transfer the quinoa to a bowl and let cool to room temperature

Add the edamame, red bell pepper, scallions, mint, cilantro, olive oil, lemon juice, lime juice, lemon zest, and lime zest and stir until well combined. Do a FASS check (see page 44); you may need to add a pinch or two of salt, a squeeze of lemon or lime juice, or a dash of olive oil.

PREP TIME: 15 minutes COOK TIME: 20 minutes
STORAGE: Store in an airtight container in the refrigerator for up to 4 days.
PER SERVING: Calories: 275; Total Fat: 9 g (1 g saturated, 4 g mono-unsaturated); Carbohydrates: 37 g; Protein: 10 g; Fiber: 14 g; Sodium: 236 mg

COOK'S NOTE: Color is key when it comes to quinoa. When cooked, white quinoa has the subtlest flavor. Red has an earthy flavor and is a bit chewier and nuttier. Black quinoa is the most striking in appearance and is perfect for salads because it retains its shape and crunchy texture best.

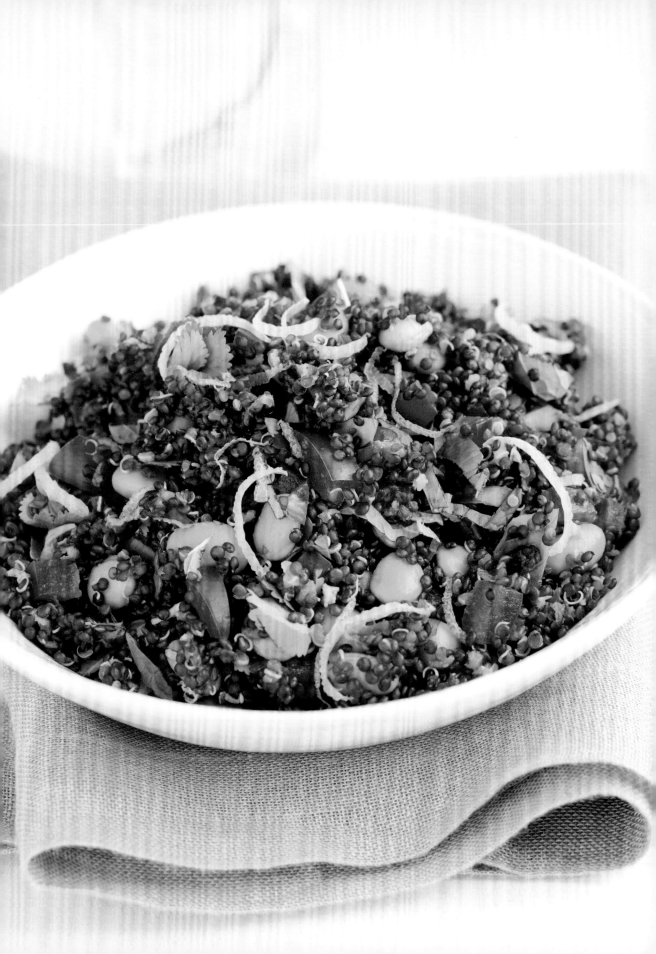

Not Your Typical Tabouli

I like the way certain words taste in my mouth, and *tabouli* is one of them. It's way more fun than saying "Middle Eastern salad with grains, parsley, and mint." In this recipe, I've replaced the traditional bulgur wheat with buckwheat for a gluten-free take on the classic. Buckwheat is one of the few foods that contain high levels of rutin, which kicks up vitamin C's antioxidant capacity. The blast of herbaceous freshness from parsley and mint brings in a host of other phytonutrients, and lemon zest, black pepper, coriander, and cumin all add to the kaleidoscope of tastes in this dish.

Prepare ahead: Soak the buckwheat in cool water with the juice of half a lemon for 8 hours or overnight before cooking; this will make its nutrients more available and decrease the cooking time. If you don't have time to soak the buckwheat, add an extra $^1/_2$ cup of broth and cook for an additional 20 minutes. MAKES 6 SERVINGS

2 tablespoons plus 2 teaspoons
   extra-virgin olive oil
1 cup buckwheat groats, soaked,
   rinsed, and drained well
1$^1/_2$ cups water or vegetable
   broth, homemade (page 55)
   or store-bought
1 teaspoon ground cumin
$^1/_2$ teaspoon ground coriander
$^1/_2$ teaspoon sea salt
3 tablespoons freshly squeezed
   lemon juice
1 tablespoon grated lemon zest
Freshly ground black pepper
$^1/_4$ cup chopped fresh parsley
3 tablespoons finely chopped
   fresh mint

WHO KNEW? A three-year prospective study of over 220 postmenopausal women with cardiovascular disease, published in the *American Heart Journal*, showed that eating six $^1/_2$-cup servings of whole grains each week slowed both atherosclerosis, the build-up of plaque that narrows blood vessels, and stenosis, the narrowing of arterial passageways. Interestingly, intake of fiber from fruits, vegetables, and refined grains wasn't associated with slowed disease progression.

Heat the 2 teaspoons of olive oil in a small saucepan over medium heat. Add the buckwheat and cook, stirring constantly, for 1 to 2 minutes to toast the buckwheat. Add the water, cumin, coriander, and salt. Decrease the heat to low, cover, and simmer for about 10 minutes, until the buckwheat is tender and the water is absorbed.

Transfer to a bowl and stir in the lemon juice and zest, the 2 tablespoons of olive oil, and a few grinds of pepper. Let cool to room temperature. Stir in the parsley and mint. Taste; you may want to add a pinch of salt.

Variations: Substitute quinoa for the buckwheat groats, cooking 1 cup of quinoa in 1$^3/_4$ cups of water for 15 minutes, until the water is absorbed. You can also use this salad as a foundation and add more raw vegetables, such as chopped cucumbers, tomatoes, and basil, or roasted summer vegetables, such as roasted eggplant, zucchini, and red bell peppers.

PREP TIME: 10 minutes (after soaking the buckwheat)
COOK TIME: 10 minutes
STORAGE: Store in an airtight container in the refrigerator for up to 4 days.
PER SERVING: Calories: 200; Total Fat: 7 g (1 g saturated, 5 g monounsaturated); Carbohydrates: 34 g; Protein: 5 g; Fiber: 11 g; Sodium: 180 mg

Farro with Kale-Basil Pesto

In days of yore, no one was fed finer than the Roman Emperor's warriors. And what, pray tell, did the legion dine upon between conquests? The same nutritious grain featured in this recipe: farro. However, I doubt they ever quite had it served up in this manner. The magic topping here is the pesto, a vivacious blend of kale, pistachios, and basil—all ingredients with remarkable healing properties. An Italian medical journal noted that pistachios might be effective against cancer, inflammatory diseases, cardiovascular disease, and free radical damage. Regarding kale, some folks avoid it because of its natural bitterness, but here the pistachios balance out its flavor. The pesto makes a bit more than needed for the recipe, but that's a good thing. It's so delicious that you'll find many other uses for it.

Prepare ahead: Soak the farro in cool water and the juice of half a lemon for 8 hours or overnight before cooking; this will make its nutrients more available and decrease the cooking time. If you don't have time to soak the farro, add an extra $1/2$ cup of broth and cook for an additional 20 minutes. MAKES 4 SERVINGS

KALE-BASIL PESTO
4 cups stemmed and chopped
    lacinato kale
1 cup loosely packed fresh basil
    leaves
$1/2$ cup chopped fresh parsley
$1/2$ cup shelled pistachios
$1/2$ cup extra-virgin olive oil
$1/4$ cup vegetable broth, homemade
    (page 55) or store-bought,
    or water
2 teaspoons finely chopped garlic
1 tablespoon freshly squeezed
    lemon juice
1 teaspoon grated lemon zest
$1/4$ teaspoon sea salt

FARRO
3 cups water
$1/2$ teaspoon sea salt
1 cup farro, soaked, rinsed, and
    drained well
$1/4$ cup freshly grated Parmesan
    or Pecorino-Romano cheese
    (optional)
1 cup cooked white beans, drained,
    rinsed, and mixed with a spritz
    of lemon juice and a pinch of salt
    if using canned beans
$1/4$ cup diced sun-dried tomatoes
    (optional)

To make the pesto, bring a large pot of salted water to a rapid boil over high heat. Add the kale and cook for 30 seconds, until it becomes bright green. Drain and rinse under cold water to stop the cooking. Squeeze the kale to remove excess water.

Put the kale, basil, parsley, pistachios, olive oil, broth, garlic, lemon juice, lemon zest, and salt in a food processor and process until well blended. Taste; you may want to add a spritz of lemon juice and a bit more lemon zest.

To prepare the farro and assemble the dish, put the water and salt in a pot and bring to a boil over high heat. Stir in the farro. Decrease the heat to medium and cook for 20 minutes. Drain the farro and return it to the pot. Add 1 cup of the pesto, and the Parmesan cheese, beans, and sun-dried tomatoes. Do a FASS check (see page 44); you may want to add a squeeze of lemon juice. Serve hot or at room temperature.

PREP TIME: 15 minutes (after soaking the farro) COOK TIME: 20 minutes
STORAGE: Store in an airtight container in the refrigerator for up to 4 days.
PER SERVING: Calories: 260; Total Fat: 14 g (2 g saturated, 9 g monounsaturated); Carbohydrates: 28.5 g; Protein: 9 g; Fiber: 6 g; Sodium: 162 mg

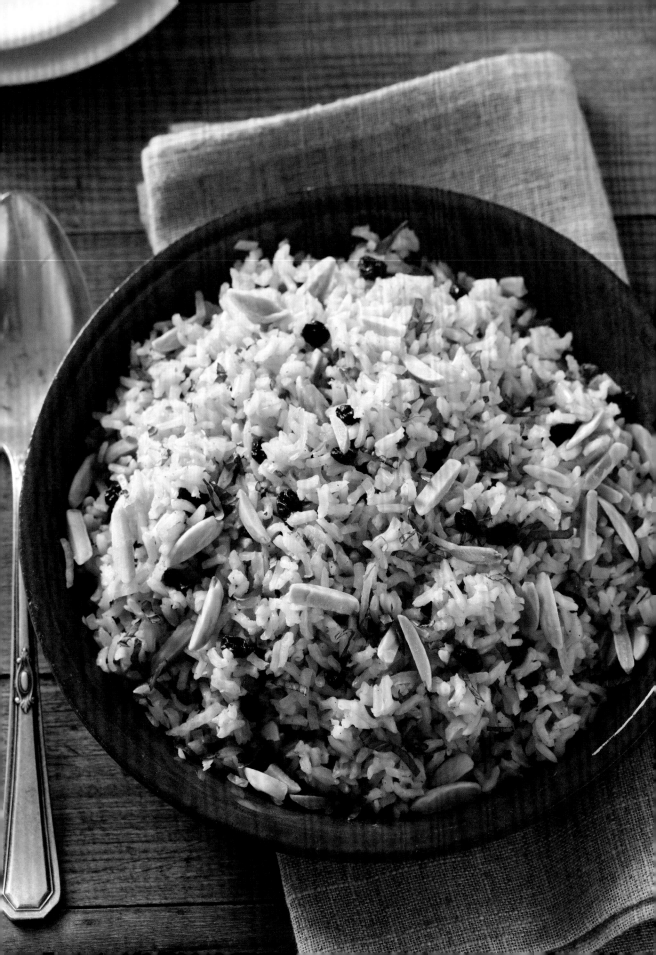

Brown Rice Pilaf with Saffron and Ginger

Healers have touted saffron's medicinal properties since the days of Hippocrates, and Cleopatra claimed that it was an aphrodisiac. Its scarcity (it takes some four thousand crocus blossoms to create an ounce of saffron) and the belief that it could be used to treat everything from wounds to the plague even caused the Austrians to go to war over the spice during the Dark Ages. This is at least one feudal folk myth that modern science has corroborated. Studies have shown that saffron has outstanding antibacterial and antiviral properties and also aids digestion. People sometimes balk at saffron's cost, but it isn't unreasonable when you consider its potency; this recipe calls for only $1/8$ teaspoon, and as you'll see, a little goes a long way. This pilaf is a delightful and gorgeous dish. The rice is sautéed before cooking to avoid that sticky, gummy consistency, and ginger, parsley, and lemon zest add zing.

Prepare ahead: Soak the rice in cool water and the juice of half a lemon for 8 hours or overnight before cooking; this will make its nutrients more available and decrease the cooking time. If you don't have time to soak the rice, add an extra $1/4$ cup of broth and cook for an additional 15 minutes. MAKES 6 SERVINGS

1 teaspoon warm water
$1/8$ teaspoon saffron
1 tablespoon extra-virgin olive oil
1 tablespoon diced shallot
1 cup brown basmati rice, soaked, rinsed, and drained well
$13/4$ cups water or vegetable broth, homemade (page 55) or store-bought
$1/2$ teaspoon sea salt
1 (1-inch) piece unpeeled fresh ginger
1 tablespoon freshly squeezed lemon juice
1 teaspoon lemon zest
1 tablespoon finely chopped fresh parsley

Combine the warm water and saffron in a small bowl. Heat the olive oil in a saucepan over medium heat. Add the shallot and sauté until translucent, about 3 minutes. Add the rice and saffron and cook, stirring constantly, until the rice is evenly coated with the oil. Stir in the water, salt, and ginger. Increase the heat, cover, and bring to a boil. Decrease the heat to low and simmer for 20 to 25 minutes, until the water is absorbed. Check after 20 minutes; if there are steam holes on the top, it's ready. Remove ginger. Add the lemon juice, lemon zest, and parsley and fluff with a fork to combine.

Variations: Substitute quinoa for the rice (no need to soak it first). For a dolled-up version of this dish, add $1/4$ teaspoon of ground cumin, $1/4$ teaspoon of ground coriander, and $1/8$ teaspoon of ground cardamom when you add the saffron. Add 2 tablespoons of currants or raisins when you add the lemon juice, and substitute mint for the parsley. Serve topped with 3 tablespoons of toasted slivered almonds.

PREP TIME: 5 minutes (after soaking the rice) COOK TIME: 30 minutes
STORAGE: Store in an airtight container in the refrigerator for up to 2 days.
PER SERVING: Calories: 135; Total Fat: 3.5 g (0.5 g saturated, 2 g mono-unsaturated); Carbohydrates: 25 g; Protein: 3 g; Fiber: 2 g; Sodium: 184 mg

Triple-Mushroom Brown Rice Risotto

Some dishes seem downright intimidating, yet it's usually all in the name. You know the ones I'm talking about: flambé, bouillabaisse, osso buco . . . If it weren't for those tongue twists, recipes for these dishes might seem much more welcoming and accessible. Take risotto. It's actually the Italian word for something very basic: rice. Of course the Italians, known for raising even the most mundane of dishes to high art, have outdone themselves with risotto. As with all art forms, creating outstanding risotto takes some patience and practice, but it's worth the effort; when made well, risotto is a delight to all the senses. I learned to make it in Italy with traditional Arborio rice, but I wanted to find a healthier whole grain rice that would yield that incomparable creamy, not mushy texture. As it turns out, basic short-grain brown rice is spot-on for the job. In this risotto, the shiitake mushrooms are rich in vitamins B_2, B_5, and B_6 and many other nutrients and help boost the immune system.

Prepare ahead: Soak the rice in cold water and the juice of half a lemon for 8 hours or overnight before cooking; this will make its nutrients more available and decrease the cooking time. If you don't have time to soak the rice, add an extra $1/4$ cup of broth and cook for an additional 15 minutes. MAKES 4 SERVINGS

---

1 cup short-grain brown rice, soaked, rinsed, and drained well

8 cups organic vegetable or chicken broth, homemade (page 55 or 56) or store-bought

Sea salt

4 tablespoons extra-virgin olive oil

4 cups mixed mushrooms, such as chanterelle, morel, shiitake, and cremini, stemmed and sliced $1/4$ inch thick

$1/4$ teaspoon freshly ground black pepper

1 cup diced yellow onion

$1/2$ cup diced shallots

2 teaspoons minced garlic

$1/2$ cup white wine

$1/2$ cup freshly grated organic Parmesan cheese

$1/4$ cup chopped fresh parsley

1 tablespoon chopped fresh thyme

Put the rice, 2 cups of the broth, and a pinch of salt in a medium saucepan and bring to a boil over high heat. Decrease the heat to low, cover, and cook for 20 minutes. Remove from the heat, leaving the pan covered. The rice won't be completely cooked, and some water will remain in the pan.

Meanwhile, heat 2 tablespoons of the olive oil in a large skillet over medium-high heat. Add the mushrooms, pepper, and a generous pinch of salt and cook without stirring until the mushrooms begin to brown on the bottom, about 2 minutes. Stir, then sauté until well browned, about 5 minutes. Transfer to a bowl.

Heat the remaining 2 tablespoons of olive oil in the same skillet over medium heat. Add the onion, shallots, and a generous pinch of salt and sauté until the onions and shallot begin to turn golden, about 4 minutes. Add the garlic and sauté for 1 minute.

Heat the remaining broth in a saucepan over high heat just until bubbling. Decrease the heat to low to maintain a simmer.

COOK'S NOTE: The technique used for cooking the mushrooms is the key to success in this recipe. Mushrooms are usually added to the risotto at the end without being cooked first, which leaves them with a springy texture and bland flavor. It's best to sauté them on their own for a few minutes, then remove them from the pan and add the other ingredients to be sautéed, in this case onions and shallots, over the fond (that's the delicious bits of mushroom and oil still in the pan). The mushrooms are then added after the risotto is cooked; because they've already been sautéed, their texture remains perfect.

LIVE LONG AND PROSPER: Garlic has been endorsed by some pretty heavy hitters. Hippocrates, Mohammed, Pliny the Elder—all have said the medical equivalent of "Got a problem? Get garlic!" Science seems to back the idea that garlic has wide-ranging healing powers. Studies have shown that garlic is helpful for fighting (take a deep breath) inflammation, bacteria, viruses, colorectal and kidney cancer, iron deficiency, clogged arteries, high triglycerides, free radical damage, and the list goes on. Suffice to say, whether you need protection from toxins or just the vampires, garlic is the way to go.

With a slotted spoon, transfer the rice to the skillet. Reserve the cooking water. Add $1/2$ teaspoon of salt and cook, stirring constantly, for about 1 minute to toast the rice. Add wine and cook, stirring constantly, until it is almost completely absorbed. Measure the remaining rice cooking water and add more of the broth to bring the volume up to 1 cup. Cook, stirring constantly, until the liquid is almost completely absorbed.

Add the simmering broth a ladleful at a time and cook, stirring frequently, until the liquid is completely absorbed after each addition. When the rice is tender but still firm, after about 18 minutes of cooking altogether, add a final $1/4$ cup of broth and turn off the heat. Stir in the mushrooms, Parmesan cheese, parsley, and thyme and stir until well combined. Serve immediately. Risotto waits for no one!

Variations: To add a little green to your life, stir in 2 cups of coarsely chopped Swiss chard or spinach just after you add the last $1/4$ cup of broth to the risotto. Another option is to serve the risotto topped with Mediterranean Greens (page 98).

PREP TIME: 20 minutes COOK TIME: 30 minutes
STORAGE: Store in an airtight container in the refrigerator for up to 5 days.
PER SERVING: Calories: 320; Total Fat: 12.5 g (2.5 g saturated, 8 g monounsaturated); Carbohydrates: 43 g; Protein: 8 g; Fiber: 5 g; Sodium: 333 mg

Hot-and-Sour Sesame Soba Noodles

When I lived in New York City, there were so many Chinese restaurants that I sometimes imagined there was a huge underground kitchen attached to Grand Central Station. During that time, I fell in love with hot-and-sour sesame noodles. It was my first food affair in the city, and as these things are wont to do, it eventually cooled off. But here lately I've found myself missing that first love. Unfortunately, now I can't eat gluten. The answer? Gluten-free 100 percent buckwheat Japanese soba noodles. In this recipe, I've drizzled them with Sesame Miso Dressing and a touch of hot pepper oil, and then accented the dish with cilantro and mint. Miso is a major player in providing zinc to greatly boost immune health, and may also provide some benefit against breast cancer. **MAKES 4 SERVINGS**

¹/₂ cup Sesame Miso Dressing (page 187)

1¹/₄ teaspoons of hot pepper sesame oil

1 teaspoon Grade B maple syrup

1 teaspoon freshly squeezed lime juice

8 ounces 100 percent buckwheat soba noodles

1 cup peeled, seeded, and finely diced cucumber

¹/₄ cup peeled and finely diced carrot

¹/₄ cup finely diced red bell pepper

1 scallion, white and green parts, thinly sliced diagonally

2 tablespoons coarsely chopped fresh cilantro

2 tablespoons coarsely chopped fresh mint

1 tablespoon black or white sesame seeds, toasted (see note, page 83)

COOK'S NOTE: Most packages of buckwheat soba call for 8 minutes of cooking, but if you do that, you'll end with gummy, mushy noodles. Start testing after 4 minutes and have a colander ready to drain them a minute later, when the noodles are just tender.

Put the dressing, 1 teaspoon of the hot pepper sesame oil, and the maple syrup and lime juice in a small bowl and stir to combine.

Bring a large pot of water to a boil over high heat. Add the noodles and decrease the heat to medium. Cook, stirring gently on occasion, until just tender, about 5 minutes. Drain and rinse well under cold water to remove the starch. Immediately transfer to a large bowl, drizzle with the remaining ¹/₄ teaspoon of hot pepper sesame oil, and toss gently to coat. Add the cucumber, carrot, bell pepper, scallion, cilantro, and mint and toss gently to combine. Drizzle with the dressing mixture and toss gently until evenly coated. Sprinkle with the sesame seeds before serving.

Variations: For a complete meal, add shredded organic chicken, cubed tofu, or peeled and deveined shrimp. If you want to bump up the heat, add another teaspoon of hot pepper sesame oil. You can use udon noodles or brown rice pasta in place of the soba. To take the flavor over the top, try topping these noodles with a bit of Indonesian Drizzle (page 183).

PREP TIME: 15 minutes **COOK TIME:** 5 minutes
STORAGE: If you're not going to serve all of this salad at one time, dress only the amount of vegetables and noodles you'll be serving. You can store the leftover noodles and vegetables in an airtight container in the refrigerator for up to 2 days, and the dressing mixture in a separate airtight container in the refrigerator for up to 5 days.
PER SERVING: Calories: 310; Total Fat: 6 g (0.5 g saturated, 1 g monounsaturated); Carbohydrates: 56 g; Protein: 10 g; Fiber: 6 g; Sodium: 535 mg

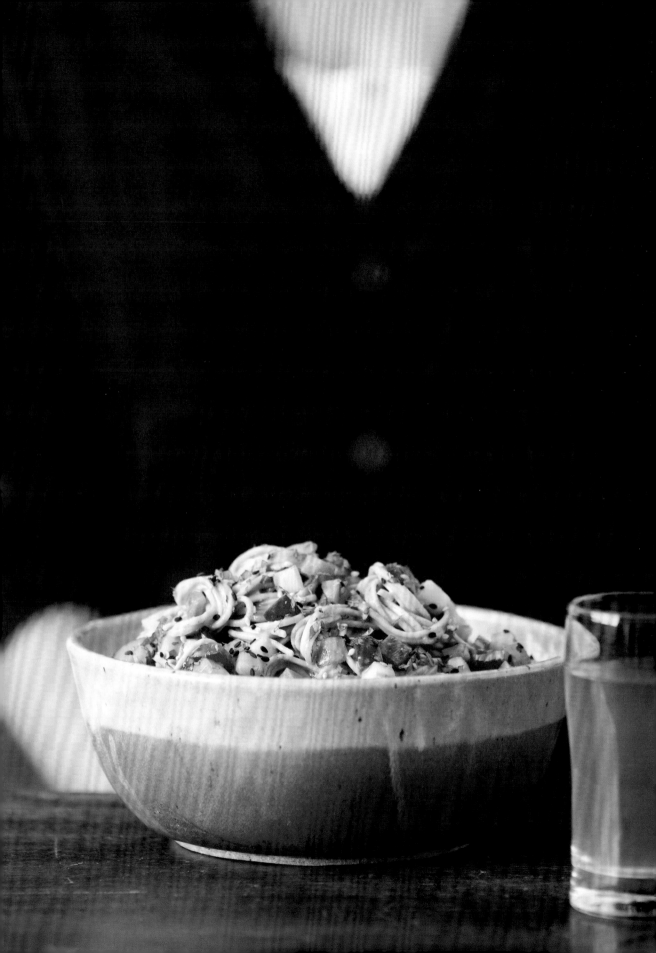

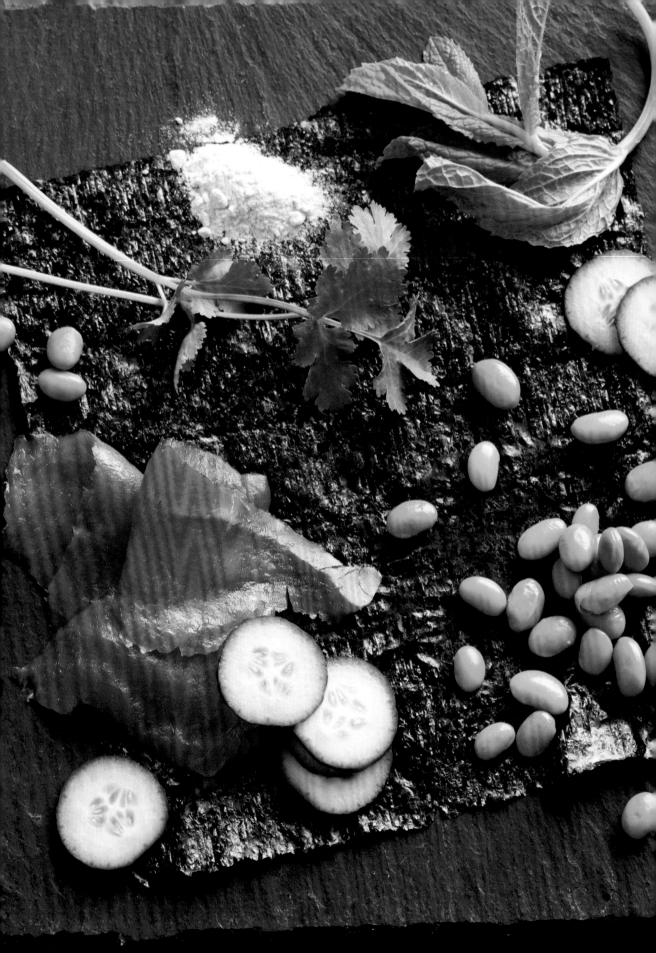

CHAPTER 7

Protein-Building Foods

When it comes to proteins, quantity, variety, and quality really matter. Let's take them in order. A little protein goes a long way, notably with animal proteins.

There's a myth that in populations noted for longevity people tend to avoid animal proteins. That isn't entirely true. However, they do generally eat far smaller portions of animal protein than the typical American belly bomb. Since meat, fowl, and fish have typically been more expensive in many of these longevity hotspots, their cuisines evolved in a very balanced manner, without single foods dominating the plate, and with proteins coming from many plant-based sources, including beans and whole grains. That's a very smart way to eat if you want to live to see your grandchildren get married, and that's why the recipes in this chapter capitalize on a wide variety of protein sources. Our bodies need that kind of variety if they are to function efficiently.

Our DNA is, in a sense, its own cook. It needs about twenty ingredients—amino acids—to whip up the proteins that create and maintain muscle, and nine of those are essential amino acids, meaning the body can't manufacture them; it can only get them from food sources. Not every protein source has all nine essential amino acids. Animal sources—fish, eggs, chicken, lamb, and beef—are usually complete proteins, meaning they contain all nine essential amino acids. Plant-based foods seldom do, with a few notable exceptions, such as quinoa and soy. The fact that individual plant-based foods lack complete protein has perpetuated another myth: that vegans (vegetarians who avoid all animal products, including dairy and eggs) don't get enough protein in their diet or must carefully combine foods to obtain complete protein. If you're living on white pasta and carrot sticks, that might be true. But if you eat a wide range of plant-based foods over the course of a day, each with its own amino acid profile, the body knows how to put those ingredients on the shelf and maintain a supply of all nine essential amino acids so that protein building can proceed uninterrupted. For example, from the body's viewpoint eating the Black Bean Skillet Cakes, with their essential amino providers of black beans and whole grains (in this case brown basmati rice), is just as fulfilling to the body's protein needs as eating beef—or better. There's cholesterol and little fiber in animal proteins, so you vitally need the abundant fiber in veggies to transport excess cholesterol out of the system.

Regardless of where you get your protein, I'd be severely delinquent in my duties if I didn't urge you, plead with you, nay, *beg* you to buy organic eggs, poultry, and meat—from pasture-raised animals whenever possible. The long list of reasons includes better treatment of the animals and more environmentally sound practices. But since the focus of this book is longevity, I'll focus on the health benefits. There's simply no comparison between the protein and overall nutritional profile of grass-fed and commercially raised animals—and between wild seafood and that produced by aquaculture. Organic beef is by definition free of antibiotics and hormones, and if it's from grass-fed animals, it's up to two-thirds leaner, so it contains far less harmful saturated fats. And what fat it does have is loaded with twice the amount of heart-healthy, cancer-fighting omega-3 fatty acids as conventional beef. Grass-fed beef also has four times more vitamin E and higher levels of thiamin, beta-carotene, calcium, and potassium. Regarding eggs, those from hens raised in pastures have less saturated fat and cholesterol, twice the omega-3s, and *seven* times the amount of beta-carotene as eggs from conventionally raised chickens. Wild salmon is similar; its ratio of omega-3 to omega-6 fatty acids is far better than that of farm-raised salmon. It's best to buy fish the day you plan to prepare it. However, life doesn't always work that way. If you must store fish longer, put it in a resealable plastic bag in the coldest part of the refrigerator, which is usually the back of the bottom shelf. It should keep for 2 days.

Not surprisingly, all organically raised foods have one other thing in common: their flavor is, in a word, *awesome*. And isn't that the best motivator for eating well? A lifetime of taste-bud titillation . . . that works for me.

Layered Frittata with Leeks, Swiss Chard, and Tomatoes

Frittatas, or baked omelets, are a delicious staple of Italian cuisine. Unfortunately, many people avoid them because they believe eggs raise cholesterol. That just ain't so. A huge study of 100,000 people proved that to be a myth, and the American Heart Association now says that eggs can be part of a healthful diet, as long as other sources of dietary cholesterol aren't excessive. Aside from being an excellent source of protein, eggs also support brain health. In this delicious frittata, the eggs frame a whirlwind of flavorful ingredients with all the colors of the Italian flag: Swiss chard, cherry tomatoes, and Parmesan cheese. MAKES 6 SERVINGS

6 organic eggs, beaten
2 tablespoons organic plain Greek yogurt
2 teaspoons chopped fresh thyme
1/4 teaspoon freshly ground black pepper
1/8 teaspoon freshly grated nutmeg
Sea salt
2 tablespoons extra-virgin olive oil
2 cups thinly sliced leeks, white and green parts
4 cups stemmed and chopped Swiss chard, in bite-size pieces (see note, page 97)
1 cup cherry tomatoes, halved
3 tablespoons almond flour, home-made (page 226) or store-bought
2 tablespoons freshly grated organic Parmesan cheese

Position one oven rack about 6 inches below the broiler and another rack in the center of the oven. Preheat the oven to 375°F.

Put the eggs, yogurt, thyme, pepper, nutmeg, and 1/2 teaspoon of salt in a bowl and whisk until the eggs are frothy and only very small lumps of yogurt remain.

Heat the olive oil in an ovenproof skillet over medium heat. Add the leeks and a pinch of salt and sauté until just golden, about 6 minutes. Put the Swiss chard on top of the leeks and sprinkle a pinch of salt over the chard. Cover and let the chard steam just until it begins to wilt, about 2 minutes. Arrange the tomatoes on top of the chard.

Pour the egg mixture over the tomatoes and make sure it seeps through the greens; you may need to gently shift the greens a bit to help with this. Sprinkle the Parmesan cheese and almond flour over the top.

Bake on the center rack of the oven for 10 to 15 minutes, until the eggs are set. Turn the oven to broil and move the skillet to the top rack. Broil for 1 minute, until the cheese and almond flours are golden brown. Serve hot or at room temperature.

Variations: Make this frittata dairy-free by substituting 2 tablespoons of water for the yogurt and omitting the cheese. Feel free to substitute spinach or kale for the chard.

PREP TIME: 10 minutes COOK TIME: 25 minutes
STORAGE: Store in an airtight container in the refrigerator for up to 3 days.
PER SERVING: Calories: 170; Total Fat: 12.5 g (3 g saturated, 5 g mono-unsaturated); Carbohydrates: 8 g; Protein: 10 g; Fiber: 2 g; Sodium: 238 mg

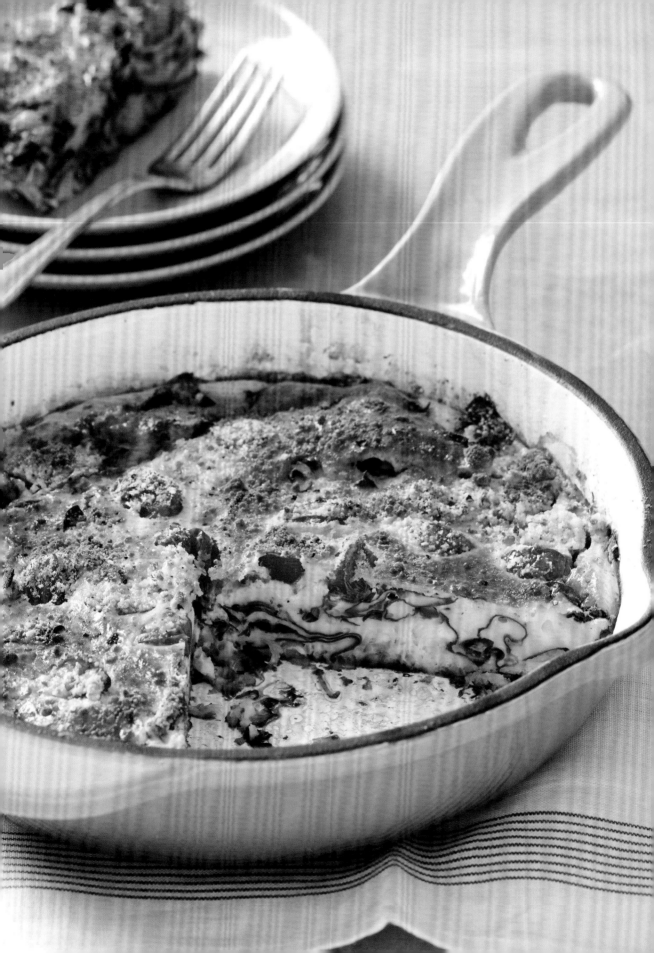

Black Bean Skillet Cakes with Poached Eggs

Some folks love poached eggs. Mat's mom loved poached eggs. Mat's dog loved poached eggs. But that's because Mat's mom gave Honey whatever she was having for breakfast, including coffee with cream. (Talk about treating the dog like family! Then again, Honey lived to 16; maybe it was the eggs.) I'm thinking my dog, Bella, would have to learn to bring in the mail (and maybe do the laundry) before she'd get anywhere near this recipe, 'cause it's just that good. The poached egg tops a super skillet cake that has a Costa Rican feel. That's the black beans at play, bringing a load of antioxidants and blood sugar regulators to the party. Instead of using wheat as a binder, we've chosen basmati rice. Add in diced onions, red bell peppers, and some lime zest and these skillet cakes really rock. The egg and the ancho-chili relish provide extra layers of lusciousness. No toast necessary; everything that doesn't make it to your mouth on the first shot gets sopped up by the skillet cake. If I could send this one back in time, Mat's mom would be first on my list. **MAKES 16 SKILLET CAKES, SERVES 8**

SKILLET CAKES

2 cups cooked black beans (see page 68), or 1 (15-ounce) can black beans, drained, rinsed, and mixed with a spritz of fresh lemon juice and a pinch of sea salt

1 1/2 teaspoons oregano

1 teaspoon ground cumin

1/2 teaspoon sea salt

1/4 teaspoon ground cinnamon

1/8 teaspoon cayenne

2 teaspoons minced garlic

3 tablespoons extra-virgin olive oil

2 tablespoons plus 1 teaspoon freshly squeezed lime juice

2 1/2 cups cooked brown basmati rice

1 beaten organic egg

1/4 cup diced red onion

1/4 tablespoons finely diced red bell pepper

1 teaspoon lime zest

1/4 cup loosely packed minced fresh cilantro

POACHED EGGS

1 tablespoon vinegar

8 organic eggs

Ancho Chili Relish (page 180), for garnish

Combine 1 cup of the black beans and the oregano, cumin, salt, cinnamon, cayenne, garlic, 1 tablespoon of the olive oil, and the lime juice in a food processor and pulse until just combined, scraping down the sides as needed. Transfer the mixture to a bowl and fold in the rice, egg, onion, bell pepper, lime zest, cilantro, and the remaining 1 cup of beans.

Moisten your hands to keep the mixture from sticking, then shape the mixture into 1/4-inch-thick patties about 2 1/2 inches in diameter. Place the prepared patties on a sheet pan lined with parchment.

Heat the remaining 2 tablespoons of the olive oil in a skillet over medium heat and cook the patties for about 3 minutes on each side, until golden brown.

To poach the eggs, pour 6 inches of water into a large saucepan and place over medium-high heat. When the water is almost boiling, add the vinegar. One by one, crack each egg into a small dish, then gently slide the egg in the water. Maintain the water temperature just below a simmer, turning the heat down to low, if necessary. Cook until the egg whites are set and the centers are still soft, about 3 minutes. Remove with a slotted spoon and place on a paper towel to drain off excess water.

Place an egg on top of a skillet cake, then top with a tablespoon of the Ancho-Chili Relish or a drizzle of your favorite hot sauce.

COOK'S NOTE: If you want to cook just a few patties, pop them in your toaster oven. To freeze these skillet cakes cooked or uncooked, stack them with parchment paper between the patties. Wrap the entire stack first in plastic wrap, then in foil. The parchment paper makes it easy to remove the desired number of skillet cakes from the bundle. Once thawed, they can be reheated at 350°F for 15 minutes, and uncooked cakes can be baked as above, at 375°F for 22 to 25 minutes. They don't need to be turned.

Variation: To stuff roasted bell peppers, cut 4 red bell peppers in half, then remove the seeds and the core. Rub 1 teaspoon of olive oil on each half and sprinkle with sea salt. Stuff each half with 1 cup of the rice and bean mixture and place in a glass or ceramic baking dish. Place the peppers in a 425°F oven and bake 15 to 20 minutes or until tender.

PREP TIME: 15 minutes COOK TIME: 25 minutes
STORAGE: Store in a covered container in the refrigerator for 3 to 5 days. The patties can also be frozen (in cooked or uncooked form) for 2 months. However, the poached eggs should be made fresh.
PER SERVING: (2 skillet cakes) Calories: 100; Total Fat: 3.5 g (0.5 g saturated, 2 g monounsaturated); Carbohydrates: 15 g; Protein: 3 g; Fiber: 3 g; Sodium: 223

Good Mood Sardines

At heart, many cooks secretly fancy themselves to be magicians. Maybe it's because people so often ask, "How *did* you do that?" But unlike, say Houdini, I always tell the tale behind the magic. Take sardines. I love them because they're extremely high in omega-3s and vitamin D, both of which tend to be in short supply in people's diets. Thanks to those mood-boosting nutrients, sardines are like little antidepressants in a can. That said, some culinary wizardry will be required to turn sardine skeptics into wild-eyed fans. Take my kitchen assistants, Jen and Katie. They swore they couldn't stand sardines. I simply said, "You haven't had them the way *I* make them" and sent them out of the kitchen so I could perform my feat of prestidigitation. (No rabbit and top hat; just red onion, basil, parsley, mint, olive oil, and lemon juice). *Voilà!* They eagerly devoured the sardines and asked for more. Now *that's* the kind of magic I like to practice. MAKES 2 SERVINGS

4 teaspoons freshly squeezed lemon juice
2 teaspoons grated lemon zest
1 tablespoon finely diced red onion
2 teaspoons finely chopped fresh parsley
2 teaspoons finely chopped fresh basil
2 teaspoons finely chopped fresh mint
1 teaspoon extra-virgin olive oil
1 teaspoon Dijon mustard
1/8 teaspoon sea salt
1 (4.35-ounce) can sardines, packed in water or olive oil

Put the lemon juice, lemon zest, red onion, parsley, basil, mint, thyme, olive oil, mustard, and salt in a bowl and stir to combine. Add the sardines and flake them into chunky pieces with a fork. Stir gently to combine. Taste; you may want to add a pinch of salt or a generous squeeze of lemon juice.

PREP TIME: 5 minutes
STORAGE: Store in an airtight container in the refrigerator for up to 3 days.
PER SERVING: Calories: 135; Total Fat: 9 g (2 g saturated, 4.5 g monounsaturated); Carbohydrates: 2 g; Protein: 12.5 g; Fiber: 0.5 g; Sodium: 593 mg

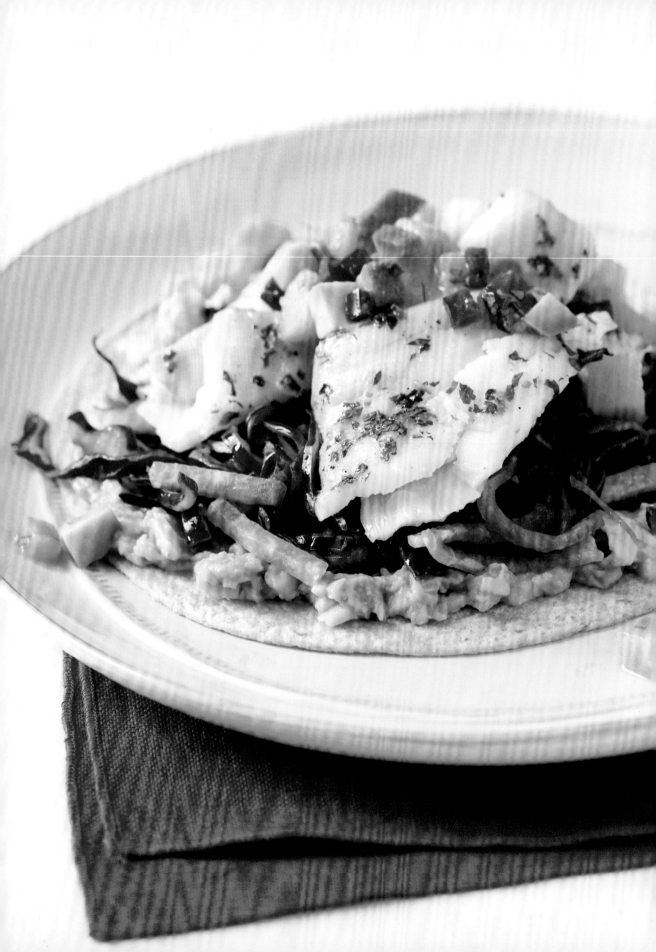

Roasted Halibut with Lime and Papaya and Avocado Salsa

This recipe is bold and pretty enough that it could be served in a Mexican restaurant, especially when made into tacos or tostadas, as in the variation. Halibut is rich in beneficial omega-3s; plus, it has a meaty texture and mild flavor, which makes it great for kids or anyone who's a little leery of fish. The marinade contains lime zest, cumin, cilantro, and cayenne, bathing the halibut in a sea of yum, and the Papaya and Avocado Salsa provides a tasty crescendo. **MAKES 4 SERVINGS**

3½ tablespoons freshly squeezed lime juice
1 teaspoon grated lime zest
¼ teaspoon sea salt
¼ teaspoon ground cumin
Pinch of cayenne
1 tablespoon extra-virgin olive oil
2 teaspoons finely chopped fresh cilantro
4 (6-ounce) halibut fillets
Papaya and Avocado Salsa (page 191)

COOK'S NOTE: Instead of baking, you can grill the halibut. Marinate as directed, then wipe off the marinade. Rub ¼ teaspoon of light sesame oil over each fillet, then grill over low, even heat for about 4 minutes per side, until the flesh is opaque and flakes easily and the center of each fillet registers 135°F. This marinade is also great with other fish, such as sea bass, black cod, and wild salmon.

WHO KNEW? Bigger isn't always better. Randy Hartnell, a veteran Alaskan fisherman and owner of Vital Choice, a purveyor of wild seafood, says that it's best to buy fillets of wild tuna and halibut cut from smaller fish (twenty pounds and under). These fish are younger and, according to Hartnell, "have the highest levels of omega-3s and the lowest levels of contaminant levels."

Combine the lime juice, lime zest, salt, cumin, cayenne, olive oil, and cilantro in a small bowl and whisk until thoroughly blended. Spread 3 tablespoons of the marinade evenly over both sides of the fillets. Reserve the remaining marinade. Cover and refrigerate for 30 minutes.

Preheat the oven to 400°F. Lightly oil an ovenproof pan large enough to accommodate all of the fillets in a single layer.

Pat the fillets dry with paper towels and put them in the prepared pan. Bake for 10 to 12 minutes, until the flesh is opaque and flakes easily. To be certain the fish is cooked through, push a two-pronged kitchen fork straight down into the flesh; the fish is done when it is no longer translucent.

Drizzle the reserved marinade over the fillets and top each with a generous dollop of the salsa. Serve immediately.

Variations: I love transforming this recipe into soft tacos or tostadas. For each soft taco, put a corn tortilla in a warm skillet and heat it through, then spread 1 tablespoon of Avocado Cream with Basil (page 58) on one side of the tortilla. Top with 2 to 4 ounces of flaked halibut, ¼ cup of Mexican Cabbage Crunch (page 86), and 1 tablespoon of Papaya and Avocado Salsa, then fold the tortilla over the fillings and enjoy. To make crisp tortillas for tostadas, bake corn tortillas in a 350°F oven for 15 minutes. Layer all of the toppings evenly over the tortillas.

PREP TIME: 5 minutes COOK TIME: 12 minutes
STORAGE: Store in an airtight container in the refrigerator for up to 5 days.
PER SERVING: Calories: 230; Total Fat: 8.5 g (2 g saturated, 5 g monounsaturated); Carbohydrates: 4 g; Protein: 35 g; Fiber: 0 g; Sodium: 240 mg

Black Cod with Miso-Ginger Glaze

Here's what happens when the Far East meets the Not-So-Far East. My Russian great-grandmother Rebecca adored sablefish, aka black cod, a key ingredient in her "white meal": sablefish (which has alabaster flesh), sour cream, and steamed red potatoes. My fond memories of her sablefish cravings inspired this recipe, and then I took a left turn courtesy of Okinawa-born Yoshi Tome, owner of Sausalito's Sushi Ran restaurant, who has an outrageously tasty and healthy black cod dish. I opted to re-create some of the flavors from his dish, using miso, mirin, ginger, and toasted sesame oil. MAKES 4 SERVINGS

¼ cup mirin

3 tablespoons light miso

3 tablespoons freshly squeezed lime juice

1½ teaspoons grated fresh ginger

1 teaspoon toasted sesame oil

4 (4-ounce) black cod fillets, bones removed

2 tablespoons chopped fresh cilantro, for garnish

1 tablespoon slivered scallion, white and green parts, for garnish

COOK'S NOTE: The Asian-style marinade in this dish is great with other fish too, including sea bass, wild salmon, and halibut. Whatever type of fish you use, Asian Cabbage Crunch (page 87) or Sweet-and-Sour Asian Cabbage and Kale (page 96) would be a nice accompaniment.

WHO KNEW? Talk about longevity! The oldest sablefish on record lived to be ninety-four years old. It's common for sablefish to reach their nineties.

Lightly oil an ovenproof pan large enough to accommodate all of the fillets in a single layer. Put the mirin, miso, lime juice, ginger, and sesame oil in a small bowl and whisk until well combined. Rinse the fillet and pat them dry. Put them in the prepared pan and brush 1 tablespoon of the miso mixture on each fillets, spreading it evenly on both sides. Reserve the remaining mixture. Cover and refrigerate for 30 minutes.

Position one oven rack about 4 inches below the broiler and another rack in the center of the oven. Preheat the oven to 375°F.

Bake the fillets on the center rack of the oven for 5 to 6 minutes or, if they are thick, until the flesh looks opaque and is beginning to flake. Turn the oven to broil, move the fillets to the top rack of the oven, and broil for 3 to 4 minutes, until brown and caramelized on top.

Meanwhile, heat the reserved miso mixture in a small saucepan over medium heat just until it starts bubbling. Drizzle over the fillets, sprinkle with the cilantro and scallion, and serve immediately.

Variation: If you want some extra gingery heat, add another teaspoon of freshly grated ginger to the reserved miso mixture when you heat it in the saucepan. Don't add it before marinating the fish, because ginger has strong enzymatic activity and will break down the fish, giving it a mealy texture—not good.

PREP TIME: 5 minutes, plus 30 minutes for marinating
COOK TIME: 7 minutes
STORAGE: Store in an airtight container in the refrigerator for up to 1 day.
PER SERVING: Calories: 195; Total Fat: 15.5 g (2 g saturated, 8.5 g monounsaturated); Carbohydrates: 14 g; Protein: 4 g; Fiber: 2.5 g; Sodium: 287 mg

Roasted Wild Salmon with Olive and Mint Vinaigrette

The source of certain foods can make a huge difference in how healthful they are. Salmon is my favorite example of this. It has an absolutely incredible nutritional profile, but only if you get wild salmon, not the farm-raised variety. My friend Randy Hartnell, owner of Vital Choice, a company that sells wild seafood, explained why. (Randy has been fishing for wild salmon in the Pacific Northwest for thirty years, and he's an expert on this.) Wild salmon eventually return from the ocean to the river they were born in to spawn. You probably know that. But what you may not know is that these salmon don't eat anything while they're in the river, and they don't spawn until they've the reached river's headwaters. In some cases that can be as long as a two-week journey against the current, so they have to store up a ton of energy garnered from the ocean for the trip. That energy is in the form of extra fat—fat that yields both fantastic taste and quantities of heart-healthy omega-3s that you simply won't find in farmed-raised salmon. This wild salmon recipe is simple, light, and tasty, with the fat from the fish blending perfectly with the mint and olive vinaigrette. I like to serve this dish with Roasted Asparagus Salad with Arugula and Hazelnuts (page 88).

MAKES 4 SERVINGS

2 teaspoons extra-virgin olive oil
2 teaspoons grated lemon zest
2 teaspoons Dijon mustard
4 (4-ounce) wild salmon fillets, pinbones removed
2 tablespoons water
1/4 teaspoon sea salt
Freshly ground black pepper
1/4 cup Olive and Mint Vinaigrette (page 181)

Put the olive oil, lemon zest, and mustard in a small bowl and stir to combine. Put the salmon in an ovenproof baking pan in which it fits in a single layer without overlapping. Spread the olive oil mixture evenly over both sides of the fillets. Cover and refrigerate for 20 minutes.

Preheat the oven to 400°F.

Remove the salmon from the refrigerator and add the water. Sprinkle the salt over the fillets and season with pepper. Bake just until an instant-read thermometer registers 127°F, 7 to 9 minutes depending on the thickness of the fillets; the salmon should be opaque and beginning to flake.

Whisk the vinaigrette to ensure that it's evenly blended, then drizzle over the fillets and serve immediately.

Variation: You can also top the fish with Indonesian Drizzle (page 183) or Yogurt Sauce with Citrus and Mint (page 195) rather than the Olive and Mint Vinaigrette.

PREP TIME: 5 minutes, plus 20 minutes for marinating
COOK TIME: 10 minutes
STORAGE: Store in an airtight container in the refrigerator for up to 1 day.
PER SERVING: Calories: 215; Total Fat: 13.5 g (2g saturated, 9 g monounsaturated); Carbohydrates: 1 g; Protein: 23 g; Fiber: 0 g; Sodium: 255 mg

Smoked Salmon Nori Rolls

Leave it to the Japanese to help me come up with a healthy version of my favorite bagel topping, lox with a *schmeer* (that's Yiddish for a slathering of cream cheese). Instead of a bread bomb, I start with a wrap made of nori, the dried seaweed sheets often used to wrap sushi rolls. Nori contains nutrients that support thyroid function and provide many other health benefits. The lox—smoked wild salmon—stays the same (thank heavens!), and the *schmeer* is something I'm quite proud of: a creamy spread made with edamame and wasabi. It's a lot more healthful than a chunk of cream cheese, and it tastes a lot better too. Thin slices of avocado, red bell pepper, and cucumber up the vegetable factor. Roll it up, slice it up, and eat it up and you won't need to nap fifteen minutes later, which is what usually happened to me in my bagel-eating days. MAKES 4 SERVINGS

8 sheets of nori

1 cup Edamame Wasabi Spread (page 172)

8 pieces (4 ounces) of smoked wild salmon, spritzed with lime juice

1 English cucumber, thinly sliced lengthwise into 16 pieces

1 large red bell pepper, thinly sliced lengthwise into 16 pieces

2 avocados, thinly sliced lengthwise into 16 pieces

24 fresh mint leaves

24 fresh cilantro leaves

WHO KNEW? The avocado is a fruit—and not just any old fruit. *Guinness World Records 2008* ranks avocados as the world's most nutritious fruit.

Place a sheet of nori on a work surface with the rough side facing up. Carefully spread 2 tablespoons of the edamame wasabi mixture over the nori, leaving $1^1/2$ inches bare along the bottom edge of the nori (the edge facing you) and $1/2$ inch bare along the top edge. Place 1 piece of the salmon, 2 slices of cucumber, 2 slices of bell pepper, and 2 slices of avocado about $1^1/2$ inches from the bottom edge. Top with 3 mint leaves and 3 cilantro leaves. Starting with the bare edge, roll the nori around the fillings, pressing gently to make a compact roll. Moisten a finger with warm water and run it along the inside edge of the flap that remains at the top of the roll, then press the moistened edge against the roll to seal. Repeat with the remaining ingredients. Cut each roll into eight pieces using a sharp serrated knife.

Variations: For a vegetarian nori roll, substitute thinly sliced tofu for the salmon (use baked tofu for better flavor and texture). For a more exotic flavor blast, substitute Indonesian Pesto (see variation, page 183) for the Edamame Wasabi Spread.

PREP TIME: 20 minutes
STORAGE: Store in an airtight container in the refrigerator for up to 1 day.
PER SERVING: Calories: 305; Total Fat: 17.5 g (3 g saturated, 10.5 g monounsaturated); Carbohydrates: 9 g; Protein: 30 g; Fiber: 5 g; Sodium: 180 mg

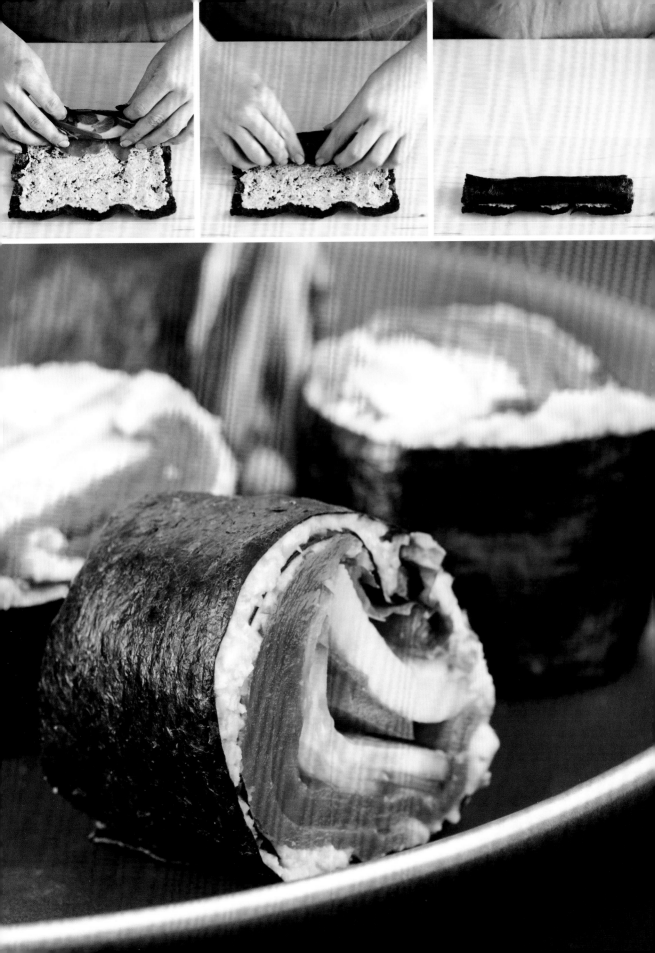

Wild, Wild Salmon Burgers

If you want to put a frown on a native Marylander's face (that would be me), make a fish cake crammed with filler. Maybe it comes from growing up near the Chesapeake Bay, but everyone in Baltimore knew which restaurants actually delivered on the promise to make crab cakes with 90 percent crab and who took the cheap way out with a fifty-fifty mix of crab and breadcrumbs. That's a no-fly zone in my book, no matter what sea dweller you're serving up. In this case, it's omega-3 powerhouse wild salmon. That's the first wild. The second wild is for wild rice, used here to hold these burgers together. Wild rice is filled with B vitamins, fiber, and zinc. This recipe is super for anyone who enjoys fish cakes but wants to avoid the gluten they usually contain, and the yogurt sauce is a heady, healthy topper.

MAKES 4 SERVINGS

1 pound wild salmon fillet, cut into
 1/2-inch chunks
1 cup cooked wild rice (see note)
1/4 cup finely chopped scallion,
 white and green parts
1 tablespoon grated lemon zest
1/2 teaspoon sea salt
1/8 teaspoon cayenne
1/4 cup chopped fresh parsley
1 tablespoon chopped fresh mint
1 tablespoon extra-virgin olive oil
Yogurt Sauce with Citrus and Mint
 (page 195)

COOK'S NOTE: Wild rice, which is actually a type of marsh grass, isn't as fussy as other types of rice. To cook it, simply bring a large saucepan of water to a boil, stir in the rice and a bit of salt, and then decrease the heat to medium-low and simmer vigorously until the grains are tender but still firm. Cooking time can vary depending on the variety of wild rice and how it's processed, but it's usually between 40 and 60 minutes. To yield 1 cup cooked, use about 1/3 cup of wild rice. If you don't have wild rice on hand, substitute a long-grain brown rice, such as jasmine or basmati.

Put the salmon, wild rice, scallion, lemon zest, salt, and cayenne in a food processor and pulse about six times, just until well combined; don't overprocess, or you'll end up with a paste.

Transfer to a bowl and gently fold in the parsley and mint. Shape the mixture into four 4-ounce patties.

Heat the olive oil in a large skillet over medium-high heat. When the oil starts to shimmer, add the salmon patties and cook until golden brown on the bottom, about 3 minutes. Gently flip them over and cook until golden brown on the other side, about 3 more minutes.

Variation: Substitute cooked long-grain brown rice, such as brown basmati or brown jasmine rice, for the wild rice.

PREP TIME: 15 minutes COOK TIME: 6 minutes
STORAGE: Store in an airtight container in the refrigerator for up to 5 days.
PER SERVING: Calories: 210; Total Fat: 8 g (1.5 g saturated, 4.5 g monounsaturated); Carbohydrates: 10 g; Protein: 25 g; Fiber: 1 g; Sodium: 283 mg

Shrimp Via My Ma

Is there really such thing as an original recipe? You know there's gotta be a hieroglyphic version of tomato sauce entombed in some pyramid. The best we can hope to do is improve on the long line of recipes that evolved into the most current version. So it goes here. The DNA of this shrimp dish ends with Mrs. John Eager, who contributed her favorite dish to a cookbook my mother stumbled across circa 1973, courtesy of the Women's Committee of Baltimore's Walters Art Museum. Mom riffed on that and came up with the Shrimp Elizabeth she made on many a Friday nights. I loved its fresh flavor, thanks to the lemon zest kicker, and I messed with the recipe for years myself. It even became my standard offering on first dates. (Love me, love my food. No exceptions—at least back then.) Paradoxically, sometimes the more you play with a recipe, the harder it is to pin down on paper. When I finally nailed it, I called Mom. She had no idea I'd been so enamored with her recipe. As I read her my latest version, I could feel her nodding in approval. By the way, shrimp is a protein dynamo, with just 4 ounces providing nearly 24 grams of protein, along with a blast of revitalizing vitamin B12 and omega-3s. I like serving this dish over Brown Rice Pilaf with Saffron and Ginger (page 123), with a side of Broccoli with Red Onion, Feta, and Mint (page 104). MAKES 4 SERVINGS

3 tablespoons extra-virgin olive oil
1 cup diced onion
1/2 cup diced fennel
1/2 cup diced red bell pepper, raw
   or roasted
Sea salt
2 teaspoons minced garlic
1/4 teaspoon red pepper flakes
1 tablespoon tomato paste
1 (14.5-ounce) can diced tomatoes
2 teaspoons chopped fresh thyme,
   or 1/2 teaspoon dried
1 teaspoon chopped fresh oregano,
   or 1/4 teaspoon dried
1 pound shrimp, peeled and deveined
2 teaspoons freshly squeezed
   lemon juice
2 teaspoons grated lemon zest
2 tablespoons finely chopped fresh
   parsley

COOK'S NOTE: You can make the sauce in advance, omitting the shrimp, lemon juice, lemon zest, and parsley. Reheat it, add the shrimp, and cook for 3 minutes, until the shrimp are cooked, right before you're ready to begin serving.

Heat olive oil in a heavy skillet over medium heat. Add the onion, fennel, bell pepper, and a generous pinch of salt and sauté until the onion is golden, about 8 minutes. Add the garlic and red pepper flakes and sauté for 1 minute. Stir in the tomato paste, then add the juice from the tomatoes to deglaze the skillet, stirring to loosen any bits that have stuck to the pan. Cook until the liquid is reduced by one-quarter. Stir in the tomatoes, thyme, oregano, and a pinch of salt and cook until the liquid has reduced by another one-quarter. Add the shrimp and a pinch of salt and stir gently to combine. Cover and cook until the shrimp is just done, about 3 minutes; it should be opaque. Gently stir in the lemon juice, lemon zest, and parsley. Taste; you may want to add another pinch of salt or lemon zest or spritz of lemon juice. Serve immediately.

PREP TIME: 10 minutes COOK TIME: 15 minutes
STORAGE: Store in an airtight container in the refrigerator for up to 5 days.
PER SERVING: Calories: 195; Total Fat: 8 g (1 g saturated, 6 g monounsaturated); Carbohydrates: 12.5 g; Protein: 18.5 g; Fiber: 3 g; Sodium: 758 mg

Pan-Seared Scallops with Citrus Drizzle

Whether it's comedy or cooking, great timing makes all the difference. That's especially true of scallops, which can go from righteous to rubbery in the length of a telephone solicitation. I think the best timer is actually an instant-read thermometer. I must have a dozen scattered around the kitchen, and they've saved many a meal. Scallops are at their best when cooked to a temperature between 150°F and 155°F. If they get to 165°F, they turn into oversized pencil erasers—definitely not good. That's really the only complication in this simple recipe, so check their temperature frequently while they're sizzling, and whatever you do, don't answer the phone. That's why there's voice mail. MAKES 4 SERVINGS

2 cups tightly packed baby spinach
   or arugula
12 dry-packed sea scallops
   (see note)
1 tablespoon extra-virgin olive oil
1 tablespoon organic butter or ghee
1 teaspoon sea salt
$\frac{1}{2}$ teaspoon freshly ground black
   pepper
1 tablespoon freshly squeezed
   orange juice, preferably blood
   orange juice
2 tablespoons freshly squeezed
   lemon juice, preferably Meyer
   lemon juice
1 tablespoon Many-Herb
   Gremolata (page 181)

COOK'S NOTE: Buy dry or dry-packed fresh or frozen scallops. The color should be translucent, white, or almost a light orange. Avoid those that look like big puffy marshmallows; they've been dipped in a solution of sodium tripolyphosphate (say that three times fast) to extend their shelf life and will be mushy and less flavorful. Also avoid bay scallops, which are about one-third of the size of sea scallops. According to the Environmental Defense Fund, bay scallops are less plentiful than sea scallops. Most bay scallops sold in the United States come from China, where they are farmed.

Divide the greens among four plates. Rinse the scallops then pat until very dry with paper towels. This step is very important, especially if you're using frozen scallops; if they aren't dry, you'll be boiling them instead of searing.

Heat the olive oil and butter in a large skillet over medium-high heat. Season the scallops with the salt and pepper, then add them to the pan one at a time in a single, uncrowded layer, cooking them in two batches if necessary. Let sear, undisturbed, until deep golden brown on the bottom, about 2 minutes. Turn and sear on the other side until golden and the internal temperature registers between 150°F and 155°F; the scallops should be almost firm to the touch. Remove from the heat, and place 3 scallops atop the greens on each plate.

Put the skillet over medium-low heat and add the orange juice, lemon juice, and a pinch of salt to deglaze the skillet, stirring to loosen any bits stuck to the pan. Cook the sauce until bubbly and slightly thickened, about 1 minute. Spoon the mixture over the scallops and sprinkle with the gremolata.

PREP TIME: 10 minutes COOK TIME: 5 minutes
STORAGE: Store in an airtight container in the refrigerator for up to 2 days.
PER SERVING: Calories: 135; Total Fat: 7 g (2.5 g saturated, 3 g monounsaturated); Carbohydrates: 5 g; Protein: 14 g; Fiber: 1 g; Sodium: 575 mg

Greek Chicken Salad

In the summer, my kitchen gets hot. At times like that, all a girl can do is fantasize about cool Mediterranean breezes, tall frosted pitchers of ice-cold concoctions, and maybe a Greek god of the mortal variety serving her a supernaturally cool Greek salad. I'm still working on the Greek god part—I'm not sure I can convince my husband to parade around the house in a toga—but I've got the salad down cold. (Sorry, couldn't resist.) What makes this dish so refreshing is generous amounts of hydrating cucumbers and tomatoes, along with a light trill of parsley and mint to tingle the taste buds. Throw in traditional Mediterranean ingredients such as feta cheese, olives, and capers, and you'll swear a cool front just passed over your house. It sure beats fanning yourself with a potholder! MAKES 4 SERVINGS

1 cup diced cooked organic chicken

12 cherry tomatoes, halved

1 small cucumber, peeled, seeded, and diced small

6 kalamata olives, sliced lengthwise

1 tablespoon extra-virgin olive oil

2 teaspoons freshly squeezed lemon juice

1 teaspoon capers, rinsed and minced

Pinch of sea salt

6 cups loosely packed arugula

1/4 cup crumbled organic goat's milk or sheep's milk feta cheese

1 tablespoon chopped fresh flat-leaf parsley

1 tablespoon chopped fresh mint

Freshly ground black pepper

COOK'S NOTE: Left over Flat-Out Good Chicken (page 148) works perfectly in this dish.

Put the chicken, tomatoes, cucumber, olives, olive oil, lemon juice, capers, and salt in a bowl and stir until well combined.

Divide the arugula among individual plates. Put a mound of the chicken salad on top, and sprinkle with the feta cheese, parsley, mint, and a few grinds of pepper.

Variations: This also makes a great sandwich filling; try it in whole wheat pita pockets, or go Latin by mixing the chicken, tomatoes, and olive oil with 1/4 avocado (diced), 1/4 cup of black beans, 1 tablespoon freshly squeezed lime juice, and 1/8 teaspoon salt. Omit the feta cheese, and substitute 1 tablespoon of chopped fresh cilantro for the mint. Another option is to swap out the lemon, olive oil, and capers and toss the chicken with Olive and Mint Vinaigrette (page 181) or Lime Vinaigrette with Toasted Cumin Seeds (page 184).

PREP TIME: 15 minutes

STORAGE: Store in an airtight container in the refrigerator for up to 2 days.

PER SERVING: Calories: 220; Total Fat: 14 g (3.5 g saturated, 7 g mono-unsaturated); Carbohydrates: 15 g; Protein: 9.5 g; Fiber: 3.5 g; Sodium: 433 mg

Braised Chicken with Artichokes and Olives

I didn't think it was possible to love artichokes more than I already did until I lived in Italy. There they harvest artichokes in both spring and fall, and that abundance graces their cuisine. Artichokes also enhance their health, as they stimulate the gallbladder to produce bile, which escorts toxins out of the body and also helps break down fats in the diet. Here, artichoke hearts are combined with chicken, chickpeas, and olives to create a rich, nourishing stew seasoned with a potpourri of heady and healthful spices, including turmeric, cumin, coriander, and mint. For a wonderful pairing, serve it over Brown Rice Pilaf with Saffron and Ginger (page 123). MAKES 4 SERVINGS

8 organic boneless, skinless chicken thighs (about 1 1/2 pounds), trimmed of excess fat
Sea salt
Freshly ground black pepper
3 tablespoons extra-virgin olive oil
1 yellow onion, diced
3 cloves garlic, thinly sliced
1 teaspoon turmeric
1/2 teaspoon ground cumin
1/2 teaspoon ground coriander
Generous pinch red pepper flakes
1 cinnamon stick, or 1/4 teaspoon ground cinnamon
1 bay leaf
2 cups organic chicken broth, homemade (page 56) or store-bought
2 teaspoons grated lemon zest
3 tablespoons freshly squeezed lemon juice
1 cup canned chickpeas, drained, rinsed, and mixed with a spritz of lemon juice and a pinch of salt
8 thawed frozen or jarred artichoke hearts (see note), quartered
1/2 cup pitted green olives, such as picholine or manzanilla
2 teaspoons lemon zest
2 tablespoons chopped fresh mint or cilantro

Pat the chicken dry and season salt and pepper. Heat the olive oil in a Dutch oven or heavy soup pot over medium-high heat. Add the chicken, working in batches if necessary, and cook until well browned on each side, about 3 minutes per side. Transfer to a plate.

Decrease the heat to medium. Add the onion and a pinch of salt and sauté until soft and slightly golden, about 5 minutes. Add the garlic and sauté for 1 minute. Add the turmeric, cumin, coriander, red pepper flakes, cinnamon stick, and bay leaf and cook, stirring constantly, until fragrant, about 1 minute. Pour in 1/4 cup of the broth to deglaze the pot, stirring to loosen any bits stuck to the pot. Stir in a pinch of salt and cook until the liquid is reduced by half. Stir in the remaining 1 3/4 cups of broth, the lemon zest, and 2 tablespoons of the lemon juice. Decrease the heat to medium-low, cover, and simmer for 15 minutes.

Add the chicken, chickpeas, artichoke hearts, and olives and stir gently to combine. Increase the heat to medium-high and simmer uncovered, stirring occasionally, until the chicken is heated through, about 5 minutes. Stir in the remaining tablespoon of lemon juice. Taste; you may want to add another squeeze of lemon juice or pinch of salt. Garnish with the mint.

Variation: This dish would work well using a firm white fish, such as 1 pound halibut, cut into 4 ounces pieces, in place of the chicken. Begin the recipe by sautéing the onion. Proceed as directed, but substitute vegetable broth, homemade (page 55) or store-bought,

continued

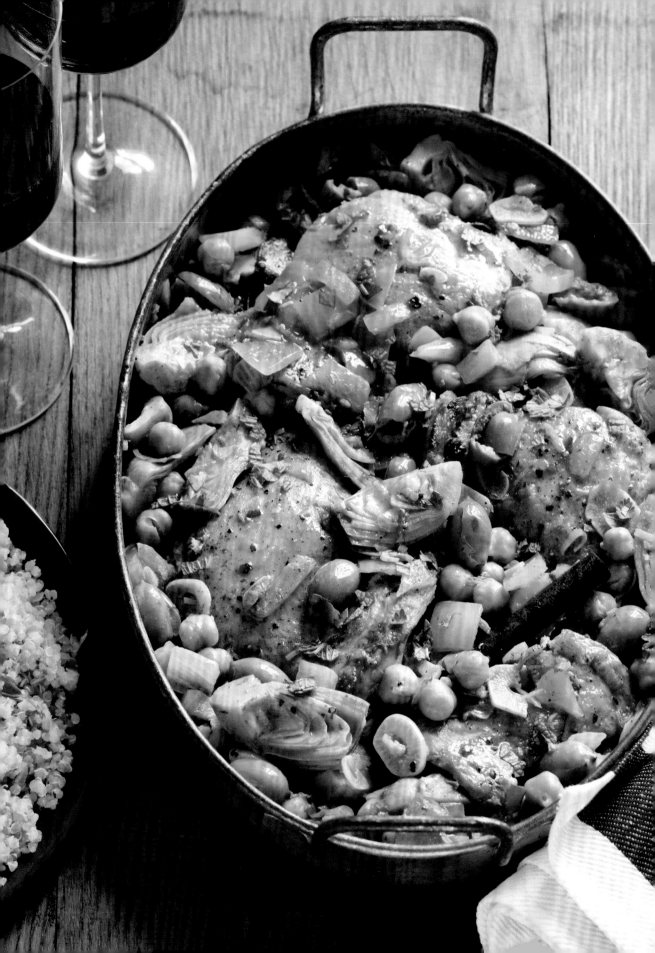

Braised Chicken with Artichokes and Olives, *continued*

COOK'S NOTE: The artichokes hearts can be fresh, frozen and thawed, or packed in water in a jar. Whichever type you use, rinse them well. If using fresh artichoke hearts, add them right after adding the garlic.

for the chicken broth. Add the fish during the last 5 minutes of cooking.

PREP TIME: 20 minutes COOK TIME: 30 minutes
STORAGE: Store in an airtight container in the refrigerator for up to 3 days or in the freezer for up to 1 month.
PER SERVING: Calories: 395; Total Fat: 21.5 g (5 g saturated, 12 g mono-unsaturated); Carbohydrates: 16 g; Protein: 33.5 g; Fiber: 3.5 g; Sodium: 498 mg

WHO KNEW? Digestion begins long before you put food in your mouth. According to nutrition expert Kathie Madonna Swift, MS, RD, LDN, our other senses, notably smell and sight, can jump-start the production of saliva and enzymes that promote better digestion. This so-called cephalic digestion—*cephalic* being Greek for "in the head"—explains why the appearance and aroma of food goes beyond mere aesthet-ics. According to Swift, attractive presentation, pleasing odors, and a relaxed mood improve digestion. So do yourself a favor and set the table with attractive dinnerware and light a candle or two.

Flat-Out Good Chicken

Anyone who thinks that cooking isn't physical should see the tennis forearms I've developed from years of lifting, chopping, stirring, and so forth. It's actually a great stress release, which brings me to Flat-Out Good Chicken. As the name suggest, the recipe involves pounding chicken breasts until they're flat. I could tell you that whenever you begin to break some of the structural proteins in meat in this way, it reduces the time required for the marinade to soak in. And that's true. And I could tell you that chicken prepared in this way really holds on to any herbs in the marinade, such as the Simon and Garfunkel blend in this recipe (for those of you born after 1970, that's parsley, sage, rosemary, and thyme). This is also true. But the real reason to make this is best summed up by a friend who asked for the recipe. When I told her that she could get the butcher to do the pounding if she didn't want to do it her-self, she laughed and said, "No, this is the perfect job for my perpetually annoyed teenager." Think of it as kitchen therapy. MAKES 4 SERVINGS

4 organic skinless, boneless chicken breast halves
1 tablespoon extra-virgin olive oil
4 cloves garlic, minced
1 tablespoon grated lemon zest
1 tablespoon chopped fresh thyme
1 teaspoon chopped fresh sage
1 teaspoon chopped fresh rosemary

Working with one chicken breast at a time, put it between several layers of parchment paper and pound with a meat pounder until about $1/4$ inch thick. Put the pieces in a pan in which they fit without overlapping.

Put the olive oil, garlic, lemon zest, thyme, sage, rose-mary, salt, and pepper in small bowl and whisk until well

1/4 teaspoon sea salt

1/4 teaspoon freshly ground black pepper

2 tablespoons finely chopped fresh parsley, for garnish

Parsley Mint Drizzle (page 189) or Artichoke, Basil, and Olive Tapenade (page 169), for garnish

COOK'S NOTES: No two pieces of chicken are alike. Some will be thicker and require a little extra pounding. Don't get carried away with your mallet though, as the thinner parts of the chicken will tear if they're pounded too much.

This recipe is a great candidate for doubling. Leftovers can be used to add protein to salads, such as Greek Chicken Salad (page 145), soups, such as Chicken Tortilla Soup (page 70), or other dishes, such as Hot-and-Sour Sesame Soba Noodles (page 126).

blended. Spread the mixture evenly over both sides of the chicken. Cover and refrigerate for 30 minutes.

Heat a grill or grill pan to medium-high heat. Remove the chicken from the marinade and pat dry with paper towels. Grill until firm to the touch and the juices run clear, 1 to 2 minutes on each side. Serve garnished with the parsley and the Parsley Mint Drizzle.

Variations: There are many ways to infuse flavor into chicken. Using this recipe as a template, try marinating the pounded chicken in the yogurt mixture used in Mediterranean Kebabs (page 150) and serving it topped it with Yogurt Sauce with Citrus and Mint (page 195). Another option is to marinate in Lime Vinaigrette with Toasted Cumin Seeds (page 184) and serve it topped with Papaya and Avocado Salsa (page 191). It's also great when marinated in My Go-To Marinade (page 188) or topped with Basil Pistachio Pesto (page 179) or Kale-Basil Pesto (page 121). Or, for a hit of umami, drizzle with Pomegranate Glaze (page 194) or pomegranate molasses, homemade (page 192) or store-bought.

PREP TIME: 20 minutes, plus 30 minutes for marinating
COOK TIME: 5 minutes
STORAGE: Store tightly wrapped in the refrigerator for up to 2 days.
PER SERVING: Calories: 180; Total Fat: 7 g (1.5 g saturated, 4 g monounsaturated); Carbohydrates: 1.5 g; Protein: 27 g; Fiber: 0.5 g; Sodium: 165 mg

WHO KNEW? How we prepare food can sometimes be just as important as the foods we choose to eat. Joseph Pizzorno, one of the world's foremost researchers into natural and integrative medicine and an adviser to presidents Bill Clinton and George W. Bush, estimates that "about 60 percent of the aging in our bodies comes from how we prepare foods." A key culprit, says Pizzorno, is how long and how directly meat is exposed to high heat, as prolonged high-heat cooking can create glycated proteins, which can build up in the body and cause oxidative stress. One way to limit the development of these proteins is to marinate any meat or fish you intend to grill. Not only does this reduce cooking time by tenderizing the food in advance, it also provides a protective barrier between the food and the flame. Marinades also happen to make food taste great. That's what I call a win-win-win.

Mediterranean Kebabs

In the United States, we never think of yogurt as a marinade for meat, but for the Turks and their neighbors, using it for that purpose is second nature. Folks throughout the Eastern Mediterranean (and notably Turkey's neighbor Cyprus) are renowned for longevity, and also big fans of yogurt. Is there a connection? Perhaps. Aside from yogurt's ability to support digestion and tummy wellness, the acids in yogurt tenderize meat and protect it from the formation of carcinogens during high heat cooking, particularly over an open flame. Here's where marinades come to the rescue. In addition to tasting great, they can decrease the formation of heat-related chemicals by a whopping 95 percent. So marinate early and often (especially when grilling). **MAKES 6 SERVINGS**

---

1 cup organic plain yogurt or goat's milk yogurt
Sea salt
$1/2$ cup grated onion
2 tablespoons freshly squeezed lemon juice
1 teaspoon lemon zest
$1 1/2$ teaspoons chopped fresh oregano, or $3/4$ teaspoon dried
2 teaspoons minced garlic
1 teaspoon ground cumin
$1/2$ teaspoon ground cinnamon
$1/4$ teaspoon cayenne
2 tablespoons extra-virgin olive oil
4 organic skinless, boneless chicken breasts, cut into 1-inch cubes
Freshly ground black pepper
Grapeseed oil, for the grill
6 tablespoons Yogurt Tahini Sauce (page 195), for garnish
6 tablespoons Parsley Mint Drizzle (page 189), for garnish

Put the yogurt, a pinch of salt, onion, lemon juice, lemon zest, oregano, garlic, cumin, cinnamon, cayenne, and the olive oil in a nonreactive bowl and whisk until well combined. Add chicken and stir gently until evenly coated. Cover and refrigerate for 1 hour.

If using wooden skewers for the kebabs, soak them in water for at least 30 minutes before grilling. Preheat an outdoor grill or a grill pan to medium-high heat.

Remove the chicken from the marinade and wipe off the excess marinade with paper towels. Thread the chicken onto metal or soaked wood skewers, using 6 cubes of chicken per skewer. Put the skewers on a rimmed baking sheet and sprinkle with salt and pepper. Discard any leftover marinade.

Oil the grate or grill pan with 1 tablespoon of grapeseed oil. Put the skewers on the grill and cook until an instant-read thermometer register 155°F, about 5 minutes per side. Serve topped with the Yogurt Tahini Sauce and Parsley Mint Drizzle.

Variations: Drizzle with Pomegranate Glaze (page 194) or pomegranate molasses, homemade (page 192) or store-bought, and omit the Yogurt Tahini sauce. You can substitute organic lamb for the chicken; for medium rare, cook the lamb until instant-read thermometer registers 145°F, about 10 minutes altogether.

If you don't have any skewers on hand, cook the chicken on the grill or under the broiler in larger pieces, or leave the chicken breasts intact and grill, broil, or bake them whole. (Instructions for broiling and baking follow.)

To broil, set the oven to the broil setting. Brush the assembled skewers with 1 tablespoon of olive oil, then sprinkle with salt and pepper. Put the skewers on a generously oiled broiler pan or on a generously oiled wire rack atop a large, rimmed baking sheet. Broil turning once, until an instant-read thermometer registers 155°F, about 5 minutes per side.

To bake, preheat the oven to 425°F. Arrange the assembled skewers on a large, rimmed nonstick baking sheet in a single layer. Brush with 1 tablespoon of olive oil, then sprinkle with salt and pepper. Bake, turning once, until an instant-read thermometer registers 155°F, about 10 minutes altogether.

PREP TIME: 20 minutes, plus 1 hour for marinating
COOK TIME: 10 minutes
STORAGE: Store in an airtight container in the refrigerator for up to 5 days.
PER SERVING: Calories: 190; Total Fat: 10.5 g (2.5 g saturated, 7 g monounsaturated); Carbohydrates: 4.5 g; Protein: 20 g; Fiber: 1 g; Sodium: 102 mg

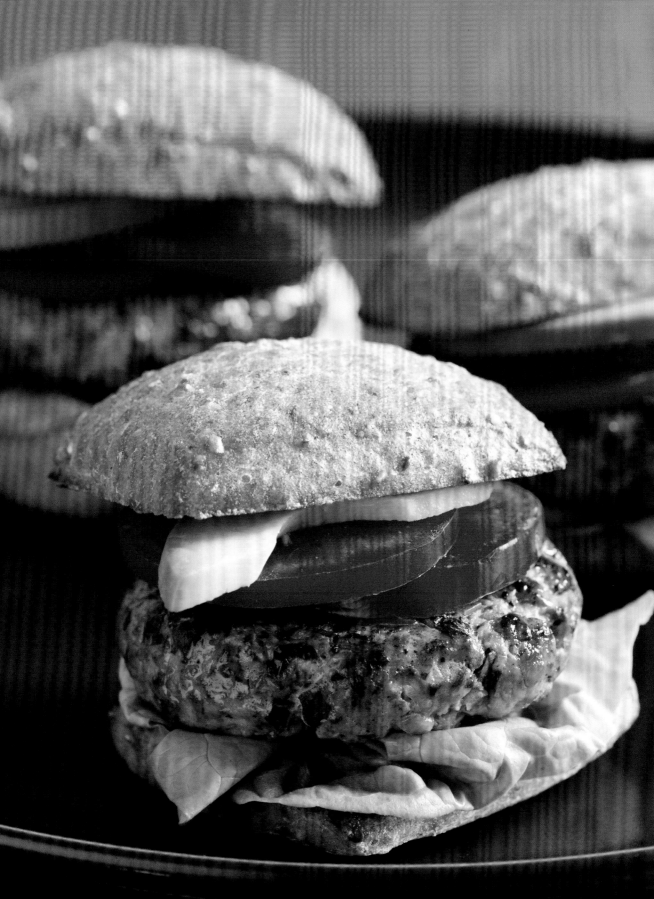

Herby Turkey Sliders

Every once in a while a girl has to do what a girl has to do. Many years ago, I was working fourteen hours a day as a cook in a vegetarian restaurant in northern California. Let's just say the owner was a tad obsessed with keeping his restaurant "pure." I swear that if you had a tuna fish sandwich in your car, an alarm would go off in his office. Every once in a while I got a hankering for something that required a field trip. There weren't many choices in town, but one place we all escaped to had awesome mini burgers made with grass-fed beef. A few bites was all it took to satisfy my cravings, and back I could go to the land of milk and honey (and tofu, polenta, and brown rice). In this recipe, I opted for dark meat turkey because it's so flavorful, and because the tryptophan in turkey is a natural stress buster—and isn't that what indulging a yen is all about? Serve these with pita pockets or buns. MAKES 8 PATTIES, 4 SERVINGS

¼ cup minced red onion
¼ cup finely chopped fresh basil
¼ cup finely chopped fresh parsley
1 tablespoon tomato paste
1 tablespoon minced garlic
1½ teaspoons fennel seeds, toasted (see note, page 83) and crushed
1½ teaspoons dried oregano
1 teaspoon grated lemon zest
½ teaspoon sea salt
¼ teaspoon red pepper flakes
⅛ teaspoon freshly ground black pepper
1 pound ground dark-meat turkey meat or ground turkey breast
Lettuce leaves, for serving
Sliced tomato, for serving
Sliced avocado, for serving

COOK'S NOTE: When mixing the turkey with the other ingredients, use a light hand. If you overwork the turkey, the burgers will be tough. That may seem counterintuitive, but trust me, it's true.

Put the onion, basil, parsley, tomato paste, garlic, fennel seeds, oregano, lemon zest, salt, red pepper flakes, and pepper in a large bowl and stir to combine. Add the turkey and gently mix with your hands or a spatula until well combined (see note). Shape the mixture into eight 2-ounce patties (about the size of your palm).

Heat a grill pan to medium heat. Brush with olive oil, then put the patties on the grill and cook until browned on both sides, about 3 minutes on each side. Cover and cook for 3 more minutes, or until an instant read thermometer registers 165°F. Alternatively, heat a skillet over medium heat. Add just enough oil to coat the skillet, then put the patties in the skillet and cooked until browned on both sides, about 3 minutes on each. Decrease the heat to medium low, add 1 tablespoon of water, cover, and cook for about 3 minutes. to steam the inside about 3 more minutes.

Serve with lettuce, tomato, and avocado.

Variations: For a "burger" look, use mini whole grain burger buns. Substitute grass-fed beef for the turkey, and top with a dollop of Ancho Chile Relish (page 180) or Kale-Basil Pesto (page 121).

PREP TIME: 15 minutes COOK TIME: 10 minutes
STORAGE: Store in an airtight container in the refrigerator for up to 3 days or in the freezer individually wrapped for up to 3 months.
PER SERVING: Calories: 195; Total Fat: 10 g (2.5 g saturated, 4 g monounsaturated); Carbohydrates: 3.5 g; Protein: 23 g; Fiber: 1 g; Sodium: 274 mg

Moroccan Mint Lamb Chops

Somewhere along the line, Americans became enamored with beef, whereas Europeans and Middle Easterners still favored lamb, an ancient food with great health benefits. Lamb is packed with protein; just 3 satiating ounces provides more than 40 percent of the average person's daily protein needs. Lamb is also a great source of vitamin B12, which is a huge energy booster. I love lamb's leanness, natural tenderness, and exceptional flavor, which is heightened here thanks to a marinade featuring mint, cumin, coriander, cayenne, and cinnamon. To round out the meal, serve this dish with Mediterranean Greens (page 98) or Walnut, Date, and Herb Salad (page 92). MAKES 4 SERVINGS

1/4 cup extra-virgin olive oil, plus more for the grill
1/4 cup chopped fresh cilantro or basil
2 tablespoons chopped fresh mint
2 teaspoons minced garlic
1 teaspoon chopped fresh ginger
1 teaspoon ground cumin
1/2 teaspoon ground coriander
1/4 teaspoon ground cinnamon
1/4 teaspoon cayenne
Sea salt
8 grass-fed organic lamb chops
2 tablespoons freshly squeezed lemon juice
Freshly ground black pepper
Pomegranate Glaze (page 194), for garnish

COOK'S NOTE: To broil, after removing the lamb from the marinade and patting dry, brush it with 1 tablespoon of olive oil and sprinkle with salt and pepper. Place the chops on a generously oiled broiler pan or a generously oiled wire rack set atop a large, rimmed baking sheet. Broil, turning once, until an instant-read thermometer registers an internal temperature of 140°F, about 3 minutes on each side, for medium rare. Let rest for 5 minutes before serving as directed.

Put the olive oil, cilantro, mint, garlic, ginger, cumin, coriander, cinnamon, cayenne, and 1/2 teaspoon of salt in a blender or food processor and process until smooth. Place the lamb in a pan so it fits in a single layer. Pour in half of the marinade and spread it evenly over the lamb. Stir the lemon juice into the remaining marinade set aside. Cover the lamb and refrigerate for 2 hours.

Preheat an outdoor grill or grill pan to medium-high heat.

Remove the lamb from the marinade, wipe off the excess marinade with paper towels, and sprinkle with salt and pepper. Generously oil the grate or grill pan with olive oil. Put the lamb on the grill and cook until an instant-read thermometer registers 140°F, about 4 minutes on each side depending on thickness, for medium rare. Transfer to a platter and let rest for 5 minutes before serving with a generous drizzle of the lemony reserved marinade or Pomegranate Glaze.

Variation: For added indulgence, serve topped with Yogurt Tahini Sauce (page 195). This marinade works well with chicken and fish.

PREP TIME: 10 minutes, plus 2 hours for marinating
COOK TIME: 8 minutes
STORAGE: Store in an airtight container in the refrigerator for up to 5 days.
PER SERVING: Calories: 315; Total Fat: 22 g (5 g saturated, 14 g monounsaturated); Carbohydrates: 1.5 g; Protein: 27.5 g; Fiber: 0.5 g; Sodium: 336 mg

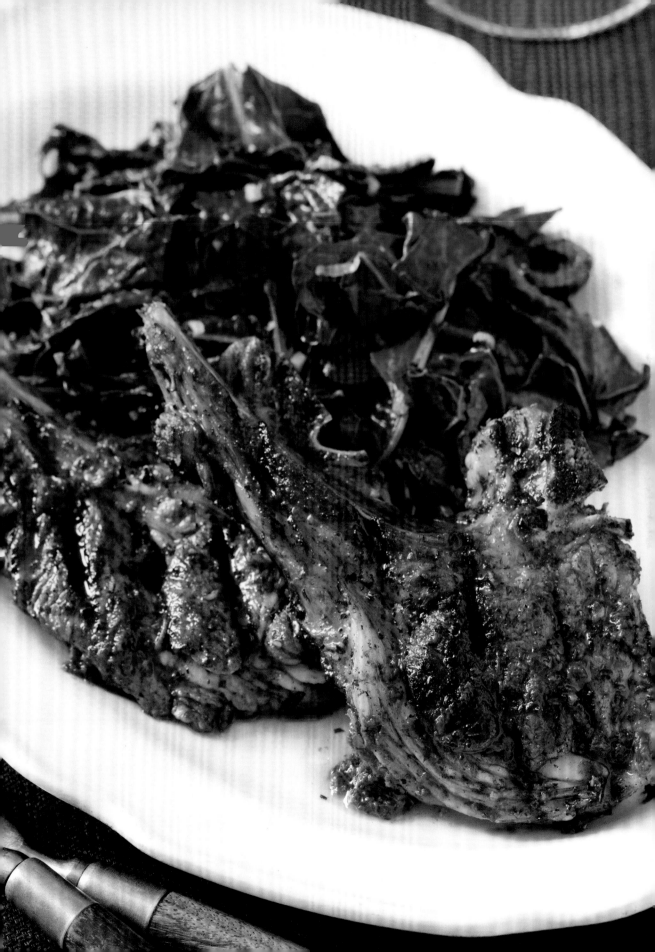

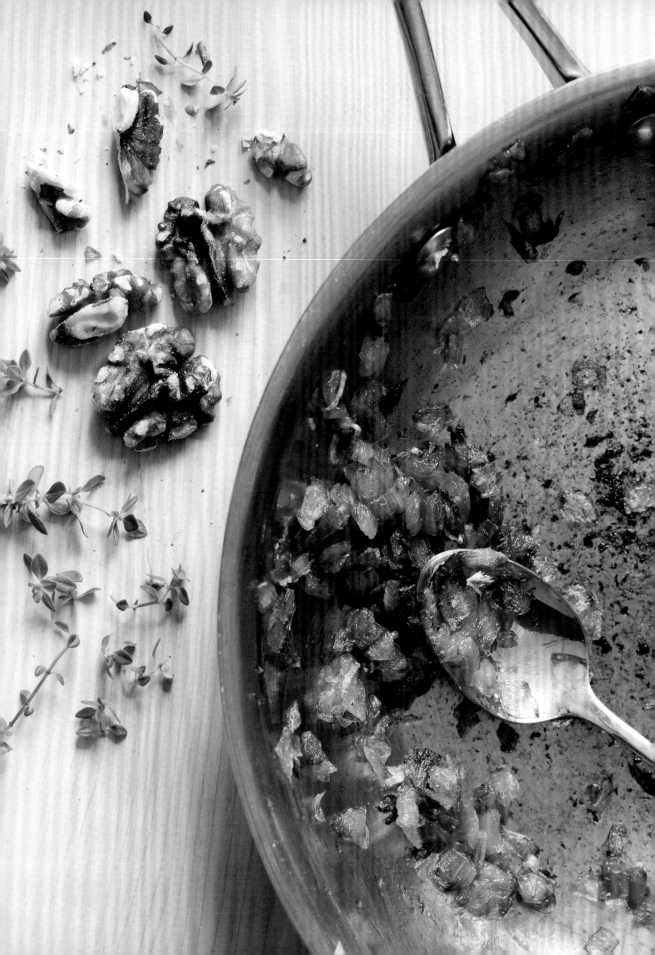

CHAPTER 8

Nibbles and Noshes

If you've learned the secret to eating three squares a day, drop me a line, will ya?

I'm not sure if it's work, life, kids, picking up the dry cleaning, out-of-town meetings, or what, but no one I know, not even yours truly, fuels up as often as they should. That's a real problem, and not just in terms of feeling cranky when your blood sugar plummets. While mood isn't inconsequential, serious, long-term health issues can also result, including insulin resistance and metabolic syndrome, both of which can lead to type 2 diabetes, which in turn raises the risk of stroke and heart attack.

There's plenty of debate about how often we should eat. For my part, I think having access to healthy, appealing noshes and nibbles throughout the day sets the body up to feel satisfied with smaller portions during major meals. Maybe it's just my sense of rhythm, but I see the ideal eating pattern for well-being as a series of gentle waves to be enjoyed, rather than thunderous surf that tosses us hither and yon. There's a reason while the latter so often causes a wipeout, while the former brings satiation and sustained energy.

The tiny bites in this chapter appeal to a wide range of taste preferences, and all are highly portable and contain no empty calories. I created them for eating on the go whenever those first hunger pangs hit. They are nutritionally powerful treats that you can pop into a little bag or containers and keep wherever you spend your time. That's what I do: in my desk drawer, my shoulder bag, the glove box in my car, they're never out of arm's reach. From spiced walnuts to mini muffins to bars that are petite and sweet, they'll blow away anything you can find on a supermarket shelf, in terms of both taste and nutrition.

Of course, these little bundles of joy don't need to leave the kitchen to do their thing. I often put them out when I'm having friends over; there's nothing like creative finger foods to set a mood. After noshing on a few roasted olives, a deviled egg, or whole grain crackers with a tasty spread, everyone's troubles suddenly are in the rearview mirror, and laughter and comfort fill the house. Who could ask more?

Apple Slices with Banana and Almond Butter

What people tell me, time and again, is that they're looking for a great balance of taste and texture. That's why, when it comes to sweet cravings, I love to use apples. They provide that crunch that folks desire, they're sweet, and best of all, they're a good source of fiber, which allows fruit to deliver its sweetness slowly, preventing insulin spikes that can lead to diabetes and damage to the blood vessels. And when fruit is dressed up with other healthful ingredients that are also a little decadent, well, what's not to like? In this simple nosh, sliced apple is topped it with a smidge of almond butter, banana, cinnamon, and dark cocoa powder. Why settle for a cookie when you can nibble on this? MAKES 1 SERVING

1 apple, cored and sliced into
 $1/2$-inch rounds
1 tablespoon almond butter
$1/2$ banana, thinly sliced
$1/8$ teaspoon ground cinnamon
$1/4$ teaspoon unsweetened cocoa
 powder

Put the apple slices on a plate and spread the almond butter on each slice. Arrange the bananas on top and sprinkle with the cinnamon and cocoa powder.

Variation: If you're a coconut lover, add a sprinkling of unsweetened shredded dried coconut.

PREP TIME: 10 minutes
STORAGE: Not applicable.
PER SERVING: Calories: 245; Total Fat: 9.5 g (1 g saturated, 5 g mono-unsaturated); Carbohydrates: 42 g; Protein: 4.5 g; Fiber: 8 g; Sodium: 37 mg

Sweet Potato Bars

These bars remind me of the lemon bars I used to make as a kid, probably because this is a treat any youngster would like. Thankfully, this treat is a little more healthful, with a nutty, gluten-free crust and a filling based on nutritionally outstanding sweet potatoes, which are loaded with antioxidants and can help regulate blood sugar levels. These bars are so nutrient dense that a small portion will leave you completely satiated, and the flavors are so delightful that you'll be blissfully aware of every bite. MAKES 16 BARS

CRUST
3/4 cup rolled oats
1/4 cup teff flour or brown rice flour
1/4 cup shelled unsalted pistachios
1/4 cup pecans
1/2 teaspoon ground cinnamon
1/2 teaspoon grated orange zest
1/4 teaspoon sea salt
2 tablespoons Grade B maple syrup
2 tablespoons extra-virgin olive oil

FILLING
1 pound orange-fleshed sweet
    potatoes, such as garnet yams,
    baked until tender
2 organic eggs, beaten
1/3 cup organic plain yogurt
3 tablespoons Grade B maple syrup
1/2 teaspoon grated orange zest
1/2 teaspoon ground cardamom
1/2 teaspoon ground ginger
Freshly grated nutmeg, for dusting

COOK'S NOTES: You can bake the sweet potatoes in advance and store them in the refrigerator for up to 3 days.

If you're sensitive to gluten, you'll love this recipe. Both teff and brown rice are gluten-free, so the flour isn't an issue. Technically, oats are also gluten-free; however, they are subject to cross-contamination in the field and during processing. If you're extremely sensitive to gluten, I recommend using Bob's Red Mill Gluten-Free Rolled Oats.

To make the crust, preheat the oven to 375°F. Lightly oil an 8-inch square baking pan.

Put the oats, teff flour, pistachios, pecans, cinnamon, orange zest, and salt in a food processor and pulse until the texture resembles coarse cornmeal. Add the maple syrup and olive oil and pulse until the ingredients are evenly combined but the mixture is still crumbly looking. Transfer the mixture to the prepared pan and press it evenly and firmly into the bottom of the pan. No need to clean out the food processor. Bake for about 15 minutes, until set. Keep the oven on.

Meanwhile, make the filling. Scoop the sweet potato flesh into a bowl and mash it. Put 1 1/2 cups of the mashed sweet potatoes in the food processor (reserve any leftovers for another use). Add the eggs, yogurt, maple syrup, orange zest, cardamom, and ginger and process until smooth.

To assemble and bake the bars, pour the filling over the crust and smooth the top with a spatula. Sprinkle with nutmeg. Bake for about 25 minutes, until the filling is set and just beginning to pull from the sides of pan. Let cool completely on a wire rack, then cover and refrigerate for at least 2 hours before cutting into 16 squares.

PREP TIME: 15 minutes COOK TIME: 40 minutes, plus 2 hours for chilling
STORAGE: Store in an airtight container in the refrigerator for up to 4 days or tightly wrapped in the freezer for up to 2 months.
PER SERVING: (2 bars per serving) Calories: 120; Total Fat: 5 g (1 g saturated, 2 g monounsaturated); Carbohydrates: 16 g; Protein: 3 g; Fiber: 2 g; Sodium: 55 mg

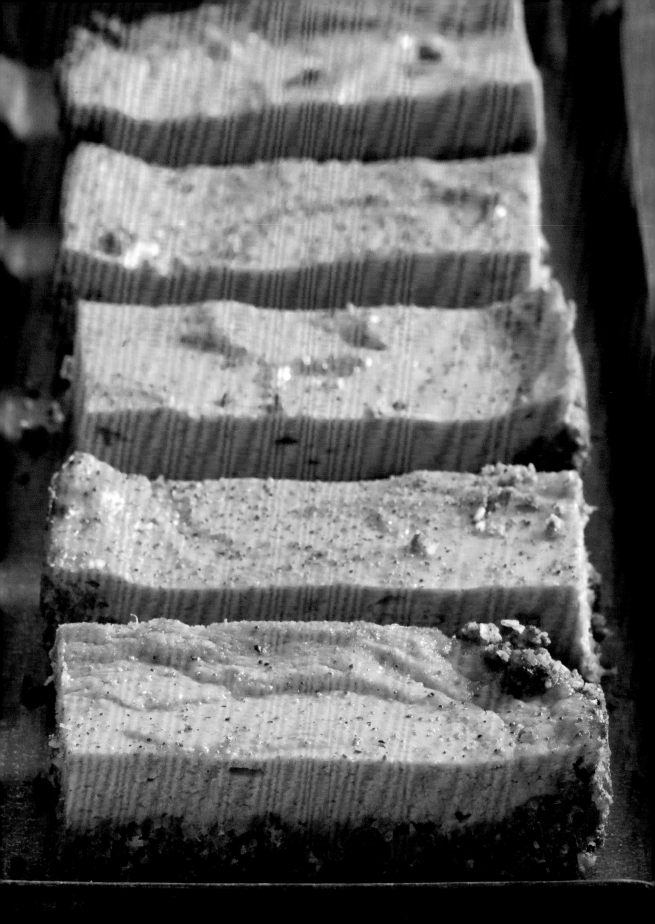

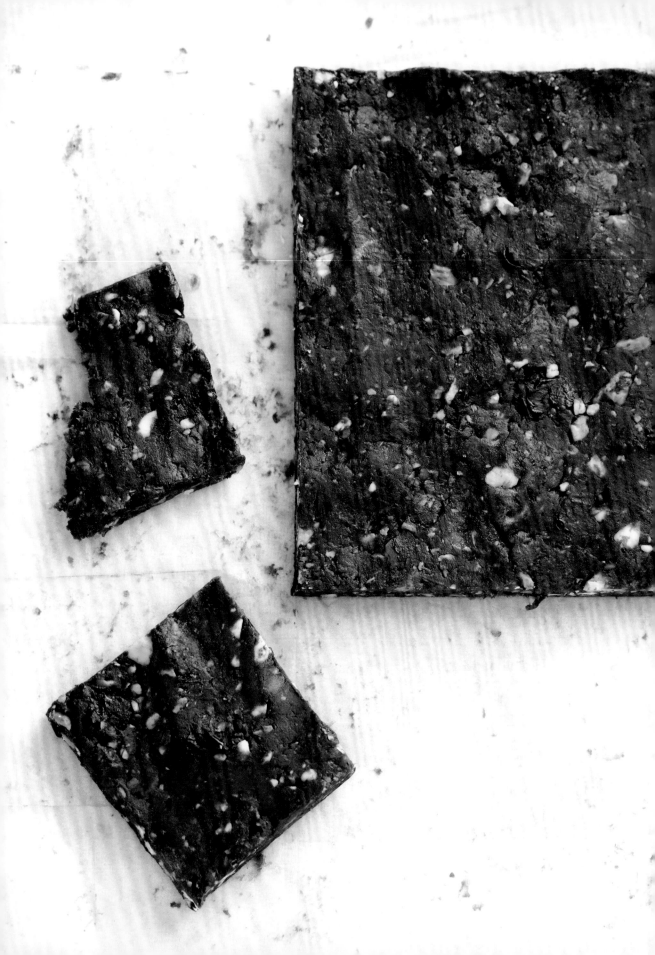

Wendy's Wunderbars

My brother Jeff is in a line of work where he can't exactly run out to the nearest coffee shop when he needs quick energy. Take his last job: photographing the construction of a subway tunnel ninety feet below Manhattan. It's not a place where you want to suddenly feel faint from hunger, or even cranky, as tends to happen when blood sugar plummets. Fortunately, Jeff has a secret weapon when he needs a quick recharge: Wendy's Wunderbars. Despite its out of the world flavor, this bar isn't a nutritional nightmare. Dark chocolate, pistachios, almonds, and dates are all healthful in moderation. When you want energy without missing a beat, this bar is the way to go. **MAKES 16 BARS**

2 ounces dark chocolate (60 to 72% cacao content), finely chopped

1 ounce unsweetened baking chocolate, finely chopped

1/3 cup shelled pistachios

1/3 cup almonds, toasted (see note, page 83)

8 ounces Medjool dates, halved and pitted

1/2 teaspoon vanilla extract

1/8 teaspoon sea salt

1/3 cup dried cherries

Very lightly oil an 8-inch square baking pan. Cut two pieces of waxed paper to the same width as the pan and long enough to go up the sides and overlap across the top of the pan. Place one piece in the pan, then place the second piece on top in the other direction.

Put all of the chopped chocolate in a heatproof bowl and set over a saucepan of simmering water. Heat, stirring often, just until the chocolate is melted and smooth. Remove from the heat.

Put the pistachios and almonds in food processor and pulse three or four times to coarsely chop. Add the dates, melted chocolate, vanilla, and salt. Pulse until the ingredients begin to hold together, almost like dough. Add the cherries and pulse a few more times, until the cherries are coarsely chopped and evenly distributed.

Transfer to the prepared pan and press in an even layer using your hands. Smooth the top with a spatula.

Cover with a piece of parchment or waxed paper and chill until firm, about 1 hour. Remove from the pan by lifting the edges of the waxed paper, and place on a cutting board, still atop the waxed paper. Using an oiled knife to prevent sticking, cut into 16 squares. Put the bars in a container, with waxed paper between the layers if stacked, or wrap the bars individually in foil. Store in the refrigerator or freezer. Warm to room temperature before eating.

PREP TIME: 25 minutes COOK TIME: 1 hour for chilling
STORAGE: Store in an airtight container in the refrigerator for up to 4 days or tightly wrapped in the freezer for up to 2 months.
PER SERVING: (1 bar per serving) Calories: 115; Total Fat: 5 g (1.5 g saturated, 2 g monounsaturated); Carbohydrates: 16.5 g; Protein: 2 g; Fiber: 2 g; Sodium: 14 mg

Gluten-Free Blueberry Mini Muffins

These mini muffins provide a nice energy boost and are easy on the constitution because they're made with almond flour, so they're gluten-free. Gluten is inflammatory and can mess with the gut and digestion, and many folks can't tolerate it, especially as they get older. MAKES 24 MINI MUFFINS

2 cups almond flour, homemade (page 226) or store-bought
¼ cup maple sugar
½ teaspoon baking soda
¼ teaspoon sea salt
2 organic eggs, beaten
2 tablespoons extra-virgin olive oil
2 tablespoons honey
½ teaspoon vanilla extract
½ teaspoon almond extract
½ cup frozen blueberries, preferably wild blueberries

LIVE LONG AND PROSPER: The healing powers of blueberries aren't new news. Native Americans have long utilized them to fight coughs and other ailments. More recently, clinical studies found that regular blueberry consumption improved brain performance in the elderly. A lot of the research on blueberries has focused on the phytonutrients responsible for their rich blue color. These antioxidants, known as anthocyanins, can help protect the eyes (notably the retina). There's also a body of evidence showing that the overall high levels of antioxidants in blueberries can help lower cholesterol, keep the blood vessels healthy, and help regulate blood sugar.

Preheat the oven to 375°F. Prepare a 24-cup mini muffin tin by generously oiling each muffin cup, or line each cup with two paper liners to make it easier to remove.

Put the almond flour, maple sugar, baking soda, and salt in a large bowl. Toss with your fingers until completely combined and the mixture is lump free.

Put the eggs in a separate bowl. Slowly add the oil and honey while whisking constantly. Add the vanilla and almond extract and whisk until well combined. Pour into the almond flour mixture and fold in with a rubber spatula. Gently fold in the blueberries. Spoon the batter into the prepared muffin cups, dividing it evenly among them; the batter should come almost to the top of each cup.

Put the muffin tin on a baking sheet and bake for about 15 minutes, until the tops are golden brown and a toothpick comes out clean when inserted in the center.

Let cool in the pan on a wire rack. If you didn't use paper liners, gently run a knife or small offset spatula around the edges of the muffins to help release them.

Variation: For a blast of antioxidant-rich chocolate, omit the blueberries and, before spooning the batter into the muffin tin, transfer ¼ cup of the batter to a small bowl. Stir in 2 teaspoons unsweetened cocoa powder, then add 2 tablespoons chopped dark chocolate. Put a heaping teaspoon of the chocolate mixture in the bottom of each muffin cup, then fill the cups with the remaining batter. Bake and cool as directed.

PREP TIME: 5 minutes COOK TIME: 15 minutes
STORAGE: Store in an airtight container in the refrigerator for up to 5 days or in the freezer for up to 3 months.
PER SERVING: (2 muffins per serving) Calories: 330; Total Fat: 25 g (2.5 g saturated, 15.5 g monounsaturated); Carbohydrates: 21 g; Protein: 10 g; Fiber: 5 g; Sodium: 214 mg

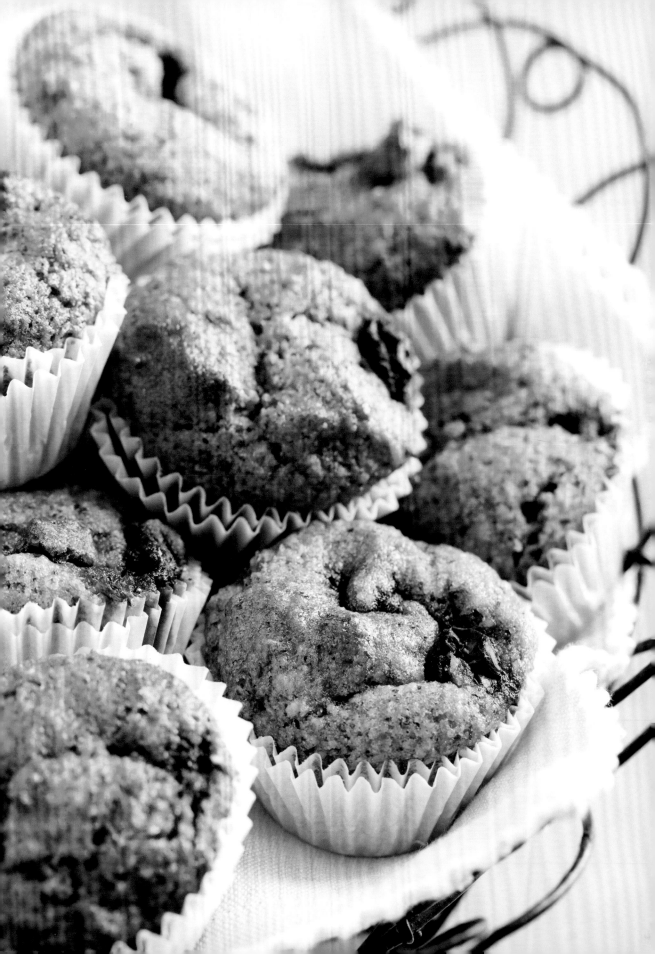

Thyme Onion Muffins

I bet when you think of muffins, vegetables aren't the first ingredient that comes to mind. But if we'd all been fed a few of these as kids, our parents might not have had to bribe us to eat our veggies. These savory morsels reminded my friend Stan of a Thanksgiving treat, and I can understand why. The nutty flavors of teff and spelt flour serve as the perfect canvas for the cozy flavors of walnuts, thyme, and sweet caramelized onion. MAKES 24 MINI MUFFINS

4 tablespoons extra-virgin olive oil
2 cups finely diced onions
3/4 teaspoon sea salt
2 tablespoons chopped fresh thyme, or 2 teaspoons dried
2 teaspoon grated lemon zest
1/8 teaspoon freshly ground black pepper
3/4 cup whole wheat pastry flour
1/3 cup teff flour or brown rice flour
1/3 cup spelt flour
2 teaspoons baking powder
1/2 teaspoon baking soda
1/2 teaspoon sea salt
2 organic eggs, beaten
2/3 cup organic buttermilk or plain yogurt
1/4 cup water
2 tablespoons extra-virgin olive oil
1 tablespoon Grade B maple syrup
1 tablespoon Dijon mustard
3/4 cup finely chopped walnuts

LIVE LONG AND PROSPER: Thyme and medicine have been intertwined since Galen, a physician in ancient Greece, gave the thymus gland its name based on the fact it looked like a bundle of thyme. The name *thyme* may derive from the Greek word for courage, and it certainly entices other nutrients to act boldly. Thyme increases the amount of beneficial omega-3 fatty acids working in the body, and its antimicrobial and antibacterial properties make it an invading bug's worst nightmare. It also stands fast in defending the health of the brain and heart.

Preheat the oven to 400°F. Prepare one 24-cup mini muffin tin by generously oiling each muffin cup, or line each cup with a paper muffin liner.

Heat 2 tablespoons of the olive oil in a large skillet over medium heat. Add the onions and 1/4 teaspoon of the salt. Decrease the heat to medium-low and cook, stirring occasionally, until the onions are very soft and just starting to turn golden brown, 20 to 25 minutes. Stir in the thyme, lemon zest, and pepper and remove from the heat.

Put the flours, baking powder, baking soda, and the remaining 1/2 teaspoon salt in a bowl and stir with a whisk to combine.

In separate bowl, combine the eggs, buttermilk, water, olive oil, maple syrup, and mustard and whisk to combine. Pour into the flour mixture and stir gently. Before the flour is completely moistened, gently fold in the onion mixture and walnuts. Spoon the batter into the muffin cups, dividing it evenly among them.

Bake for 25 to 30 minutes, until the tops are golden brown and a toothpick inserted in the center of a muffin comes out clean. Let the muffins cool in the pan for a few minutes, then turn out onto a wire rack and let cool for 15 minutes. Serve warm or at room temperature.

PREP TIME: 15 minutes COOK TIME: 55 minutes
STORAGE: Store in an airtight container at room temperature for up to 4 days or in the freezer for up to 2 months.
PER SERVING: (2 muffins per serving) Calories: 170; Total Fat: 11 g (1.5 g saturated, 5 g monounsaturated); Carbohydrates: 15 g; Protein: 5 g; Fiber: 2 g; Sodium: 286 mg

Silk Road Spiced Walnuts

Walnuts are, indisputably, the grooviest nuts. In fact, that groovy surface gives them an advantage when it comes to holding on to seasonings. This recipe includes cumin and coriander, two spices with outstanding antioxidant and anticancer properties, and lets the walnuts take a quick skinny dip with orange juice. Then it's into the oven for a rapid bake and dry. You'll know when these nuts are ready because of the delightful aroma that fills the kitchen. MAKES 8 SERVINGS

2 tablespoons freshly squeezed
    orange juice
1/4 teaspoon orange zest
2 teaspoons extra-virgin olive oil
1 teaspoon Grade B maple syrup
1/2 teaspoon ground cumin
1/2 teaspoon ground coriander
1/4 teaspoon sea salt
1/4 teaspoon ground ginger
Pinch of cayenne
1 cup walnuts
1/4 cup unsweetened dried
    cranberries

LIVE LONG AND PROSPER: It's easy to go nuts over nuts, and in moderation they're great for you. Yes, they do contain quite a bit of fat, but it's predominantly healthful monounsaturated fat—the kind you want in your diet. In fact, despite their fat content, studies have shown that people who eat nuts are far less likely to gain weight than those who generally abstain from them. Almonds, walnuts, pecans, pistachios, hazelnuts—all are loaded not just with monounsaturated fat, but also with a wealth of other nutrients, including vitamin E, potassium, magnesium, and calcium, all of which benefit the body. Regular nut consumption has been shown to lower levels of LDL (bad cholesterol) and reduce the risk of heart disease. In addition, nutrients in nuts have been shown to raise serotonin levels (hello, happiness!) and help prevent metabolic syndrome, a precursor to diabetes.

Preheat the oven to 350°F. Line a rimmed baking sheet with parchment paper.

Put the orange juice, orange zest, olive oil, maple syrup, cumin, coriander, salt, ginger, and cayenne in a small bowl and whisk to combine. Add the walnuts and cranberries and toss until evenly coated. Spread the mixture evenly on the lined baking sheet.

Bake for 10 to 15 minutes, until liquid is bubbly and has mostly cooked off and the walnuts are aromatic and slightly browned. Let cool to room temperature, then use a metal spatula to loosen the mixture.

Variations: Substitute raisins for the cranberries. Substitute almonds for some or all of the walnuts or use pistachios in place of some of the walnuts; you could even use a combination of all three nuts. For a high-powered antioxidant trail mix, after the mixture has cooled, add 1 tablespoon of dark chocolate chips and 1/4 cup of dried blueberries.

PREP TIME: 5 minutes COOK TIME: 15 minutes
STORAGE: Store in an airtight container in the refrigerator for up to 5 days.
PER SERVING: Calories: 120; Total Fat: 11 g (1 g saturated, 2 g monounsaturated); Carbohydrates: 6 g; Protein: 2 g; Fiber: 1.5 g; Sodium: 54 mg

COOK'S NOTE: As soon as you start to smell that heavenly aroma wafting from the stove, it's time to remove the nuts from the oven. They will continue to cook as they cool.

Roasted Olives with Citrus and Herbs

I thought I'd experienced olives every which way possible until a dinner party years ago, when I watched as Carolyn Brady, an incredible artist, popped a bunch of olives in the oven and *roasted* them. It seemed so exotic, and the results were incredible. The brininess was replaced by a sweet flavor heightened by the oven's heat. In my version, I've surrounded the olives with garlic, fennel seeds, rosemary, red pepper flakes, and Meyer lemon. You're not going to find anything like this at a supermarket olive bar. MAKES 12 SERVINGS

2 cups assorted olives, rinsed
1 Meyer lemon, cut into quarters
2 tablespoons freshly squeezed
  Meyer lemon juice
2 tablespoons extra-virgin olive oil
4 cloves garlic, slivered
1 teaspoon fennel seeds
1/2 teaspoon dried oregano
1/4 teaspoon red pepper flakes
1 sprig fresh rosemary

COOK'S NOTE: If you don't have access to Meyer lemons, omit the quartered lemon and replace the Meyer lemon juice with the juice of 1 regular lemon and 1/2 orange.

Preheat the oven to 400°F.

Put the olives in an 8-inch square nonreactive baking pan. Squeeze the juice from the lemon quarters over the olives and add the lemon quarters to the pan, along with the lemon juice, olive oil, garlic, fennel seeds, oregano, red pepper flakes, and rosemary. Stir until well combined.

Bake for 30 minutes. Serve warm.

PREP TIME: 5 minutes COOK TIME: 30 minutes
STORAGE: Store in an airtight container in the refrigerator for up to 5 days.
PER SERVING: Calories: 80; Total Fat: 7.5 g (1 g saturated, 6 g monounsaturated); Carbohydrates: 3 g; Protein: 0.5 g; Fiber: 1 g; Sodium: 370 mg

LIVE LONG AND PROSPER: The ancient Romans and Greeks put a lot of thought into olives, from seed to table. Harvesting them was considered a delicate matter and brought out the tender side of Pliny the Elder (a man perfectly capable of delivering a hammer blow, being commander of the Roman Empire's military). "Do not shake and beat your [olive] trees," he advised, appalled by the common practice of whacking a rod against olive trees to get the olives to fall. "Gathering by hand ensures a good harvest." Given the many ways ancients used them, for everything from peace laurels for Olympic champions to a cleaner, olives were always in demand, but never more so than for their healing properties. Hippocrates claimed olive oil could heal dozens of ailments. Ear infections, gynecological issues, skin contusions, you name it—out came the olive oil. Modern studies back up the Father of Medicine's faith in olives: their phytonutrients have been shown to fight cancer (notably breast cancer) and bone loss. They are rich in monounsaturated fats, which can help improve the ratio of LDL (bad cholesterol) to HDL (good cholesterol), decrease blood pressure, and reduce the risk of heart disease.

Artichoke, Basil, and Olive Tapenade

When people snack, they tend to unconsciously consume a lot of empty calories. I get it; we all have a lot on our minds. A great way to turn this dynamic around is to choose snacks that are loaded with flavor When you wake up the taste buds, the mind tends to follow. To that end, let me suggest this tapenade. It's super with crackers or toasted bread or as a sandwich spread. The olives and artichokes play wonderfully off of each other, and the basil provides a nice caress of freshness across the tongue—a pleasant reminder that mindful snacking brings its own rewards. MAKES 1 CUP

1/2 cup prepared artichoke hearts, quartered (rinsed and spritzed with lemon juice if canned)
20 pitted kalamata olives
3/4 cup loosely packed fresh basil leaves
2 tablespoons extra-virgin olive oil
1 tablespoon freshly squeezed lemon juice
1 teaspoon grated lemon zest
1 clove garlic, minced
1/4 teaspoon sea salt

Put all the ingredients in a food processor and pulse about 15 times, scraping down the sides of the work bowl once or twice, until mixture is well blended but still has some texture.

PREP TIME: 10 minutes
STORAGE: Store in an airtight container in the refrigerator for up to 2 days.
PER SERVING: (2 tablespoons per serving): Calories: 65; Total Fat: 6 g (1 g saturated, 5 g monounsaturated); Carbohydrates: 3 g; Protein: 1 g; Fiber: 1 g; Sodium: 290 mg

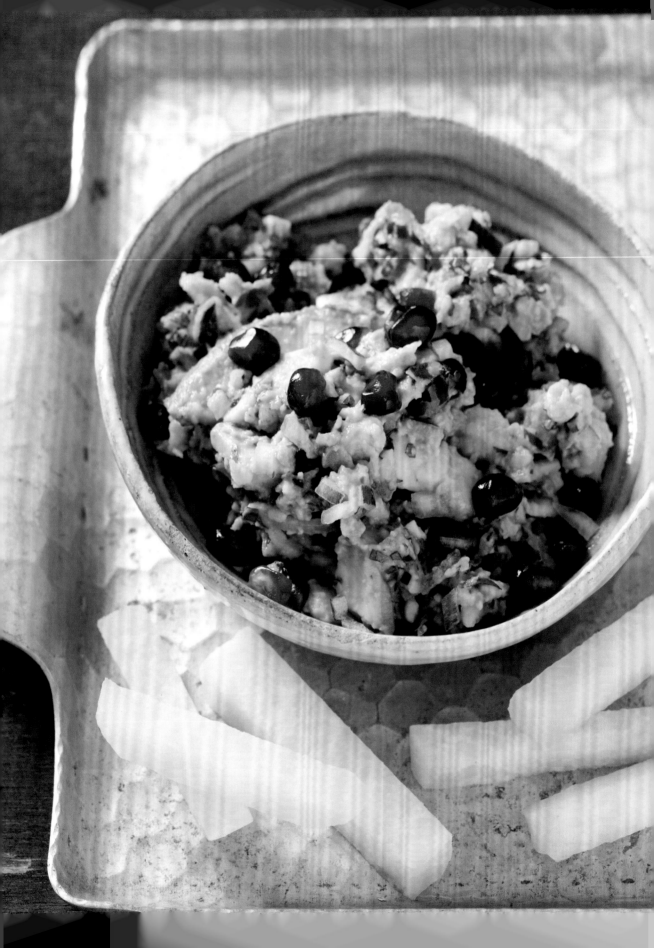

Minted Guacamole with Pomegranate Seeds

Cooks get their inspiration in the strangest places . . . like old ghost towns. No lie. For my fiftieth birthday, I met up with my best friend from back East in Jerome, Arizona. Once an abandoned copper mining town, it has transformed itself into a hip arts community with a hole-in-the-wall Southwestern restaurant that we serendipitously stumbled upon. We ordered guacamole, and it arrived studded with pomegranate seeds. Our eyes lit up, and then our tongues. As I recall, Jill said something like "Oh my! This is so good . . . and it looks like Christmas!" I took a mental snapshot of both the appearance and the flavor, and I've re-created it here. MAKES 1 CUP

2 avocados, halved and flesh scooped out

2 tablespoons finely diced red onion

1 tablespoon finely chopped fresh cilantro

1 tablespoon finely chopped fresh mint

1 tablespoon freshly squeezed lime juice

1/4 teaspoon sea salt

Pinch of cayenne

3 tablespoons pomegranate seeds (see note)

Put the avocado in a bowl and mash with a fork until mostly smooth. Add the onion, cilantro, mint, lime juice, salt, and cayenne and stir until well combined. Stir in 2 tablespoons of the pomegranate seeds and garnish with the remaining tablespoon of pomegranate seeds.

PREP TIME: 10 minutes

STORAGE: Store in an airtight container in the refrigerator for up to 3 days.

PER SERVING: (2 tablespoons per serving) Calories: 85; Total Fat: 7.5 g (1 g saturated, 5 g monounsaturated); Carbohydrates: 5.5 g; Protein: 1 g; Fiber: 4 g; Sodium: 57 mg

COOK'S NOTES: Here's a quick trick for removing pomegranate seeds from the fruit. Cut the pomegranate in half crosswise. Then, working over a large bowl, hold one half with the cut side facing down, into the bowl. Give the uncut side of the fruit a few good whacks with the back of a large wooden spoon to release the seeds. When pomegranates are in season, I buy several and store the seeds in an airtight container in the freezer to use throughout the year. They make any dish pop with color and flavor.

I like to serve this guacamole with jicama sticks. Take a vegetable peeler to the jicama, then cut it in half with a sharp knife. Cut the halves into 1/2-inch-wide strips, then turn the strips onto their side and repeat the process, cutting them into 1/2-inch-wide strips. To store the jicama strips, put them in a bowl, add cold water to cover, and mix in the juice of 1 lime or lemon. Cover and store in the refrigerator for up to 3 days.

Edamame Wasabi Spread

Remember how you felt when you first heard that dark chocolate or red wine was good for you? That elation hit me when I was listening to a lecture by friend and nutritionist extraordinaire Jeanne Wallace, PhD. As Jeanne was listing ways to consume more cruciferous vegetables, she noted that many people already get one particular cruciferous vegetable without realizing it. She leaned forward on the podium, we leaned forward in our seats, and she whispered one long, drawn-out word: "*Waaaasaaaahbeeee*." To which we responded as one, as if a giant, gorgeous firework had just exploded: "Ooooooooooohhh!" The edamame here is no nutritional slouch either; it's soy in its fresh, whole form. Put them together and you have a kick guaranteed to clean out any brain fog on contact. MAKES 1 CUP

1 cup fresh or frozen shelled edamame, mixed with a spritz of lime juice and a pinch of salt

1/4 cup water

3 tablespoons extra-virgin olive oil

2 tablespoons freshly squeezed lime juice

1 tablespoon chopped fresh cilantro or parsley

2 teaspoons wasabi powder mixed with 1 teaspoon water, or 2 teaspoons wasabi paste

1/2 teaspoon sea salt

Put all the ingredients in a food processor and process until smooth. Do a FASS check (see page 44); you may want to add a squeeze of lime juice or a pinch of salt.

Variation: If you're up for it, go the extra mile and add another 1/4 teaspoon of wasabi powder to amp up the *zowie* factor in this dip.

PREP TIME: 5 minutes COOK TIME: Not applicable

STORAGE: Store in an airtight container in the refrigerator for up to 2 days.

PER SERVING: (2 tablespoons per serving) Calories: 70; Total Fat: 6 g (1 g saturated, 4.5 g monounsaturated); Carbohydrates: 2.5 g; Protein: 2 g; Fiber: 1 g; Sodium: 100 mg

Curried Deviled Eggs

People have been deviling eggs for almost as long as there have been eggs to devil. Recipes can be found in writings from ancient Rome, thirteenth-century Andalusia, and current culinary blogs worldwide. I'm into deviled eggs both for their flavor and for practical reasons. They keep well in the fridge, and they're an ideal protein-packed snack. Grandma might have spiked them with a little paprika on top, but the flavors I've come up with are a lot more interesting: mint, cilantro, curry powder, and turmeric. Nana will either be astounded or appalled, depending upon whether she considers you to be inspired or heretical. I'm betting she'd go with inspired. MAKES 4 SERVINGS

4 organic eggs
2 tablespoons organic plain yogurt
1 tablespoon chopped fresh cilantro
2 teaspoons chopped fresh mint
½ teaspoon curry powder
¼ teaspoon turmeric
¼ teaspoon freshly ground black
   pepper
¼ teaspoon sea salt

COOK'S NOTE: If you bring the eggs to room temperature before cooking them, you'll shave a few minutes off the cooking time and also decrease the chance of the eggs cracking in the hot water. To bring them to room temperature more quickly, put them in a bowl of warm water. And if you'd like to boil them in advance, it's fine to store them in their shells in the refrigerator for up to 3 days.

Put the eggs in saucepan and add enough cold water to cover them by about 1 inch. Bring to a boil over medium-high heat, then cover and immediately remove from the heat. Let sit for 15 to 18 minutes, until the water is tepid.

Transfer the eggs to a bowl of cool water. When they're cool enough to handle, peel them under cold running water. Cut the eggs in half lengthwise. Scoop out the yolks and put them in a small bowl. Add the yogurt, cilantro, 1 teaspoon of the mint, curry powder, turmeric, pepper, and salt and stir with a fork until smooth. Spoon the mixture into the egg whites and sprinkle with the remaining mint.

PREP TIME: 15 minutes COOK TIME: 20 minutes
STORAGE: Store in an airtight container in the refrigerator for up to 2 days.
PER SERVING: Calories: 80; Total Fat: 5 g (2 g saturated, 2 g monounsaturated); Carbohydrates: 2 g; Protein: 7 g; Fiber: 0 g; Sodium: 189 mg

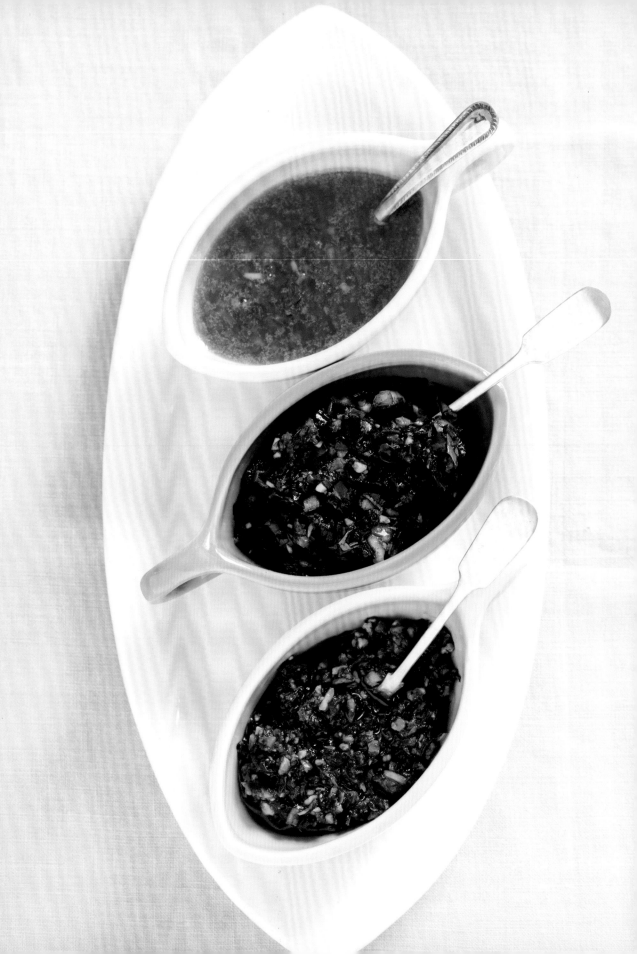

CHAPTER 9

Dollops of Yum!

Dollops might seem like a flourish: a nice but hardly necessary accessory for finishing a dish. I beg to differ.

Flavorful dollops are essential. So much so that if you told me you only had time to make recipes from one chapter of the book, dollops would be the chapter I'd pick.

Here's my reasoning: while most of the recipes in this book don't take long to make, if you're short on time the dollops are the fastest, yet because they're concentrated, their health benefits rival those of many of the recipes in other chapters. For example, the phytochemicals in just five peppermint leaves (about ¼ teaspoon chopped) can be effective in cancer prevention. That's what I call serious bang for the buck! And it's not an isolated case. Basil, parsley, lemon zest, pomegranate, pistachios, cinnamon, cayenne—pick a dollop and you'll find ingredients chock-full of nutrients that regulate blood sugar, protect the heart, help improve memory, fight infection, keep bones strong, and much more.

DOLLOP	GOES WITH...
Ancho Chile Relish (page 180)	Costa Rican Black Bean Soup with Sweet Potato (page 68), Chicken Tortilla Soup (page 70), White Bean and Chicken Chili (page 76), Black Bean Skillet Cakes (page 134), Herby Turkey Sliders (page 153)
Basil Pistachio Pesto (page 179) and Kale-Basil Pesto (page 121)	Peppino's Cowboy Minestrone with Herb Mini Meatballs (page 78), Tuscan Beans and Greens (page 100), Sicilian Green Beans (page 101), Roasted Fingerling Potatoes (page 103), Lemony Lentil and Quinoa Salad (page 117), Flat-Out Good Chicken (page 148), Herby Turkey Sliders (page 153), and as a sauce for pasta dishes
Chive Oil (page 178)	Summer's Sweetest Corn Bisque (page 60), Julie's "Spring Is Busting Out All Over" Soup (page 61), Vampire Slayer's Soup (page 64), Ridiculously Good Split Pea Soup (page 73), and almost any vegetable, grain, or fish dish
Greener Than Green Goddess Dressing (page 186)	Avocado Lover's Salad (page 83) and your favorite salads.
Indonesian Drizzle and pesto variation (page 183)	Quinoa with Edamame, Ginger, and Lime (page 118), Hot-and-Sour Sesame Soba Noodles (page 126), Roasted Wild Salmon (page 139), Smoked Salmon Nori Rolls (page 140)
Lemon Dijon Vinaigrette (page 185)	Lemon Chive Potatoes (page 102), Flat-Out Good Chicken (page 148), and as a marinade for chicken and fish
Lemony Balsamic Vinaigrette (page 185)	Strawberry, Fennel, and Arugula Salad (page 91), Walnut, Date, and Herb Salad (page 92), and as an all-purpose salad dressing
Lime Vinaigrette with Toasted Cumin Seeds (page 184)	Mexican Cabbage Crunch (page 86), Greek Chicken Salad (page 145), Flat-Out Good Chicken (page 148), as all-purpose marinade for chicken and fish, and as an all-purpose salad dressing

But that's just the start. These dollops have so much flavor and visual appeal that they're irresistible, whether you're new to cooking or highly experienced. Spoon or drizzle them over your go-to recipes to take them to a whole new level of flavor and nutrition. You'll find them invaluable in motivating people to joyfully savor every nutritious morsel on their plates. That's the kind of positive feedback cooks thrive on.

The concoctions in this chapter are also extremely versatile. With just a few tweaks, you can transform a glaze into a marinade or dressing. They also store extremely well, so you can make enough to last a while and store them in the refrigerator or freezer. I always have a few dollops on hand. That way, no matter what I choose to make for dinner, I can dress it up any way I please. That kind of flexibility makes both cooking and dining fun, creating positive connections that turn healthy eating from a novelty into an embraceable, sustainable way of life.

Below you'll find a chart—I call it my "dollop cheat sheet"—which will give you an idea of how to pair dollops with recipes in the book. Of course you're free to create your own pairings . . . and do let me know when you hit one out of the park; those kinds of emails make my day!

DOLLOP	GOES WITH . . .
Many-Herb Gremolata (page 181)	Pan-Seared Scallops with Citrus Drizzle (page 144), and just about any other savory dish
My Go-To Marinade and dressing variation (page 188)	Not Your Typical Tabouli (page 120), Flat-Out Good Chicken (page 148), Mediterranean Kebabs (page 150), and drizzled on vegetables
Olive and Mint Vinaigrette (page 181)	Sicilian Green Beans (page 101), Roasted Wild Salmon (page 139), and as a drizzle on chicken, fish, and vegetables.
Papaya and Avocado Salsa (page 191)	Roasted Halibut with Lime (page 137), Flat-Out Good Chicken (page 148), and as a topping for chicken or fish
Parsley Mint Drizzle (page 189)	Curried Butternut Squash Soup (page 65), Flat-Out Good Chicken (page 148), Mediterranean Kebabs (page 150), stirred into grains, and drizzled on chicken and fish
Pomegranate Molasses (page 192) and Pomegranate Glaze (page 194)	Cozy Roasted Vegetable Soup (page 63), Curried Butternut Squash Soup (page 65), Flat-Out Good Chicken (page 148), Mediterranean Kebabs (page 150), Moroccan Mint Lamb Chops (page 154), and other chicken or lamb dishes
Sesame Miso Dressing (page 187)	Asian Cabbage Crunch (page 87), Hot-and-Sour Sesame Soba Noodles (page 126), and drizzled on chicken and fish
Yogurt Sauce with Citrus and Mint (page 195)	Not Your Typical Tabouli (page 120), Roasted Wild Salmon (page 139), Wild, Wild Salmon Burgers (page 142), Flat-Out Good Chicken (page 148)
Yogurt Tahini Sauce (page 195)	Mediterranean Kebabs (page 150) and Moroccan Mint Lamb Chops (page 154)

Chive Oil

If you believe, as I do, that ancient ingredients have generally stood the test of time because they possess elements important for well-being, let me introduce you to chives, which have been used in recipes for about five thousand years. I'm so partial to chives that I grow them in my garden for both their wonderful flavor and the beautiful purple flowers the plant produces. They're members of the genus *Allium*, making them cousins to onions, garlic, shallots, and leeks. The sulfur in chives is believed to help the liver detoxify the body, but you won't taste any of that sulfur in this drizzle. Instead, their volatile oils impart an almost sweet onion fragrance. This oil adds a bright, fresh-green pop to soups, salads, and fish. As for whether it also imparts the wisdom of the ancients, well, there's only one way to find out. (Pictured on page 174; top bowl.) MAKES ½ CUP

½ cup chopped fresh chives
½ cup extra-virgin olive oil
Pinch of sea salt

Put all the ingredients in a blender and process until smooth.

PREP TIME: 5 minutes
STORAGE: Store in an airtight container in the refrigerator for up to 2 weeks.
PER SERVING: (2 tablespoons per serving) Calories: 120; Total Fat: 14 g (2 g saturated, 11 g monounsaturated); Carbohydrates: 0 g; Protein: 0 g; Fiber: 0 g; Sodium: 5 mg

Basil Pistachio Pesto

Talk about longevity: Pistachio trees can bear fruit for two hundred years, and they've been doing that for a long, long time. Pistachios are even mentioned in the Bible. Pistachios are a little wellness center unto themselves, rich in potassium and B6. Their buttery taste is also extremely addictive, and I have pictures of my green hands to prove it. That's one reason why I've chosen to use them in this pesto, rather than the traditional pine nuts. When I prepare this for guests, it seldom makes it to the dining room table, but instead ends up on crackers, carrots, pinkies . . . whatever people can find for dipping when they wander into the kitchen. (Pictured on page 174; bottom bowl.) MAKES ²/₃ CUP

1 cup tightly packed fresh basil leaves
¹/₂ cup shelled raw pistachios
¹/₃ cup extra-virgin olive oil
1 tablespoon freshly squeezed lemon juice
¹/₄ teaspoon sea salt
¹/₄ teaspoon freshly ground black pepper
1 tablespoon water (optional)

Put the basil, pistachios, olive oil, lemon juice, salt, and pepper in a food processor and process until well blended. For a thinner pesto, add the water and briefly process again. Do a FASS check (see page 44); you may want to add a squeeze of lemon juice or a pinch of salt.

PREP TIME: 5 minutes
STORAGE: Store in an airtight container in the refrigerator for up to 5 days or in the freezer for up to 2 months.
PER SERVING: (1 tablespoon per serving) Calories: 90; Total Fat: 9 g (1 g saturated, 7 g monounsaturated); Carbohydrates: 2 g; Protein: 1 g; Fiber: 1 g; Sodium: 37 mg

LIVE LONG AND PROSPER: Basil has come a long way over the centuries. In Socrates's time, Greeks believed basil would bring poor fortune and enmity from others. That vibe lasted well into the seventeenth-century, when a noted English physician and herbalist announced that basil must surely bode ill health, because it refused to grow near rue, "as great an enemy to poison as any that grows." Thank heavens attitudes finally turned around—and that someone finally put basil under the microscope. As it turns out, basil wards off infection, inflammation, and free radicals intent on harming the walls of blood vessels. It may even keep radiation from harming chromosomes. To paraphrase Paul Harvey, now you know the *rest* of basil's story. Glad I could set the record straight.

Ancho Chile Relish

Wilbur Scoville should be the patron saint of chile pepper fans. In 1912, he invented a scientific scale that forever settled the question of which chile pepper is hottest. Not that settling bar bets was his intent; as a pharmacist, he was probably more interested in the medicinal aspects of capsaicin—the active ingredient in chiles that not only provides the heat, but also increases metabolic rate and fights inflammation. Ancho chiles come in at around 1,000 Scoville heat units, which could seem frightening until you compare them to habaneros, which top out at 350,000. So, all things considered, this relish is more sultry than steaming. Garlic, onion, lime juice, herbs, spices round out the flavor. (Pictured on page 174; middle bowl.) MAKES ³/₄ CUP

2 dried ancho chiles
¹/₃ cup finely diced red onion
¹/₃ cup chopped fresh cilantro
1 teaspoon minced garlic
1 teaspoon dried oregano
¹/₄ teaspoon ground cumin
¹/₄ teaspoon sea salt
¹/₈ teaspoon ground cinnamon
2 tablespoons freshly squeezed
    lime juice
1 tablespoon extra-virgin olive oil
1¹/₄ teaspoons Grade B maple syrup

COOK'S NOTE: This relish is so versatile. Mix it with black beans or brown rice, serve it on top of eggs, use it as a condiment for fajitas, include it when sautéing green beans, and the list goes on. It's also great on beef, turkey, or chicken.

Soak the dried chiles in hot water for about 15 minutes. (Using a sharp knife, poke a hole in the chile so that they soak instead of float!) Drain, discarding the soaking liquid. Seed and mince the chiles, then put them in a small bowl. Add the onion, cilantro, garlic, oregano, cumin, salt, cinnamon, lime juice, olive oil, and maple syrup and stir to combine. Taste; you may want to add a spritz of lime juice.

PREP TIME: 20 minutes
STORAGE: Store in an airtight container in the refrigerator for up to 5 days.
PER SERVING: (1 tablespoon per serving) Calories: 25; Total Fat: 1.5 g (0 g saturated, 1 g monounsaturated); Carbohydrates: 3 g; Protein: 0.5 g; Fiber: 1 g; Sodium: 35 mg

Many-Herb Gremolata

When I told my coauthor, Mat, I was making gremolata, his response was "Gremolata? That sounds like one of those old American Motors cars." That's what I get for speaking Italian to him. Gremolata is a traditional Milanese condiment that sounds fancy, but it's merely chopped herbs, garlic, and lemon zest. MAKES ¼ CUP

¼ cup finely chopped fresh parsley
1 tablespoon finely chopped fresh mint or basil
1 tablespoon finely chopped fresh thyme
Grated zest of 1 lemon
1 teaspoon minced garlic

Put all the ingredients in a small bowl and stir to combine.

PREP TIME: 5 minutes
STORAGE: Store in an airtight container in the refrigerator for up to 5 days.
PER SERVING: (2 teaspoons per serving) Calories: 2; Total Fat: 0 g (0 g saturated, 0 g monounsaturated); Carbohydrates: 0.5 g; Protein: 0 g; Fiber: 0 g; Sodium: 1.5 mg

Olive and Mint Vinaigrette

I think of this vinaigrette as a culinary reveille. It was designed as a serious wake-up call for the taste buds. Normally I pair salty and sweet flavors because they're complementary opposites. But sometimes the combination of salty and fresh works well, as it does here with olives and mint. I love to bring this kind of mouth pop to bear on fish and chicken dishes, which always benefit from a little zing. Mint is a breath freshener, but that's only the most obvious of its charms. It also aids digestion, is packed with vitamin C, and inhibits tumor growth. MAKES ¾ CUP

¼ cup freshly squeezed lemon juice
1 teaspoon Dijon mustard
¼ teaspoon sea salt
⅛ teaspoon freshly ground black pepper
1 tablespoon minced shallot
¼ cup extra-virgin olive oil
¼ cup kalamata olives, finely chopped
2 tablespoons fresh finely chopped fresh mint

Put the lemon juice, Dijon mustard, salt, pepper, and shallot in a small bowl and stir to combine. Slowly pour in the olive oil, whisking all the while, and continue whisking until smooth. Add the olives and mint. Transfer to a small container with a fitted lid and shake well.

PREP TIME: 5 minutes
STORAGE: Store in an airtight container in the refrigerator for up to 5 days.
PER SERVING: (2 tablespoons per serving) Calories: 70; Total Fat: 8 g (1 g saturated, 6 g monounsaturated); Carbohydrates: 1 g; Protein: 0 g; Fiber: 0 g; Sodium: 75 mg

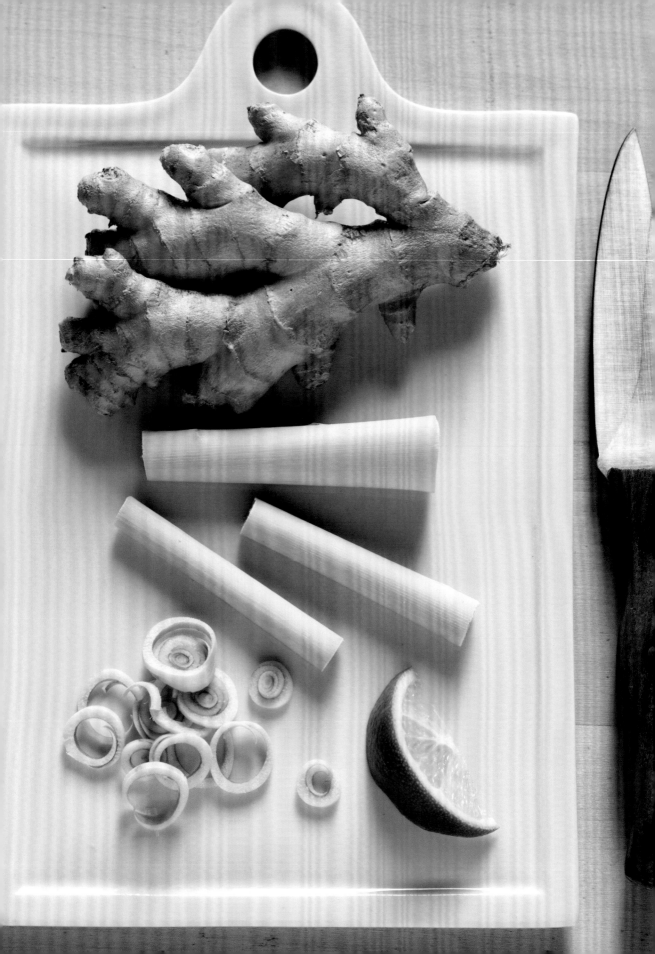

Indonesian Drizzle

This is my go-to dollop when people say, "Gee, I'm in the mood for Thai food." There's a distinct flavor profile that most people associate with Southeast Asian cuisine, and it typically includes lemongrass, so that's the launch point for this recipe. The key with lemongrass is to use it not as a diva, dominating the orchestra, but as a team player, pulling together all the other performers. Here I've given lemongrass a lot to work with—cilantro, mint, parsley, garlic, ginger, and more—and the result is a wellness waltz. This drizzle is perfect on any fish or chicken dish that calls out for an Asian accent. MAKES ½ CUP

¾ cup loosely packed fresh cilantro leaves
¼ cup loosely packed fresh mint leaves
¼ cup loosely packed fresh flat-leaf parsley leaves
1 tablespoon minced lemongrass (see note, page 76)
2 teaspoons minced fresh ginger
1 teaspoon minced garlic
3 tablespoons freshly squeezed lime juice
3 tablespoons extra-virgin olive oil
2 teaspoons fish sauce
½ teaspoon Grade B maple syrup
⅛ teaspoon sea salt
Pinch of cayenne

Combine all the ingredients in a blender or food processor and process until smooth and creamy. Do a FASS check (see page 44); if the drizzle tastes too sour, add a pinch of salt.

Variation: Add ½ cup of cashews for an irresistible, out-of-this-world pesto.

PREP TIME: 15 minutes
STORAGE: Store in an airtight container in the refrigerator for up to 2 days.
PER SERVING: (1 tablespoon per serving) Calories: 45; Total Fat: 4.5 g (0.5 g saturated, 3.3 g monounsaturated); Carbohydrates: 1.5 g; Protein: 0.5 g; Fiber: 0 g; Sodium: 98 mg

COOK'S NOTE: Lemongrass is a woody herb that looks like a baton and has an aromatic lemony flavor. You can find it in the produce section of well-stocked grocery stores or at Asian markets. To use lemongrass, cut off the root end and the grassy top. Peel away the fibrous outer layers to expose the tender layers of the inner stalk. With a sharp knife, finely slice the lemongrass crosswise starting from the bottom and working your way up the stalk.

WHO KNEW? Cilantro tends to be a love-it-or-hate-it ingredient, and it turns out your opinion depends entirely on your DNA. Some folks have a gene that makes cilantro taste like soap, which makes it hard to become a fan, even if they really wish they could on account of how healthful this herb is. If you're looking to replace cilantro in a recipe, try Italian flat-leaf parsley—it's a great power herb that will give you a similar nutritional wollop.

Lime Vinaigrette with Toasted Cumin Seeds

I can understand why our distant ancestors must have thought fire was magic. Applying heat to certain foods releases their aromas and delights the senses. That's definitely the case with cumin seeds. Toast them for a tad and their oils release a lovely fragrance. The fire also unlocks a treasure trove of well-being, making some of the beneficial compounds in cumin more available to the body to stimulate digestive enzymes, help fight cancer, and improve the absorption of other nutrients. This is a simple vinaigrette, with just a few basic ingredients. Does it fly? I'll leave you with the three words written on the recipe by Catherine, an exacting recipe tester with pitch-perfect taste buds: "Yum. Loved it." MAKES 1/2 CUP

1/4 cup freshly squeezed lime juice
1 teaspoon freshly squeezed lemon juice
1/2 teaspoon grated lemon zest
1/2 teaspoon sea salt
1/8 teaspoon cayenne
1 teaspoon cumin seeds, toasted (see note, page 83)
1 tablespoon Grade B maple syrup
1/4 cup extra-virgin olive oil

COOK'S NOTE: Although toasting the cumin seeds may seem like an unnecessary step, I assure you it's worth the few minutes it takes. Toasting unleashes the volatile oils in the cumin seeds, coaxing out their tremendous flavor and boosting their longevity benefits.

Put the lime juice, lemon juice, lemon zest, salt, cayenne, cumin seeds, and maple syrup in a small bowl and stir to combine. Slowly pour in the olive oil, whisking all the while, and continue whisking until smooth. Transfer to a small container with a fitted lid and shake well.

PREP TIME: 5 minutes
STORAGE: Store in an airtight container in the refrigerator for up to 5 days.
PER SERVING: (1 tablespoon per serving) Calories: 70; Total Fat: 7 g (1 g saturated, 5.5 g monounsaturated); Carbohydrates: 2.5 g; Protein: 0 g; Fiber: 0 g; Sodium: 110 mg

Lemony Balsamic Vinaigrette

Like Lemon Dijon Vinaigrette (page 185), this dressing lends a light, refreshing flavor to all manner of foods. Since it could hardly be easier to make, I recommend keeping some on hand at all times. I know I do. MAKES ½ CUP

2 tablespoons balsamic vinegar
2 tablespoons freshly squeezed lemon juice
½ teaspoon grated lemon zest
½ teaspoon sea salt
½ teaspoon freshly ground black pepper
¼ cup extra-virgin olive oil

COOK'S NOTE: Add the salt with the acid but *prior* to adding the oil. The reason? The acid breaks down the salt, allowing it to do its job as a flavor carrier.

Put the balsamic vinegar, lemon juice, lemon zest, salt, pepper, in a small bowl and stir to combine. Slowly pour in the olive oil, whisking all the while, and continue whisking until smooth. Transfer to a small container with a fitted lid and shake well.

PREP TIME: 5 minutes
STORAGE: Store in a glass jar in the refrigerator for up to 1 week.
PER SERVING: (2 tablespoons per serving) Calories: 130; Total Fat: 14 g (2 g saturated, 11 g monounsaturated); Carbohydrates: 2 g; Protein: 0 g; Fiber: 0 g; Sodium: 200 mg

Lemon Dijon Vinaigrette

I always have a container of this vinaigrette on hand. It's the perfect solution when just about anything I'm cooking needs a light, fresh lift. The lemon zest and juice brighten everything they touch, whether used as a marinade, a salad dressing, or a drizzle. Try it and see if it doesn't help you leave the table feeling satiated without overstuffing yourself. MAKES 1 CUP

¼ cup freshly squeezed lemon juice
1 teaspoon Dijon mustard
¼ teaspoon sea salt
⅛ teaspoon freshly ground black pepper
2 tablespoons minced shallot
½ teaspoon minced garlic
½ cup extra-virgin olive oil

Put the lemon juice, Dijon mustard, salt, pepper, shallot, and garlic in a small bowl and stir to combine. Slowly pour in the olive oil, whisking all the while, and continue whisking until smooth. Transfer to a small container with a fitted lid and shake well.

PREP TIME: 5 minutes
STORAGE: Store in an airtight container in the refrigerator for up to 5 days.
PER SERVING: (2 tablespoons per serving) Calories: 130; Total Fat: 14 g (2 g saturated, 11 g monounsaturated); Carbohydrates: 2 g; Protein: 0 g; Fiber: 0 g; Sodium: 200 mg

Greener Than Green Goddess Dressing

This one goes out to my dad, Jay, who made salad dressings for a living. In fact, he was one of the first to jump on the Green goddess bandwagon when it made a comeback in the early 1970s. It gets its name from the emerald colors of parsley and a bouquet of other herbs. In this recipe, I've replaced Dad's mayo and sour cream base with healthier but no less tasty avocados and yogurt. In addition to being luscious, avocados offer up healthy fats and glutathione, an antioxidant that works inside of cells to prevent and reverse damage, making it an essential complement to most other antioxidants that cruise around the body and neutralize free radicals before they can get into cells. MAKES 1³/₄ CUPS

³/₄ cup water
¹/₂ cup organic plain yogurt
2 tablespoons freshly squeezed
    lemon juice
2 tablespoons extra-virgin olive oil
1 avocado, halved and flesh
    scooped out
¹/₄ cup chopped fresh parsley
2 scallions, white and green parts,
    chopped
1 clove garlic, chopped
¹/₂ teaspoon sea salt

Put all the ingredients in a blender or food processor and process until smooth and creamy. Do a FASS check (see page 44); you may want to add a pinch of salt and a squeeze of lemon juice.

PREP TIME: 5 minutes
STORAGE: Store in an airtight container in the refrigerator for up to 3 days.
PER SERVING: (2 tablespoons per serving) Calories: 55; Total Fat: 4 g (1 g saturated, 3 g monounsaturated); Carbohydrates: 4 g; Protein: 1 g; Fiber: 2 g; Sodium: 110 mg

WHO KNEW? Certain nutrients are absorbed better when eaten with avocado. In one study, participants eating a salad containing avocado absorbed *five* times the amount of carotenoids (including lycopene and beta-carotene) than those who didn't consume avocado.

Sesame Miso Dressing

If the United Nations ever bottled a dressing, this would be it. Half of the countries in the General Assembly are represented. There's tahini (ground sesame seeds) from the Middle East, rice vinegar from China, miso from Japan, and cayenne from French Guiana. Sesame seeds rate a ten out of ten on the wellness scale, offering an array of minerals, including zinc, calcium, and, notably, magnesium, which promotes sound sleep. Although the ingredients are global, the flavor is distinctively Asian. In addition to using it as a salad dressing, try drizzling it over cooked fish. However you use it, you won't need a UN translator to make sense of it; just put your taste buds to work. MAKES 1/2 CUP

2 tablespoons mellow (light) miso
1 tablespoon tahini
3 tablespoons rice vinegar
1 tablespoon tamari
1 tablespoon Grade B maple syrup
1 tablespoon freshly squeezed
    lime juice
1 teaspoon freshly squeezed
    lemon juice
1/2 teaspoon grated lemon zest
2 teaspoons grated fresh ginger
Pinch of cayenne

In a small bowl, combine the miso and tahini and stir with a fork until smooth. Add the vinegar, tamari, maple syrup, lime juice, lemon juice, lemon zest, ginger, and cayenne and whisk until well combined.

PREP TIME: 5 minutes
STORAGE: Store in an airtight container in the refrigerator for up to 5 days.
PER SERVING: (2 tablespoons per serving) Calories: 30; Total Fat: 1 g (0 g saturated, 0 g monounsaturated); Carbohydrates: 4.5 g; Protein: 1.5 g; Fiber: 1 g; Sodium: 256 mg

My Go-To Marinade

This marinade is my secret weapon in the fridge, the talisman I wave over anything that needs a little oomph. Fish, chicken, potatoes, chickpeas, or roasted eggplant—it doesn't matter; this is a one-hit wonder that makes everything sing. Nutritionally, it's the marinade equivalent of Magic Mineral Broth 2.0 (page 55), chock-full of well-being from a host of aromatic ingredients. If I were stranded on a desert island, I'd want to have this marinade in my culinary survival kit. MAKES ³/₄ CUP

¹/₂ cup diced onion
¹/₄ cup chopped fresh parsley
2 tablespoons chopped fresh mint
1 tablespoon minced garlic
1 tablespoon chopped fresh thyme, or 1 teaspoon dried
2 teaspoons ground cumin
1 teaspoon ground cinnamon
¹/₄ teaspoon sea salt
Pinch of cayenne
¹/₂ cup extra-virgin olive oil

Put all the ingredients in a blender or food processor and process until smooth.

Variation: To use this marinade as a salad dressing, whisk in a squeeze of fresh lemon juice.

PREP TIME: 10 minutes
STORAGE: Store in an airtight container in the refrigerator for up to 5 days.
PER SERVING: (3 tablespoons per serving) Calories: 90; Total Fat: 9 g (1.5 g saturated, 7 g monounsaturated); Carbohydrates: 1 g; Protein: 0.5 g; Fiber: 0.5 g; Sodium: 37 mg

Parsley Mint Drizzle

This drizzle is rather self-explanatory. It's freshness to the third power (or perhaps freshness cubed is more apt for those of us who appreciate knife skills) and works wonders for kebabs or anytime you'd like to put a Mediterranean spin on a dish. Parsley and mint freshen the breath, aid digestion, and can even inhibit tumor growth. MAKES ½ CUP, 1 TABLESPOON PER SERVING

1 cup tightly packed fresh
   parsley leaves
½ cup tightly packed fresh
   mint leaves
2 tablespoons freshly squeezed
   lemon juice
¼ teaspoon sea salt
1 teaspoon Grade B maple syrup
¼ cup extra-virgin olive oil
1 tablespoon water

Combine all the ingredients in a food processor and process until well blended. For a thinner drizzle, and another tablespoon of water and briefly process again. Do a FASS check (see page 44); you may want to add a pinch of salt.

Variation: For a Latin or Asian flavor, substitute cilantro for the parsley.

PREP TIME: 5 minutes
STORAGE: Store in an airtight container in the refrigerator for up to 5 days or in the freezer for up to 2 months.
PER SERVING: (1 tablespoon per serving) Calories: 60; Total Fat: 7 g (1 g saturated, 5 g monounsaturated); Carbohydrates: 1 g; Protein: 0 g; Fiber: 0 g; Sodium: 75 mg

COOK'S NOTE: To quickly remove stems from cilantro or parsley, hold a clean, towel-dried bunch of the herbs in your nondominant hand, angling them downward 45 degrees, with the top of the bunch touching the cutting board. Scrape down along the stems with a chef's knife, using short strokes, to separate the leaves from the stems.

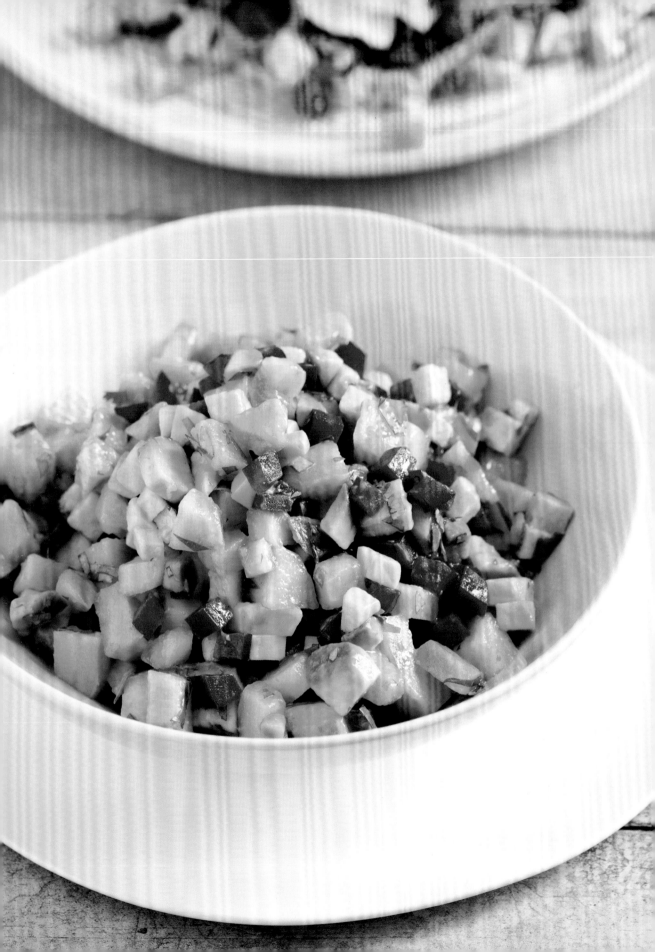

Papaya and Avocado Salsa

The name of this dollop alone is enough to make you sigh. Avocado and papaya—do I really need to say more? Papaya's key enzyme, papain, is a superb digestive aid and is often used in tenderizing blends. I designed this sweet, creamy salsa, which looks like edible confetti, to go with halibut, but it will take any fish or chicken dish from ballast to bling. MAKES 2 CUPS

1 cup diced papaya
1 cup diced avocado
3 tablespoons finely diced red bell pepper
3 tablespoons finely chopped fresh cilantro
2 tablespoons freshly squeezed lime juice
1 tablespoon extra-virgin olive oil
1/4 teaspoon sea salt
Pinch of cayenne

Put all the ingredients in a bowl and stir gently to combine. For optimal flavor, cover and let sit at room temperature for 30 minutes before serving.

Variations: Substitute mango, pineapple, or tomato for the papaya. Substitute pomegranate seeds for the red bell pepper.

PREP TIME: 10 minutes
STORAGE: Store in an airtight container in the refrigerator for up to 3 days.
PER SERVING: (3 tablespoons per serving) Calories: 55; Total Fat: 4.5 g (0.5 g saturated, 3 g monounsaturated); Carbohydrates: 4 g; Protein: 1 g; Fiber: 2 g; Sodium: 55 mg

Pomegranate Molasses

For a long time, culinary wisdom held that there were four basic flavors that the taste buds could measure—sweet, sour, salty, and fat—and that much of the art of cooking lay in learning how to balance those four basic flavors. But it turns out that there's a fifth taste at play: umami. Umami is actually less about flavor and more a certain savory sensation in the mouth (see page 47), and pomegranate has it in abundance. As a cook, I revel in the tannins in pomegranate (which echo those in red wine). It's a wake-up call for the taste buds. Concentrating pomegranate juice into pomegranate molasses only ups the ante. You may be able to find pomegranate molasses in specialty stores or ethnic markets, but as you'll see in this recipe, it's really easy to make. Just three ingredients: pomegranate juice, Grade B maple syrup, and lemon juice. It's great drizzled over soup, lamb, fish, or chicken or even added to a smoothie. MAKES 1¼ CUPS

4 cups unsweetened pomegranate juice
⅓ cup Grade B maple syrup
2 tablespoons freshly squeezed lemon juice

COOK'S NOTE: Pomegranate molasses is basically a reduction: a culinary preparation made by cooking down a liquid (usually broth, wine, or a sauce) until evaporation reduces its volume. The result is a thicker consistency and intensified flavors.

Put all the ingredients in a large saucepan over medium-high heat and stir to combine. Cook uncovered until the mixture starts to bubble. Decrease the heat to very low—just enough to maintain a simmer—and cook uncovered, stirring occasionally, until syrupy and reduced to about 1¼ cups, about 45 minutes Taste; you may want to add a bit of maple syrup or a squeeze of lemon juice.

PREP TIME: 5 minutes COOK TIME: 50 minutes
STORAGE: Store in an airtight container in the refrigerator for up to 2 weeks or in the freezer for up to 3 months.
PER SERVING: (2 tablespoons per serving) Calories: 45; Total Fat: 0 g (0 g saturated, 0 g monounsaturated); Carbohydrates: 11 g; Protein: 0 g; Fiber: 0 g; Sodium: 5 mg

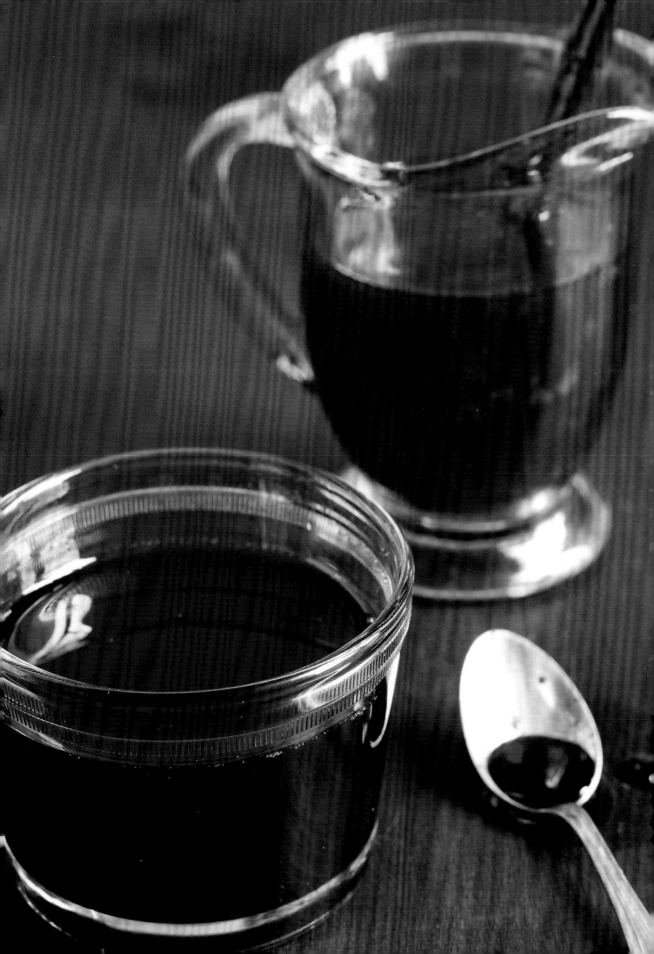

Pomegranate Glaze

When I create a new recipe, I'm looking for the "Eureka!" moment where the elements (guided, no doubt, by the muses) yield a new taste. The moment I first tasted this pomegranate glaze, I got hints of such a discovery. It was such a unique blend of ingredients; rich pomegranate, garlic, and shallots—all sautéed in olive oil. With every tweak, I got closer and closer. Turns out all it took to bring it home was a spritz of blood orange at the end. This magical glaze goes great with salmon, chicken, lamb, and especially the Moroccan Mint Lamb Chops on page 154. MAKES 3/4 CUP

1 teaspoon extra-virgin olive oil
2 cloves garlic, finely chopped
1 shallot, finely chopped
Sea salt
1/2 cup pomegranate molasses, homemade (page 192) or store-bought
1/4 cup organic vegetable or chicken broth, homemade (page 55 or 56) or store-bought
2 tablespoons Grade B maple syrup
1 tablespoon tomato paste
1 cinnamon stick
1 tablespoon freshly squeezed blood orange juice

COOK'S NOTE: If blood oranges aren't available, substitute the juice of a Valencia orange. You can take this recipe over the top if you add 1/2 teaspoon of grated orange zest.

Heat the olive oil in a small saucepan over medium-high heat. Add the garlic, shallot, and a pinch of the salt and sauté until lightly browned, about 5 minutes. Stir in the pomegranate molasses, broth, maple syrup, tomato paste, and cinnamon stick. Decrease the heat to medium and cook, stirring occasionally, until thickened, 10 to 15 minutes. Remove from the heat and stir in the orange juice. Do a FASS check (see page 44); you may want to and add a pinch of salt and a squeeze of lemon juice.

PREP TIME: 5 minutes COOK TIME: 15 minutes
STORAGE: Store in an airtight container in the refrigerator for up to 5 days.
PER SERVING: (2 tablespoons per serving) Calories: 45; Total Fat: 0 g (0 g saturated, 0 g monounsaturated); Carbohydrates: 11 g; Protein: 0 g; Fiber: 0 g; Sodium: 25 mg

Yogurt Sauce with Citrus and Mint

There's a reason no one's ever written a book called *The Joy of Tartar Sauce*. It may be the traditional condiment for many a fish dish, but really, can't we do better? Consider this sauce my humble attempt to achieve that. It's an energetic finishing touch that was designed to go with the Wild, Wild Salmon Burgers (page 142), but it will complement plenty of other recipes in the book (see the dollop chart on pages 176–77). The combination of yogurt and flourishes of citrus, cayenne, and mint will make tartar sauce seem, by comparison, like something from the Paleozoic era. This is what culinary evolution is all about. MAKES 1 CUP

1 cup organic plain Greek yogurt
1 teaspoon freshly squeezed
    orange juice
1 teaspoon grated orange zest
1 teaspoon freshly squeezed
    lemon juice
1 teaspoon grated lemon zest
1/4 teaspoon sea salt
Pinch of cayenne
2 tablespoons chopped fresh mint

Put all the ingredients in a small bowl and stir to combine. Cover and let sit at room temperature for 15 minutes for the flavors to meld.

PREP TIME: 5 minutes
STORAGE: Store in an airtight container in the refrigerator for up to 5 days.
PER SERVING: (1 tablespoon per serving) Calories: 40; Total Fat: 3 g (2 g saturated, 0 g monounsaturated); Carbohydrates: 1 g; Protein: 2 g; Fiber: 0 g; Sodium: 60 mg

Yogurt Tahini Sauce

Believe it or not, some head chefs actually hire *sauciers* just to make sauces. And believe it or not, I once saw a head chef throw a full bottle of wine at the head of a *saucier* just because the sauce wasn't up to snuff. Such needless drama! You don't have to be a graduate of the French Culinary Institute to create great sauces. In fact, it can be pretty easy, as this sauce proves. And in addition to being delicious atop chicken kebabs and veggies, it has top-notch anti-inflammatory ingredients, particularly the sesame seeds in the tahini. If you're looking for Sturm und Drang, you won't find it here. I leave that to the folks at the Food Network. MAKES 1/2 CUP

1/2 cup organic plain yogurt
1/4 cup tahini
1 tablespoon freshly squeezed
    lemon juice
1/4 teaspoon sea salt
1/4 teaspoon ground cumin
1/4 teaspoon Grade B maple syrup

Put all the ingredients in a small bowl and stir until well combined.

PREP TIME: 5 minutes
STORAGE: Store in an airtight container in the refrigerator for up to 5 days.
PER SERVING: (2 tablespoons per serving) Calories: 70; Total Fat: 6 g (2 g saturated, 0 g monounsaturated); Carbohydrates: 1 g; Protein: 3 g; Fiber: 0.3 g; Sodium: 55 mg

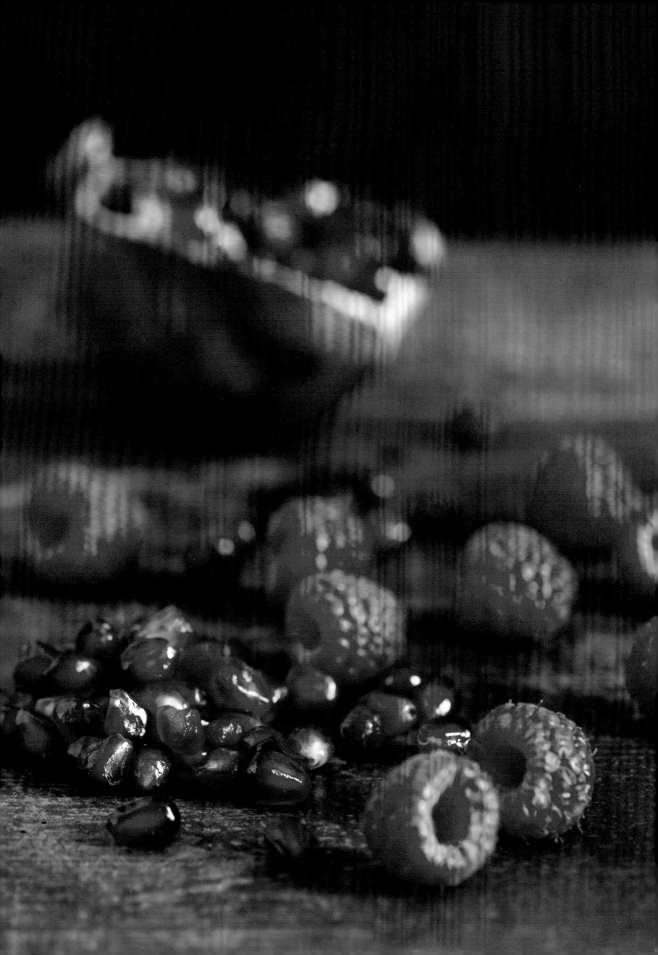

CHAPTER 10

Invigorating Tonics and Elixirs

Every one of us is a miniature estuary, a place where salts meet water to create and sustain life.

The most important way to do that is by staying hydrated. Now, I don't know about you, but every time I hear someone preaching about hydration, I imagine some poor soul getting up in the morning and trying to down a half gallon of water to meet the "quota" for the day. Actually, I know a few people who do this. Personally, I think that's nuts—and potentially dangerous too. We absolutely need water, but getting a lot of it in one big shot, and with nothing to slow the absorption of that water into the system, puts tremendous strain on the kidneys. It also puts tremendous strain on any household with just one bathroom and lots of contenders.

There's a better way, and the recipes in this chapter will provide some direction. The truth is, most of us stay a bit dehydrated, and as we age this often shows up as muscle aches and pains that never quite go away. Other signs include dry skin and constipation. In more severe chronic cases, people become fatigued and foggy, especially if they live in a warm climate and age has impacted their body's ability to adjust its internal thermostat. Fluids can address many of these issues, especially when they're infused with the nutrients and minerals, as in the recipes in this chapter.

I've tried to anticipate the times when thirst tends to strike and create drinks designed to perfectly fit the moment. If you aren't one to sit down in the morning for breakfast, Gregg's Morning Protein Shake (page 206) is an outstanding starter with more than enough sustenance to get you to lunch. Feeling a little under the weather? Simon's Most Nourishing Elixir (page 203) is just that. There are coolers and lemonade for summer, smoothies for an afternoon refresher, and even a twist on an Indian lassi for an exotic taste of the East. So sit down, take a load off, and let these tonics and elixirs transport you to a place where the ice maker is always full, berries are never out of season, and there's always a pitcher waiting in the fridge with your name on it.

Chamomile Lemonade with Green Apple

Whether it's kids, traffic, work, marriage, or any combination thereof, stress is an ever-present factor in most people's lives. I've long turned to chamomile's relaxing properties to pull some of that stress out of my system. A lot of folks like chamomile as a hot tea, but that's not exactly a summertime go-to, thus the inspiration for this lemonade that combines chamomile tea, green apples, lemon juice, and a hint of maple syrup. MAKES 5 CUPS

4 chamomile tea bags
4 1/4 cups boiling water
2 green apples, finely grated
3/4 cup freshly squeezed
   lemon juice
2 teaspoons Grade B maple syrup

Put the tea bags in a heatproof container. Pour in the boiling water and let steep for 4 minutes. Remove the tea bags, then stir in the apples, lemon juice, and maple syrup. Chill for at least 2 hours. Strain through a fine-mesh sieve before serving.

PREP TIME: 10 minutes COOK TIME: 2 hours for chilling
STORAGE: Store in an airtight container in the refrigerator for up to 2 days.
PER SERVING: (1 cup per serving) Calories: 35; Total Fat: 0 g (0 g saturated, 0 g monounsaturated); Carbohydrates: 10 g; Protein: 0 g; Fiber: 2 g; Sodium: 7 mg

Catherine's Survival Shooters

Not long ago, my recipe tester and I were trying to come up with a delicious green drink, as lots of folks are into juicing with fruits and vegetables. Truth be told, our early efforts tasted awful, going completely against my mantra, which requires that each sip deliver great health benefits *and* great flavor. Then I received a phone call from Catherine McConkie, ace recipe taster: "I've broken the code!" she exclaimed, and indeed she had. Parsley was the key, providing both a blast of freshness and antioxidant *vavavooom*. MAKES 4 CUPS

2 cups chopped pineapple
2 cups loosely packed fresh
   parsley leaves
2 cups water
1/4 cup freshly squeezed orange
   juice
1 1/2 teaspoons grated fresh ginger
1/2 teaspoon freshly squeezed
   lemon juice

Combine the ingredients in a blender and process until smooth.

Variations: Substitute mango or papaya for the pineapple. For a colder drink, replace 1 cup of the water with a heaping cup of ice cubes.

PREP TIME: 5 minutes
STORAGE: Store in an airtight container in the refrigerator for up to 1 day.
PER SERVING: (1 cup per serving) Calories: 55; Total Fat: 0.5 g (0 g saturated, 0 g monounsaturated); Carbohydrates: 13.5 g; Protein: 1.5 g; Fiber: 1 g; Sodium: 20 mg

Spa in a Pitcher

If you've ever had a Pimm's cocktail (or Pimm's Cup, as it's known among the British faithful), you know it often contains a variety of herbs and sliced fruits. I was watching a friend make his version of a Pimm's cocktail with orange, lemon, cucumber peel, and a secret herb blend when I thought, "Wow, that looks so refreshing; it's like going to a spa!" Of course, the 50 proof Pimm's had to go (sorry, folks), but I could work around that. What I wanted to create was something that would inspire people to drink, because hydration is so vital to maintaining the body's equilibrium, especially in hot weather. This tonic is like art floating in a chilled pitcher, with thin rounds of orange, lemon, and cucumber interspersed with sprigs of thyme and mint. MAKES 8 CUPS

1 orange, thinly sliced into rounds
1 Meyer lemon, thinly sliced into rounds
1 unpeeled English cucumber, thinly sliced into rounds
3 sprigs fresh thyme, tarragon, or mint or fennel fronds, or a combination
1 tablespoon freshly squeezed Meyer lemon juice
8 cups water or sparkling water

Put the orange, lemon, cucumber, herbs, and lemon juice in a large pitcher. Press the fruit, cucumber, and herbs against the bottom of the pitcher with a wooden spoon, pushing down and twisting slightly to release their juices and volatile oils. Add the water and stir to combine. Refrigerate for 1 hour before serving.

Variation: In place of the water, use a weak tea made with 8 cups of boiling water and 4 chamomile, ginger, or green tea bags. Let the tea cool to room temperature before adding it to the pitcher.

PREP TIME: 5 minutes COOK TIME: 1 hour for chilling
STORAGE: Store in an airtight container in the refrigerator for up to 4 days.
PER SERVING: (1 cup per serving) Calories: 0; Total Fat: 0 g (0 g saturated, 0 g monounsaturated); Carbohydrates: 0 g; Protein: 0.5 g; Fiber: 1 g; Sodium: 1.5 mg

WHO KNEW? According to Cynthia Geyer, MD, medical director at the Canyon Ranch health spa in Lenox, Massachusetts, there's a reason you can no longer party like it's 1999: As we age, our organs have fewer reserves. Put another way, there's less gas in our tank, which is why it's important that we fill up with the best-quality fuel out there. "There is a senescence that's programmed into our cells, a slowing down," says Geyer. "Things you could handle when you were twenty, like staying up all night and functioning the next day, are just impossible at forty or fifty. Back then you might have been able to handle it even if you weren't at your best, but now it can precipitate a health crisis. As you age, it becomes even more important to support yourself nutritionally, because you don't have those reserves anymore."

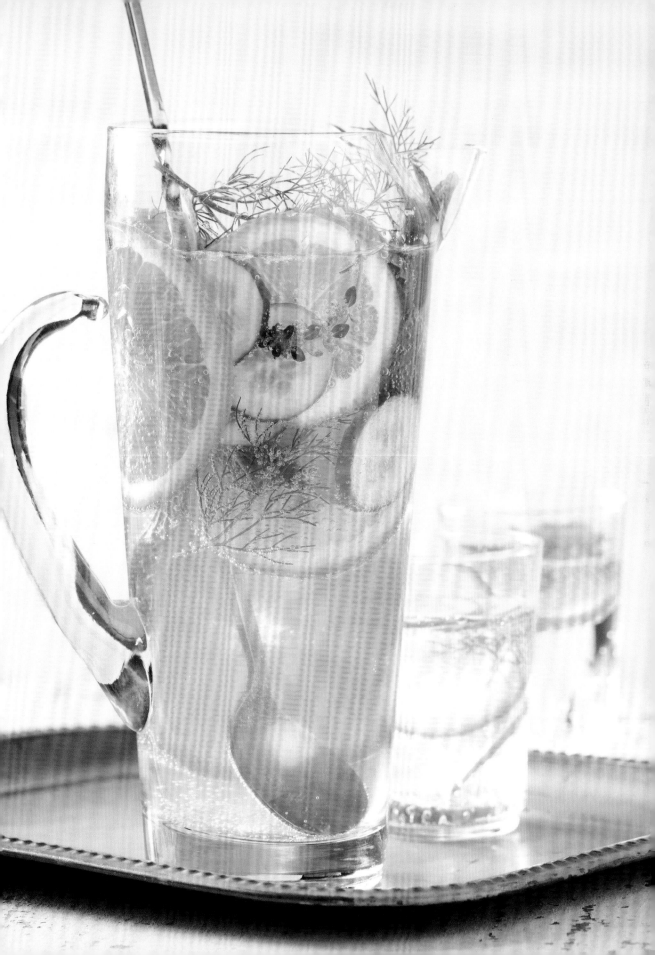

Green Tea Cooler with Ginger, Papaya, and Lime

When it comes to improving your well-being, green tea is a slam dunk. It's a phenomenal immune booster and can protect against tumor growth. But when it comes to taste, let's just say it needs a good point guard to help it set up the alley-oop. In this recipe, that would be papaya, which Columbus called "the fruit of the angels." It's a popular food in Nicoya, Costa Rica, one of the "blue zones" renowned for longevity. Papaya's sweetness balances the natural bitterness of straight green tea. The two dance nicely together in the lab as well; one study suggests that the combination of green tea and papaya may cut the risk of prostate cancer. I have to admit, I get a kick out of it when I choose ingredients based on taste and later find out that they're also great for you. MAKES 8 CUPS

6 green tea bags
3 ginger tea bags
6 cups boiling water
2 cups papaya nectar
1 tablespoon freshly squeezed
    lime juice
1 lime, sliced into rounds

Put the green tea and ginger tea bags in a large heatproof container. Pour in the boiling water and let steep for 5 minutes. Remove the tea bags and stir in the papaya nectar and lime juice. Add the lime slices and refrigerate for at least 2 hours, until well chilled.

PREP TIME: 5 minutes COOK TIME: 2 hours for chilling
STORAGE: Store in an airtight container in the refrigerator for up to 5 days.
PER SERVING: (2 cups per serving) Calories: 50; Total Fat: 0 g (0 g saturated, 0 g monounsaturated); Carbohydrates: 14 g; Protein: 1 g; Fiber: 1.5 g; Sodium: 12 mg

WHO KNEW? Green and black tea are derived from the same plant; green tea is less processed and has higher levels of phytonutrients.

Simon's Most Nourishing Elixir

My good friend Jeremy is a fantastic cook and has spent many a day in the kitchen with his knee-high understudy, his son, Simon. As Jeremy describes Simon, he's "twelve going on thirty," and he's developed quite the palate—as Jeremy discovered when he was recently a bit under the weather. He was lying in bed and suddenly got a whiff of heady smells wafting out of the kitchen. A few minutes later, in walked Simon with some tea, and I'm not talking Lipton. Simon looked at his dad, handed him the steaming homemade brew, and made a simple request: "Drink this." It was love in a cup. It was also a fantastically healing, flavorful concoction. Ginger, cloves, cardamom, two types of citrus zest, honey—what's not to like? Jeremy felt nourished in both body and heart, for here was a son to kvell over (that's Yiddish for "take pride in"). And I'm kvelling right along with him. You go, Simon!

MAKES 8 CUPS

8 cups water
1 (1-inch) piece of ginger
1 tablespoon grated Meyer
  lemon zest
2 teaspoons grated tangerine zest
1 cinnamon stick
5 green cardamom pods
4 allspice berries
2 whole cloves
Pinch of saffron
1/4 cup freshly squeezed Meyer
  lemon juice
2 tablespoons freshly squeezed
  tangerine juice
2 tablespoons honey

Put the water, ginger, lemon zest, tangerine zest, cinnamon, cardamom, allspice, cloves, and saffron in a saucepan, and bring to a boil over medium-high heat. Decrease the heat to low, cover, and simmer for 30 minutes.

Strain through a fine-mesh sieve into a clean saucepan. Add the lemon juice and tangerine juice and cook over low heat until warm. Stir in the honey. Taste; you may want to add a bit of honey.

PREP TIME: 5 minutes COOK TIME: 30 minutes
STORAGE: Store in an airtight container in the refrigerator for up to 1 week.
PER SERVING: (1 cup per serving) Calories: 0; Total Fat: 0 g (0 g saturated, 0 g monounsaturated); Carbohydrates: 0 g; Protein: 0 g; Fiber: 0 g; Sodium: 5 mg

COOK'S NOTE: The Meyer lemon is a hybrid between an orange and a Eureka lemon, which makes it milder and sweeter tasting than most store-bought lemons. If you don't have access to Meyer lemons, use 2 tablespoons of lemon juice combined with 2 tablespoons of freshly squeezed tangerine or orange juice. As for the zest, regular lemon zest is an acceptable substitute.

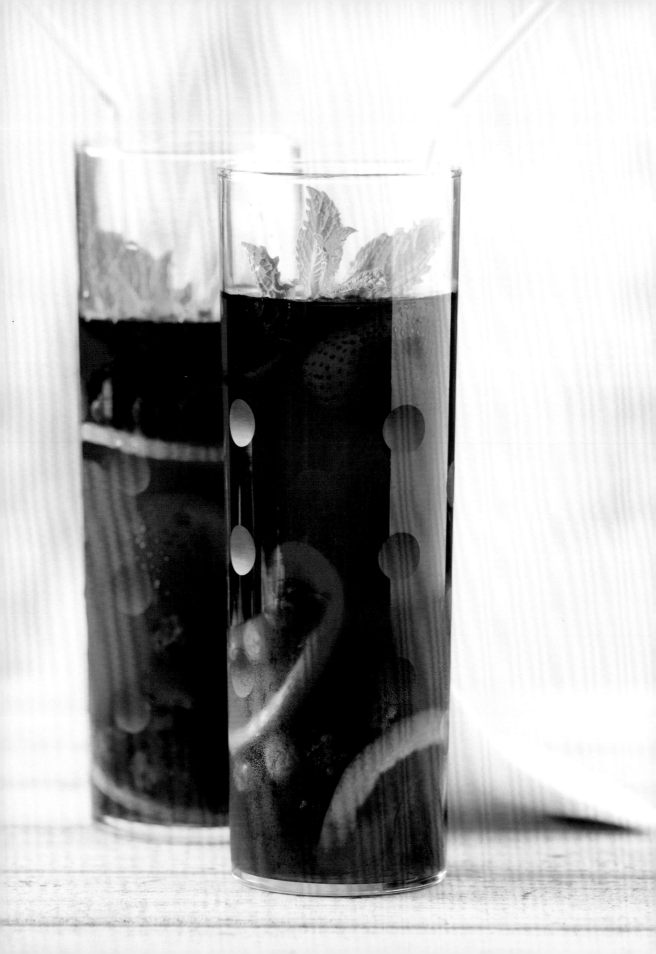

Hibiscus Pomegranate Cooler

Pomegranate juice might just be the gateway to eternal life. It has been consumed for about five thousand years and revered for nearly as long. Early Persians claimed the fruit had immortal properties, while in China it was a symbol of longevity. Contemporary science is content to say pomegranates have unusually high levels of antioxidants—more than blueberries or cranberries, and that's saying a lot. And contemporary Rebecca is content to say it has a lovely sweet-tart taste that I've enjoyed since I was a kid. In this recipe, I wanted to smooth out pomegranate's somewhat assertive flavor while pumping up the nutrition, so I turned to musky hibiscus, which has been shown to help control cholesterol and limit fatty buildup in arteries. To take it over the top, I added frozen strawberries, frozen blueberries, and orange rounds, to make something akin to Middle Eastern sangria. I think the ancients were on to something. MAKES 9 CUPS

¼ cup loose hibiscus tea, or 12 hibiscus tea bags
4 cups boiling water
4 cups cold water
1 cup unsweetened pomegranate juice
Spritz of fresh lemon juice
1 orange, sliced into rounds
3 sprigs fresh mint
16 frozen strawberries
24 frozen blueberries

Put the tea in a heatproof container. Pour in the boiling water and let steep for 5 minutes. Strain the tea into a pitcher. Stir in the cold water, pomegranate juice, lemon juice. Add the orange slices and mint and refrigerate for at least 1 hour, until well chilled. Add the frozen strawberries and blueberries to individual glasses when serving.

PREP TIME: 5 minutes COOK TIME: 1 hour for chilling
STORAGE: Store in an airtight container in the refrigerator for up to 4 days.
PER SERVING: (2 cups per serving) Calories: 40; Total Fat: 0 g (0 g saturated, 0 g monounsaturated); Carbohydrates: 9 g; Protein: 0 g; Fiber: 1 g; Sodium: 10 mg

Gregg's Morning Protein Shake

All the credit for this recipe goes to my husband, Gregg, and talented friend and integrative nutritionist Kathie Swift. The morning cold cereal and milk routine was getting old for Gregg, and he also really wanted to cut some carbs from his diet. Gregg has a big brain and works long hours at the computer, so he needed a breakfast that would be simple to make and give him hours of sustained energy, rather than amping him up for a little while prior to a late-morning crash. Enter Kathie. She came up with a tasty high-protein concoction filled with nutrient-dense ingredients, including protein powder, ground flaxseeds, rice milk, and sunflower seed butter. Most importantly, Gregg found the shake really hit the mark on taste, thanks to the berries, which also offer an abundance of healthful phytochemicals. Best of all? After this shake became his morning staple, at his next checkup his blood pressure and blood sugar levels had dropped significantly. He also credits the shake for helping him to think more clearly during the day. Those are pretty awesome results for something easily whizzed up in a blender. MAKES 2 CUPS

1½ cups unsweetened plain rice milk or almond milk
1½ cups frozen mixed berries, such as blueberries, raspberries, and blackberries
1 tablespoon rice protein powder or whey protein powder
1 heaping tablespoon sunflower butter or almond butter
1 tablespoon ground flaxseeds
1 teaspoon honey
Spritz of fresh lemon juice (optional)

Put the milk, berries, protein powder, sunflower butter, flaxseeds, and honey in a blender and process until smooth. Taste; you may want to add a spritz of lemon juice. Serve immediately.

PREP TIME: 5 minutes
STORAGE: Store in an airtight container in the refrigerator for up to 2 days. Shake well or blend again before using.
PER SERVING: (2 cups per serving) Calories: 430; Total Fat: 20 g (2 g saturated, 7 g monounsaturated); Carbohydrates: 39 g; Protein: 33.5 g; Fiber: 13 g; Sodium: 375 mg

WHO KNEW? There's something to be said for getting flaxseeds into your diet regularly. Their plethora of plant-based omega-3s appears to benefit blood vessels, possibly by counteracting inflammation and making the blood vessels more pliable, which can lower blood pressure and reduce atherosclerosis. Additionally, one study of patients with high cholesterol found that those who consumed flaxseeds daily for two months had reductions in cholesterol and triglycerides on par with those of a control group that was taking statins (cholesterol-lowering medications). Both omega-3s and lignans, another component of flaxseeds, have shown promise for inhibiting tumor growth.

Chocolate-Laced Blueberry Cherry Smoothie

When I was a kid and really needed a pick-me-up, I'd grab my friend Jill and we'd walk to Fields, the local soda shop, for a chocolate milk shake. No matter how bad the day had been, which boy had teased us, or which girl's outfit totally topped ours, by the time we finished that shake we were right as rain. As it turns out, dark chocolate is rich in antioxidants and really does have healing powers for both mood and body. The trick with this recipe was figuring out how to create a chocolate smoothie that wouldn't go straight to the thighs. There were also flavor considerations, since cocoa powder is bitter. That's where the cherries come in—and aside from providing sweetness, they also have excellent anti-inflammatory properties. When blueberries, frozen banana, yogurt, and just a touch of almond butter are blended in, the result is a healthful but decadent-tasting treat. If they had made this at Fields back in the day, Jill and I wouldn't have walked there; we would have run. MAKES 3 CUPS

1 cup organic plain full-fat yogurt
1 cup water
1 cup frozen banana pieces
1 cup frozen cherries
1 cup frozen blueberries
2 tablespoons unsweetened cocoa powder
1 tablespoon almond butter
1/8 teaspoon sea salt

Put the yogurt, water, banana, cherries, blueberries, cocoa powder, almond butter, and salt in the blender and process until smooth. Serve immediately.

Variations: For more fiber, add 1 tablespoon ground flaxseeds. For more protein, add a scoop of rice protein powder or whey protein powder.

PREP TIME: 5 minutes
STORAGE: Store in an airtight container in the refrigerator for up to 2 days. Shake well or blend again before serving.
PER SERVING: (1 1/2 cups per serving) Calories: 190; Total Fat: 6 g (2.5 g saturated, 2.5 g monounsaturated); Carbohydrates: 31 g; Protein: 6 g; Fiber: 4 g; Sodium: 119 mg

WHO KNEW? Even early scientists were beside themselves over chocolate's heavenly taste. They gave cacao the Latin name *Theobroma cacao*, *theobroma* being Greek for "food of the gods."

Mango Lassi

If you've never been to an Indian restaurant, one menu delight is in the beverage section. It's called *lassi*. In American cuisine, yogurt–based smoothies are most similar to *lassis*, though traditional *lassis* are thinner. They're often made with a variety of luscious fruits and are extremely refreshing. Here I've chosen mango, but strawberry, banana, or papaya would work just as well. The key to this *lassi* is a spice that Indian establishments offer at the cash register in place of sugary breath mints: tiny pods of cardamom. I first saw cardamom in pod form while working at the Chopra Center for Wellbeing. They put the seeds on the dining tables for people to chew after meals to sweeten the breath. In addition, cardamom oils soothe indigestion. MAKES 4 CUPS

2 cups diced fresh or frozen mango
1 cup organic plain yogurt
1¼ cups plain almond milk
1 tablespoon Grade B maple syrup
Spritz of fresh lemon or lime juice
¼ teaspoon ground cardamom
Pinch of sea salt
4 sprigs fresh mint, for garnish

Put the mango, yogurt, almond milk, maple syrup, lemon juice, cardamom, and salt in a blender and process until smooth. Taste; you may want to add a spritz of lemon or lime juice for a little extra pop. Pour into individual glasses and garnish with the mint.

PREP TIME: 10 minutes
STORAGE: Store in an airtight container in the refrigerator for up to 1 day. Shake well or blend again before serving.
PER SERVING: (1 cup per serving) Calories: 110; Total Fat: 2.5 g (1.5 g saturated, 0.5 g monounsaturated); Carbohydrates: 21 g; Protein: 3 g; Fiber: 2 g; Sodium: 77 mg

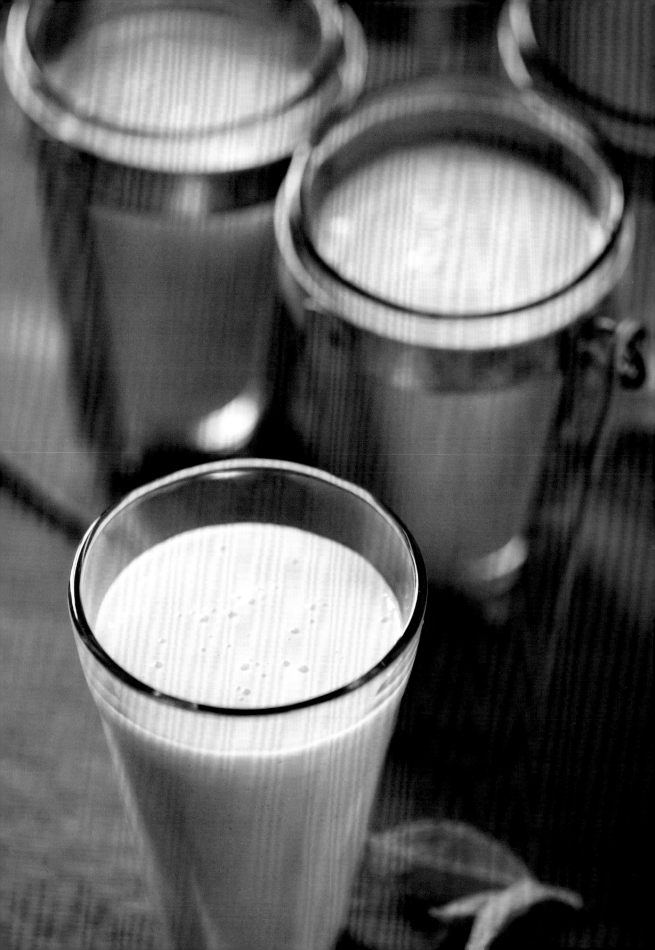

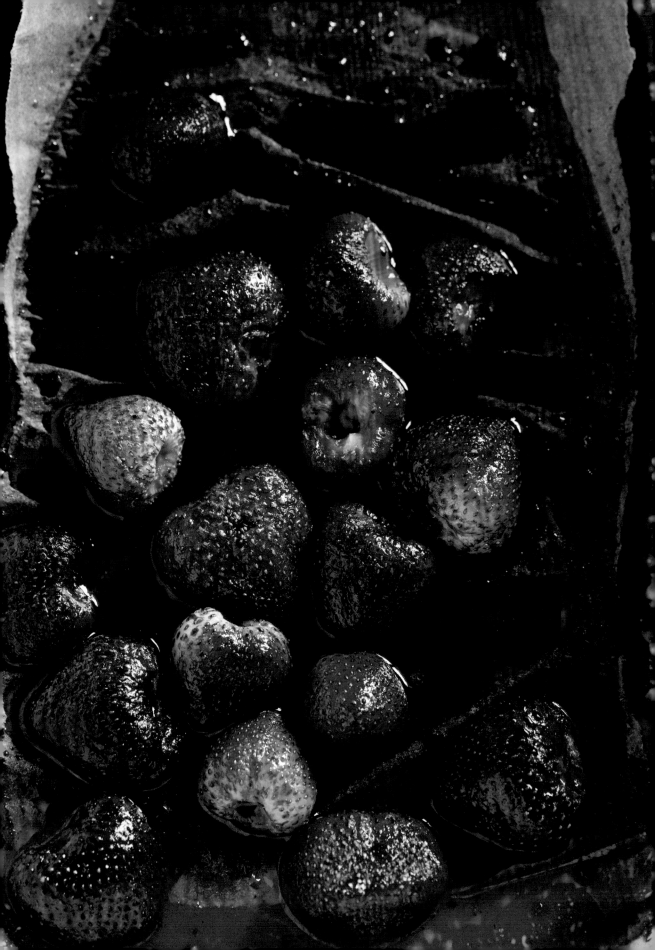

CHAPTER 11

Sweet Bites

This chapter is a small miracle. And as much as I'd like to take credit for it, no can do.

The credit goes entirely to my friend and baker extraordinaire Wendy Remer. Here's how it unfolded: I wanted to showcase Wendy's skills in this book, so I approached her with a proposition. If she'd known what was in my mind at that moment, I'm sure she'd have run for the hills. "Wendy," I said, "this is what I need from you if I'm going to be able to put sweet treats in this book."

I could see her left eyebrow begin to arch.

"No white sugar," I said. "No white flour. No butter."

Now both eyebrows were climbing toward her hairline. I knew I only had seconds before her mouth caught up with her brain.

"And by the way," I concluded, "could you come up with a few gluten-free desserts while you're at it?"

She looked at me like I was genuinely crazy. Who could blame her? I'd just ruled out the ingredients most bakers rely on. It was like asking a jockey to ride a thundering thoroughbred sans saddle, reins, and stirrups.

It's a good thing that Wendy likes a challenge, because sweets are something most of us can't do without—nor should we, because as crazy as it sounds, sweets can be nutritious and life enhancing. Coming up with recipes that accomplish that is what I tasked Wendy with, and boy did she deliver! By working with whole grains, nuts, fruits, chocolate, and a wide variety of spices, Wendy brought a ton of antioxidants and health-boosting phytochemicals to the table. As for sweeteners, she mostly stuck with maple syrup. Plus, with such delicious base ingredients, only small quantities of sweeteners are needed. The result is treats that release their sugars into the bloodstream slowly, preventing spikes in insulin.

So go forth, cook, bake, and enjoy in good conscience. Once you've tasted the wonderful offerings in this chapter, I'm sure you'll join me in saying, "Wendy, you rock!"

Chocolate-Dipped Cherry Haystacks and Chocolate-Dipped Apricots

These simple-to-make treats are a wonderful dessert that really adds the *wow* factor to a dinner party. Feel free to substitute your favorite dried fruits and nuts in the recipe, but keep in mind that it's the slivered almonds that create the haystack look. Tempering chocolate is a complex process that requires precise temperature readings and typically a great deal of practice. In this recipe, just a bit of care when melting the chocolate and the addition of a bit of neutral-flavored oil offers an easy shortcut that produces fantastic results. The trick is to have the ingredients you're going to dip at hand, because once the chocolate is ready, it waits for no one! MAKES 32 PIECES

1/2 cup dried cherries or blueberries
1/3 cup slivered almonds, toasted (see note, page 83)
2 tablespoons cacao nibs
5 ounces dark chocolate (70 to 72% cacao content), finely and uniformly chopped
1 teaspoon neutral oil, such as almond or grapeseed oil
16 dried apricots
1/2 cup chopped pistachios

WHO KNEW? Academy Award–winning actress Katherine Hepburn, who lived to be ninety-six, credited her longevity—along with her effervescence and beauty—to a lifetime of eating chocolate.

Line a baking sheet with parchment paper. Put the cherries, almonds, and cacao nibs in a bowl and stir to combine.

Set aside 1/4 cup of the chopped chocolate and put the rest in a small stainless steel bowl. Add the oil. Bring about one inch of water to a boil in a skillet, then remove it from the heat and put it on a kitchen towel or hot pad on the countertop. Put the bowl of chocolate into the hot water, being careful not to get any water into the chocolate, and stir gently and constantly with a spatula until the chocolate is melted. Remove the bowl from the hot water, add the reserved chocolate, and stir until melted. If bits remain unmelted, put the bowl back into the hot water for a few seconds and stir until all the chocolate is melted, smooth, and shiny.

One by one, dip the apricots halfway into the chocolate, then place them on the lined baking sheet. Sprinkle with the pistachios before the chocolate sets up.

Scrape the remaining chocolate into the bowl with the cherry mixture. Stir thoroughly until well combined. Using a teaspoon, scoop the mixture onto the lined baking sheet, creating 16 little mounds, or haystacks. Place the baking sheet in the refrigerator for 5 to 10 minutes to set the chocolate. Serve right away, or save for later.

PREP TIME: 10 minutes COOK TIME: 10 minutes
STORAGE: Store in an airtight container in the refrigerator for up to 3 days. Let the chocolates warm to room temperature before serving.
PER SERVING: (1 Haystack and 1 Apricot per serving) Calories: 130; Total Fat: 7 g (2.5 g saturated, 3 g monounsaturated); Carbohydrates: 13 g; Protein: 2 g; Fiber: 2 g; Sodium: 4 mg

Roasted Strawberries with Pomegranate Molasses and Basil

Roasting strawberries reminds me of Carly Simon's song "Anticipation." When you can take your time in the kitchen—or at least wait awhile for something to cook—magic happens. When you roast strawberries *slooooowly*—I'm talking for 90 minutes—the alchemy that occurs is wondrous. Their flavors become so condensed and intense as they shrink. In this recipe, the strawberries are bathed in pomegranate molasses and maple syrup before roasting, for even more flavor. The last step, post-roast, is a mouth-blast of basil (a super anti-inflammatory). These sumptuous berries are a great addition to Yogurt-Berry Brûlée with Maple Almond Brittle (page 224). MAKES 4 SERVINGS

3 tablespoons Grade B maple syrup
1 tablespoon pomegranate molasses, homemade (page 192) or store-bought
1¹/₂ teaspoons extra-virgin olive oil
¹/₄ teaspoon sea salt
Freshly ground black pepper
2 cups strawberries, hulled
2 teaspoons very thinly sliced fresh basil

Preheat the oven to 250°F. Line a rimmed baking sheet with parchment paper.

Put the maple syrup, pomegranate molasses, olive oil, salt, and a few grinds of pepper in a large bowl and whisk to combine. Add the strawberries and stir gently until the strawberries are well coated.

Spread the strawberry mixture on the lined baking sheet in a single layer. (Save any leftover juices to drizzle over the strawberries, or to slurp with great enjoyment!) Bake for about 90 minutes, until the strawberries are about half their original size, stirring and redistributing them halfway through the baking time. Let cool for 5 minutes, then transfer the berries and any remaining juices to a bowl. Gently stir in the basil, then let sit for 5 minutes for the flavors to meld. Serve warm or at room temperature.

PREP TIME: 10 minutes COOK TIME: 1 hour 30 minutes
STORAGE: Store in an airtight container in the refrigerator for up to 4 days or in the freezer for up to 3 months.
PER SERVING: Calories: 45; Total Fat: 1.5 g (0 g saturated, 1 g monounsaturated); Carbohydrates: 8 g; Protein: 1 g; Fiber: 1 g; Sodium: 100 mg

Raspberry Hibiscus Sorbet

There is a tiny ice cream and sorbet shop near my house called The Scoop, and you just know they're doing something right. I have to time my visits just right or else stand in a line a block long. Everything is handmade, and they often have raspberry concoctions to die for. I took their wizardry as a point of inspiration and added hibiscus and coconut milk to this sorbet (pictured on page 217). Some folks wonder why raspberries and not strawberries? For me, especially in this book, I generally opt for raspberries because of their nutritional profile; they have 50 percent more antioxidant power than strawberries.

Prepare ahead: you'll need an ice cream maker for this recipe. Once the sorbet mixture is prepared, it must be chilled for at least 2 hours. Be sure to put the bowl of the ice cream maker in the freezer at least 6 to 8 hours before churning the sorbet. MAKES 2¹/₂ CUPS

2 hibiscus tea bags
¹/₂ cup boiling water
³/₄ cup water
¹/₄ cup honey
1 (12-ounce) package frozen raspberries, or 2 cups fresh raspberries
¹/₂ cup coconut milk
¹/₈ teaspoon freshly squeezed lime juice

Put the tea bags in a small heatproof container or cup. Pour in the boiling water and let steep for 5 minutes. Remove the tea bags.

Meanwhile, put the water and honey in a saucepan over medium-high heat and bring to a simmer. Add the raspberries and cook, stirring constantly, until raspberries begin to fall apart, 2 to 3 minutes. Remove from the heat and whisk in the hibiscus tea and coconut milk. Let cool for about 10 minutes.

Transfer to a blender, add the lime juice, and process until smooth. Strain through a fine-mesh sieve, pressing the pulp with the back of a spoon to extract as much liquid as possible. Transfer to a storage container, cover, and chill for at least 2 hours.

Remove the bowl of the ice cream maker from the freezer. Whisk the sorbet mixture until smooth, then pour it into the bowl of the ice cream maker. Process according to the manufacturer's instructions.

Transfer to an airtight container. Place plastic wrap or waxed paper directly on the surface to prevent freezer burn, then cover with a lid. Freeze to the desired firmness.

PREP TIME: 20 minutes COOK TIME: At least 2 hours for chilling, plus churning and freezing time
STORAGE: Store in an airtight container in the freezer, with plastic wrap or waxed paper covering the top to prevent freezer burn, for up to 3 months.
PER SERVING: (about ¹/₂ cup per serving) Calories: 150; Total Fat: 6 g (5 g saturated, 0.5 g monounsaturated); Carbohydrates: 24 g; Protein: 1 g; Fiber: 4 g; Sodium: 7 mg

Coffee-Infused Chocolate Sorbet

I'm betting that this recipe will make you happy. Numerous studies have found that consuming chocolate—especially dark chocolate—can help ward off depression, high blood pressure, and cancer, and it's been shown to improve memory in mice. So, I put two different types of dark chocolate in this sorbet and combined it with other great-tasting, healthful costars, like almond milk and coffee beans—all in the name of science, of course.

Prepare ahead: you'll need an ice cream maker for this recipe. The sorbet mixture must be chilled for at least 4 hours; be sure to put the bowl of the ice cream maker in the freezer at least 6 to 8 hours before churning the sorbet. MAKES 3 CUPS

1/4 cup whole coffee beans
3/4 cup water
1/2 cup Grade B maple syrup
Pinch of sea salt
5 ounces dark chocolate
    (64 to 70% cacao content),
    finely chopped
1/3 cup unsweetened cocoa powder
1/2 teaspoon vanilla extract
1 cup plain almond milk

Put the coffee beans in a small resealable plastic bag and roll with a rolling pin to coarsely crush them.

Put the water, maple syrup, and salt in a saucepan over high heat and stir to combine. Bring to a boil, then decrease the heat to low and simmer for 1 minute. Add the coffee beans, cover, and remove from the heat. Let the coffee infuse for 5 minutes.

Put the chocolate in a heat-proof bowl. Line a sieve with a piece of cheesecloth and place it over the bowl.

Put the coffee infusion over medium heat and return to a simmer, then pour it through the lined sieve, directly into the chocolate. Let sit for 1 minute, then whisk until smooth. Add the cocoa powder and whisk until well combined and smooth, then whisk in the vanilla.

Scrape the mixture into a blender, add the almond milk, and process until smooth and frothy. Pour the blended mixture back into the bowl, cover with plastic wrap, and chill for at least 4 hours.

Remove the bowl of the ice cream maker from the freezer. Whisk the sorbet mixture until smooth, then pour it into bowl of the ice cream maker. Process according to the manufacturer's instructions.

Transfer to an airtight container. Place plastic wrap directly on the surface to prevent freezer burn, then cover. Freeze to the desired firmness.

PREP TIME: 20 minutes COOK TIME: At least 4 hours for chilling, plus churning and freezing time
STORAGE: Store in an airtight container in the freezer, with plastic wrap or waxed paper on the surface to prevent freezer burn, for up to 1 month.
PER SERVING: (3/4 cup per serving) Calories: 240; Total Fat: 10 g (5 g saturated, 3 g monounsaturated); Carbohydrates: 33.5 g; Protein: 3 g; Fiber: 4 g; Sodium: 45 mg

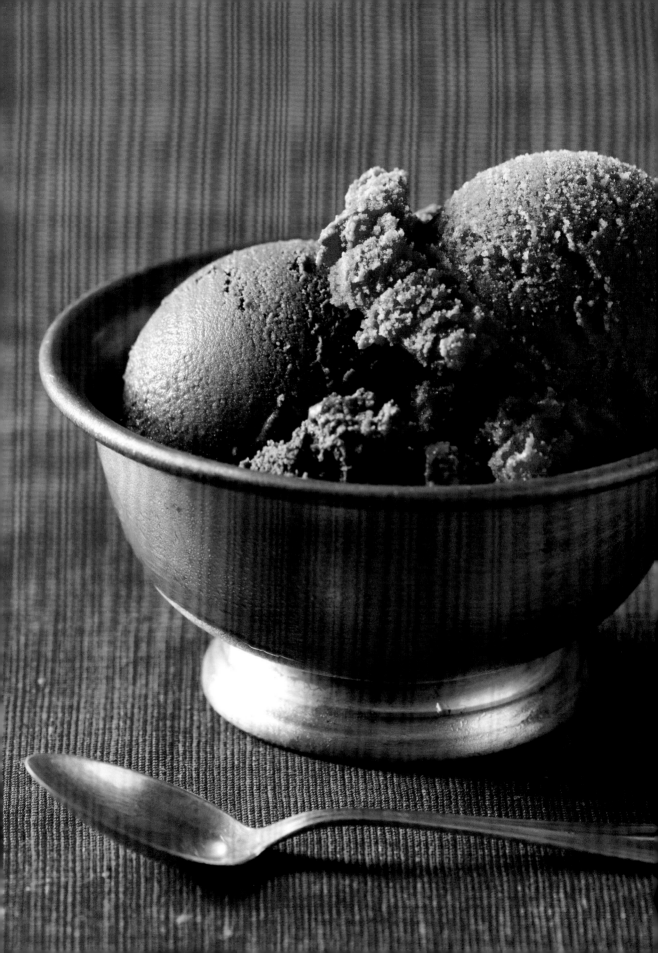

Apple-Raspberry Nut Crumble

Here's an example of equal parts observation and inspiration. I went over my friend Wendy's house because she was testing an apple crumble recipe. I was tasting it, and started dipping my bites into a slowly burbling pot of raspberry sauce and going nuts over the sauce. Wendy silently noted what was going on, and after I left she tried the combination and had her own "aha!" moment. As she pondered how nicely their flavors—tart opposite sweet—tangoed together, she eventually came up with this recipe. It's a veritable health factory: raspberries help with everything from keeping skin elastic to fighting inflammation, walnuts are high in omega-3s, and apples have pectin for soothing the tummy. Call it serendipity or just a keen eye, but either way this is a sweet bite that was meant to be.

MAKES 6 SERVINGS

FILLING
2 teaspoons extra-virgin olive oil
3 cups Granny Smith apples, peeled and sliced into ¼-inch-thick wedges
Pinch of sea salt
¼ teaspoon ground cinnamon
⅛ teaspoon ground allspice
Pinch of freshly grated nutmeg
1 cup unfiltered apple cider
1 cup fresh or frozen raspberries
½ teaspoon vanilla extract

TOPPING
½ cup coarsely chopped walnuts
¼ cup almond flour, homemade (page 226) or store-bought
¼ teaspoon ground cinnamon
3 tablespoons Grade B maple syrup
1 tablespoon extra-virgin olive oil

COOK'S NOTE: You can eat this crumble for breakfast if you like; try it with a dollop of yogurt on top.

Preheat the oven to 375°F.

To make the filling, heat the olive oil in a skillet over medium heat. (If you use an 8-inch ovenproof skillet, you can bake the crumble right in the skillet.) Add the apple slices and salt and sauté for 2 minutes. Add the cinnamon, allspice, and nutmeg and cook, stirring gently and frequently for 3 to 4 minutes. Add the apple cider and bring to a boil. Decrease the heat to low and simmer until the apples are tender, about 5 minutes. Remove from the heat and stir in the raspberries and vanilla. Transfer to a pie plate. (You can skip this step if using an ovenproof skillet.)

Meanwhile, make the topping. Put the walnuts, almond flour, and cinnamon in a small bowl and stir to combine. In a separate small bowl, whisk the maple syrup and olive oil together. Pour into the walnut mixture and stir until well combined.

To assemble and bake the crumble, spoon the topping evenly over the filling. Bake for about 35 minutes, until the topping is golden and the filling is bubbly. Let cool for at least 10 minutes. Serve warm or at room temperature.

PREP TIME: 10 minutes COOK TIME: 45 minutes
STORAGE: Store in an airtight container in the refrigerator for up to 3 days.
PER SERVING: Calories: 210; Total Fat: 13 g (1.5 g saturated, 5 g monounsaturated); Carbohydrates: 25 g; Protein: 3 g; Fiber: 4.5 g; Sodium: 15 mg

Spiced Almond Macaroon Buttons

Macaroons and Mexican food have one thing in common: the US versions bear little resemblance to their namesakes. For many of us, the word *macaroon* conjures up an image of a large, chocolate-covered, coconut-engorged belly bomb. That's nothing like the original French *macaron*. Ask for a *macaron* in Paris and you'll get an assemblage of wonderfully light almond-based meringue cookies sandwiching a creamy filling. This recipe goes back to the delightfully sinful French roots, but I modified it so that you only have to say one Hail Mary, not three, as penance. It uses just a bit of turbinado sugar instead of a heap of the refined white variety, along with almonds, cinnamon, and allspice. (As a bonus, allspice is excellent if you're feeling bloated, so here's a case where a little dessert might be called for after a big meal.) I think of this as macaroon reductionism: everything except the flavor has been scaled down, and takes just one or two of these diminutive cookies to leave you feeling pleasantly satiated. There's really no sin in that. **MAKES 20 MACAROONS**

1 cup almond flour, homemade (page 226) or store-bought
3 tablespoons turbinado sugar
1/4 teaspoon ground cinnamon
1/8 teaspoon ground allspice
Pinch of ground cardamom
1/8 teaspoon sea salt
1/4 cup organic egg whites (about 2 large eggs)
3/4 teaspoon almond extract
1/4 teaspoon vanilla extract
20 whole almonds, or 1 cup slivered almonds, for decoration

COOK'S NOTE: These treats are best when they're freshly made, though they do freeze and reheat well. Just refresh them in a 300°F oven for a few minutes after thawing.

Preheat the oven to 350°F. Line a baking sheet with parchment paper.

Put the almond flour, sugar, cinnamon, allspice, cardamom, and salt in a bowl and stir to combine.

Put the egg whites in a small bowl and beat lightly with a fork to make them easier to measure and pour. Add 3 tablespoons of the egg whites, the almond extract, and the vanilla to the almond mixture and stir with a spatula. The texture should be wet and soft, but stiff enough to form into a ball between wet hands. If the dough feels too stiff, add a bit more egg white.

Using wet palms and fingers, roll a scant teaspoonful of the dough into balls. Put them on the baking sheet, spacing them about 2 inches apart, and flatten slightly with damp finger. Press an almond or a few slivered almonds onto the top of each cookie. Bake for about 15 minutes, until the tops are dry and a very pale golden brown. Peek at the bottoms; they should be a golden brown. Immediately transfer to a wire rack and let cool before serving.

PREP TIME: 15 minutes COOK TIME: 15 minutes
STORAGE: Store in an airtight container, layered between parchment paper, at room temperature for up to 2 days or in the freezer for up to 1 month.
PER SERVING: (2 macaroons per serving) Calories: 190; Total Fat: 14 g (1 g saturated, 8 g monounsaturated); Carbohydrates: 13 g; Protein: 7 g; Fiber: 3 g; Sodium: 69 mg

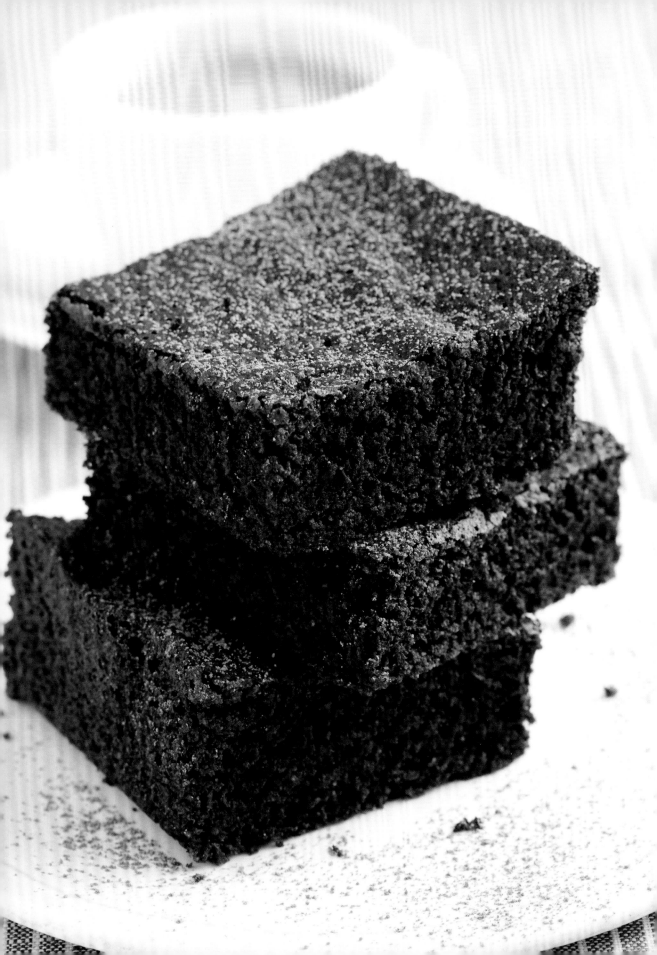

Insanely Good Chocolate Brownies

Jumbo shrimp. Airline food. Boneless ribs. Fuzzy logic. Some words just don't seem to belong together. I'm betting you'd say *healthy brownie* falls into that category. Au contraire! How do I know that isn't the case? Because there was a lot of "yumming" in my kitchen as a gaggle of brownie aficionados devoured these. Refined white sugar out; Grade B maple syrup in. See ya white flour; hello almond flour and brown rice flour. Fare-thee-well butter; come-on-down olive oil! Add dark chocolate, walnuts, and cinnamon, and the result is a decadent culinary oxymoron for the ages. MAKES 16 BROWNIES

¹/₃ cup almond flour, homemade (page 226) or store-bought

¹/₃ cup brown rice flour

2 tablespoons natural unsweetened cocoa powder

¹/₂ teaspoon ground cinnamon

¹/₂ teaspoon baking soda

¹/₈ teaspoon sea salt

8 ounces dark chocolate (68 to 72% cacao content), chopped

¹/₃ cup extra-virgin olive oil

2 organic eggs

¹/₃ cup Grade B maple syrup

¹/₃ cup maple sugar

1 teaspoon vanilla extract

¹/₂ cup coarsely chopped walnuts (optional), toasted (see note, page 83)

COOK'S NOTE: You can also use a 9 by 6-inch baking pan. If you do, the baking time will be only about 25 minutes.

WHO KNEW? Cacao content is the amount of pure cacao products (chocolate liquor, cocoa butter, and cocoa powder) used in the chocolate; the higher the percentage, the more antioxidants the chocolate contains. And if you're into addition by subtraction, higher cacao percentages mean lower sugar content.

Preheat the oven to 350°F. Line an 8-inch square baking pan (see note) with two pieces of foil long enough to overlap on all four sides. Lightly oil the foil.

Put the almond flour, brown rice flour, cocoa powder, cinnamon, baking soda, and salt in a bowl and stir with a whisk to combine.

Put half of the chocolate in a heatproof bowl and set the bowl over a saucepan of simmering water. Heat, stirring often, just until the chocolate is melted and smooth. Remove from the heat and whisk in the olive oil.

Crack the eggs into a large bowl and whisk until frothy. Slowly add the maple syrup and maple sugar, whisking all the while, and continue whisking until the mixture is smooth. Add the vanilla extract, then gradually add the chocolate, whisking vigorously all the while, and continue whisking until smooth and glossy.

Add the flour mixture and beat for about 1 minute. Stir in the remaining chocolate and the walnuts. Scrape the mixture into the prepared pan and smooth the top with a spatula.

Bake for 30 minutes or until a toothpick inserted in the center comes out clean. Let cool to room temperature in the pan, then cover and refrigerate for at least 1 hour before cutting into 16 brownies.

Variation: For brownies that are more fudgy, replace the rice flour with another ¹/₃ cup of almond flour.

PREP TIME: 20 minutes COOK TIME: 30 minutes
STORAGE: Store in an airtight container in the refrigerator for up to 5 days or in the freezer for up to 3 months.
PER SERVING: (1 brownie per serving) Calories: 130; Total Fat: 9 g (2.5 g saturated, 5 g monounsaturated); Carbohydrates: 10 g; Protein: 2 g; Fiber: 1 g; Sodium: 64 mg

Triple-Chocolate Date Torte

Here's all you need to know about dates and longevity. Somehow, someway (blame it on the pharoahs and those elaborate tombs), a Judean date palm seed was recently discovered after 2,000 years in storage. Nice note for archaeologists, but why should we care? Because someone got the rather inspired idea to cultivate the seed . . . and dang if it didn't sprout! Now that's what I call a fruit with life force. Here we surround all that power with a load of pleasure in the form of three chocolates: cocoa powder, dark chocolate, and chocolate's purest form, cacao nibs. MAKES 8 SERVINGS

$^1/_2$ cup pitted dates (about
   3 ounces), cut into quarters
$^1/_2$ cup water
2 tablespoons Grade B maple syrup
$^1/_2$ teaspoon ground cinnamon
$^3/_4$ cup walnuts
1 cup almond flour, homemade
   (page 226) or store-bought
1 tablespoon natural unsweetened
   cocoa powder
$^1/_2$ teaspoon baking soda
$^1/_4$ teaspoon sea salt
3 tablespoons extra-virgin olive oil
2 organic eggs
2 teaspoons vanilla extract
3 ounces dark chocolate
   (68 to 75% cacao content),
   finely chopped
1 tablespoon cacao nibs, sliced
   almonds, or a combination

LIVE LONG AND PROSPER: Chocolate is good for you. Really! Cross my heart. Consider that ounce for ounce, the cacao in dark chocolate has more antioxidants than blueberries. The phytochemicals in chocolate may offer cardiovascular protection to postmenopausal women, perhaps by lowering cholesterol, high blood pressure, or both. Several studies suggest that to get the most out of chocolate nutritionally, dark chocolate, without any milk, is best.

Preheat the oven to 350°F. Lightly oil the bottom and sides of an 8-inch springform pan (see note, page 223) and line the bottom with a round of parchment paper.

Put the dates, water, maple syrup, and cinnamon in a small saucepan and bring to a boil over high heat. Decrease the heat to low and simmer, stirring often, until the dates are tender and the water is absorbed, 5 to 7 minutes. Set aside to cool.

Put the walnuts in a food processor and pulse just until finely ground. Be careful not to overprocess, or the walnuts will turn into an oily, sticky paste.

Put $^1/_2$ cup of the ground walnuts in a large bowl (no need to clean out the food processor). Store any left-over walnut meal in a resealable plastic bag in the freezer for another use. Add the almond flour, cocoa powder, baking soda, and salt and toss and crumble with your fingers until the ingredients are completely combined and the mixture lump free.

Put the date mixture in the food processor and process until smooth. With the motor running, slowly add the oil, then the eggs, one at a time, and finally the vanilla, stopping to scrape down the sides of the work bowl once or twice. Add to the walnut mixture and stir with a rubber spatula. Fold in the chopped chocolate.

Pour the mixture into the prepared pan and shake gently to spread the batter evenly. Sprinkle the cacao nibs over the top. Bake for 20 to 25 minutes, until the top is be a bit puffed up and a toothpick inserted in the center comes out clean. Let the torte cool completely before removing the sides of the springform pan.

COOK'S NOTE: You can also use a 9-inch springform pan. If you do, the baking time will be shorter—about 18 minutes.

Variation: For an over-the-top dessert, drizzle 1 tablespoon of Raspberry Pomegranate Sauce (below) over each plate and place a piece of torte on top.

PREP TIME: 25 minutes COOK TIME: 20 to 25 minutes
STORAGE: Store in an airtight container in the refrigerator for up to 4 days or tightly wrapped in the freezer for up to 1 month.
PER SERVING: Calories: 330; Total Fat: 26 g (5 g saturated, 11 g monounsaturated); Carbohydrates: 22 g; Protein: 8 g; Fiber: 4.5 g; Sodium: 160 mg

Raspberry Pomegranate Sauce

This is the kind of sauce you have dreams about. It's insanely concentrated deliciousness, and simple, too: take raspberries and pomegranate molasses and cook them down into a bubbling pool of absolute yum, then pour it over anything and go nuts. I always keep some in the freezer so I can bring it out whenever a chocolate or almond torte makes its way to the table. It's healthy, too. Enough said. MAKES 1 CUP

1 (12-ounce) bag frozen raspberries, or 2 cups fresh raspberries
2 tablespoons Grade B maple syrup
2 teaspoons pomegranate molasses, homemade (page 192) or store-bought
Pinch of sea salt
2 tablespoons freshly squeezed orange juice

Put the raspberries, maple syrup, pomegranate molasses, and salt in a small, heavy saucepan and stir to combine. Bring to a boil over medium-high, stirring frequently. Decrease the heat to low and simmer until most of the berries have fallen apart, 1 to 2 minutes. Remove from the heat and let cool for about 10 minutes.

Transfer to a blender, add the orange juice, and process until smooth. Strain through a fine-mesh sieve, pressing the pulp with the back of a spoon to extract as much liquid as possible. Do a FASS check (see page 44); you may want to add a bit more maple syrup.

PREP TIME: Not applicable COOK TIME: 15 minutes
STORAGE: Store in an airtight container in the refrigerator for up to 1 week or in the freezer for up to 2 months.
PER SERVING: (2 tablespoons per serving) Calories: 35; Total Fat: 0 g (0 g saturated, 0 g monounsaturated); Carbohydrates: 10 g; Protein: 0 g; Fiber: 2 g; Sodium: 7 mg

Yogurt-Berry Brûlée with Maple Almond Brittle

You may think that making crème brûlée requires blowtorches, welder's glasses, and asbestos gloves. But I've come up with an alternative method that doesn't involve having to whip out the torch. Instead, a sweet, crunchy brittle is made in the oven, with only one requirement: keeping a very close eye on it as it cooks. The brittle is perched atop a delectable bowl of berry-studded sweetened Greek yogurt, which is just as creamy as the egg-, dairy-, and sugar-laden custard typical in crème brûlée, and it also brings a host of health benefits to the table. MAKES 4 SERVINGS

BRITTLE
1 teaspoon extra-virgin olive oil
3 tablespoons Grade B maple syrup
2 tablespoons sliced almonds
1/8 teaspoon ground cardamom

MAPLE-SCENTED YOGURT
2 cups organic plain Greek yogurt
1 1/4 cups fresh berries, any type
1 teaspoon Grade B maple syrup

To make the brittle, preheat the oven to 375°F and turn the oven light on. Line a rimmed baking sheet with parchment paper.

Spread the oil on the parchment paper with a paper towel or brush, covering the parchment with a thin, even film of oil.

Combine the maple syrup, almonds, and cardamom in a small bowl. Pour the mixture onto the oiled parchment paper, then tilt the pan to spread it evenly. Bake for 5 to 7 minutes, staying close to the oven. The syrup will first become bubbly, then, after another 2 or 3 minutes, the almonds will take on a nice golden color and the syrup will have a deep amber color. At this point, remove the brittle from the oven and let cool to room temperature. To make it easier to break into pieces, you can pop it into the freezer for about 5 minutes. Using a thin metal spatula, lift the hardened brittle and break it into randomly sized pieces. Use immediately or store in an airtight container.

To make the yogurt mixture and assemble the dish, put the yogurt, 1 cup of the berries, and the maple syrup in a bowl and stir gently to combine.

Just before serving, spoon the yogurt mixture onto dessert dishes, top with the brittle, and scatter the remaining 1/2 cup berries around the edges.

Variation: Elevate this recipe by incorporating Roasted Strawberries (page 214) and their juices as a layer.

PREP TIME: 10 minutes COOK: 12 minutes
STORAGE: Store the brittle in an airtight container in the refrigerator for 5 days or in the freezer for up to 1 month.
PER SERVING: Calories: 240; Total Fat: 14 g (9 g saturated, 2 g mono-unsaturated); Carbohydrates: 21 g; Protein: 8.5 g; Fiber: 2 g; Sodium: 35 mg

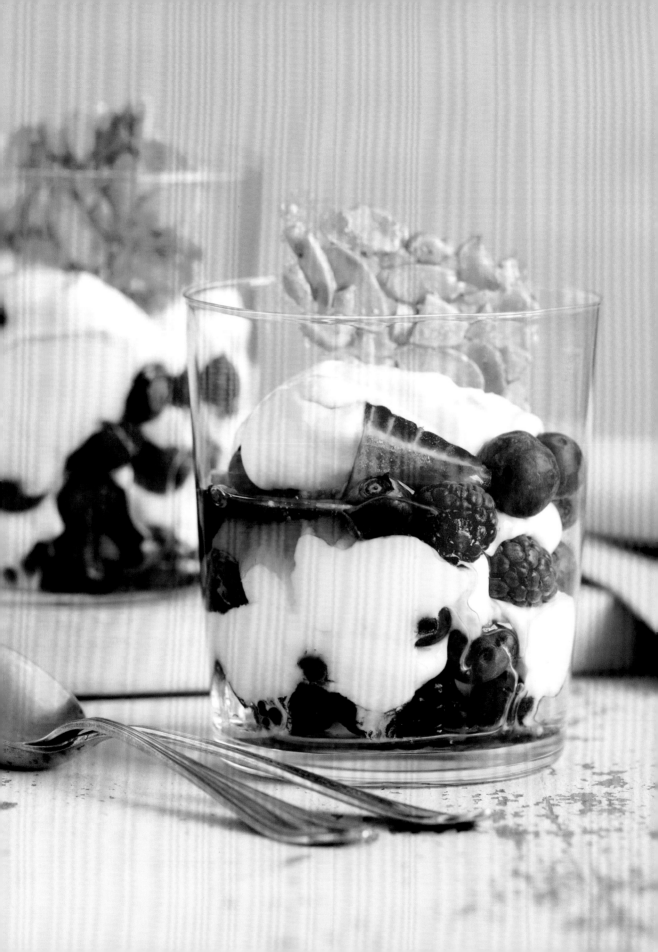

Almond Flour

I call for almond flour, aka almond meal, in many recipes in this book because it's just what I'm looking for in an ingredient. It's tasty and healthful, and it often works just as well as refined white flour, if not better. Plus, it's gluten-free, so it's much easier for many people to digest, and when used in sweetened baked goods, its high fiber content keeps blood sugar levels in check. It's a great flour to work with, and as you'll see, it's also very easy to make. MAKES 1¼ CUPS

1 cup raw almonds

Put ½ cup of the almonds in a food processor and process until coarsely chopped. Then pulse until a medium-fine meal forms and just starts to cling to the sides of the work bowl. (See photo page 38.) Be careful to not over-process, or you'll end up with almond butter. Transfer to a bowl or storage container and repeat with the remaining ½ cup of almonds. If not using immediately, store the almond flour in an airtight container in the refrigerator or freezer to preserve freshness and prevent the delicate nut oils from becoming rancid.

PREP TIME: 10 minutes
STORAGE: Store in an airtight container in the refrigerator for up to 1 week or in the freezer for up to 6 months.
PER SERVING: (¼ cup per serving) Calories: 210; Total Fat: 18 g (1.5 g saturated, 11 g monounsaturated); Carbohydrates: 8 g; Protein: 8 g; Fiber: 4 g; Sodium: 0 mg

Resources

Where can you find everything from a big, 16-quart stockpot to heirloom rice to information on local farmers' markets?

The Internet, of course. Here's a list of websites you might find useful in stocking your longevity kitchen and staying well informed.

Kitchen Equipment Suppliers

Bed Bath & Beyond: www.bedbathandbeyond.com

Chef's Resource: www.chefsresource.com

Cooking.com: www.cooking.com

Cutlery and More: www.cutleryandmore.com

Instawares Restaurant Supply: www.instawares.com

MetroKitchen: www.metrokitchen.com

Snapware (for airtight glass storage containers): www.snapware.com

Sur La Table: www.surlatable.com

Vitamix (for excellent high-speed blenders): www.vitamix.com

Williams-Sonoma: www.williams-sonoma.com

Sources for Specialty Ingredients

Bob's Red Mill (for a variety of flours and gluten-free products): www.bobsredmill.com

Celtic Sea Salt (for sea salt): www.selinanaturally.com

Eden Foods (for 100% buckwheat soba noodles, hot pepper sesame oil, and many other high-quality ingredients): www.edenfoods.com

Hodgson Mill (for a variety of whole grains and gluten-free grains): www.hodgsonmill.com

Lava Lake Lamb (for outstanding grass-fed lamb): www.lavalakelamb.com

Living Tree Community Foods (for raw, organic, and kosher nut butters, tahini, pestos, oils, honey, and grains) www.livingtreecommunity.com

Lotus Foods (for heirloom and alternative varieties of rice): www.lotusfoods.com

MaraNatha (for organic nut and seed butters): www.maranathafoods.com

Maine Coast Sea Vegetables: (for kombu and nori sheets) www.seaveg.com

Maple Valley (for organic Grade B maple syrup from an organic maple cooperative): www.maplevalleysyrup.com

Real Salt (for natural, kosher-certified sea salt): www.realsalt.com

Republic of Tea (for a wide variety of herbal teas, including hibiscus): www.republicoftea.com

San-J (for tamari, Asian cooking sauces, and Japanese salad dressings): www.san-j.com

Spectrum (for healthful cooking oils): www.spectrumorganics.com

Spicely Organic Spices (for a wide variety of spices and herbs in small packages): www.spicely.com

Smith & Truslow (for freshly ground spices and spice combinations): www.smithandtruslow.com

Traditional Medicinals (for certified organic herbal and medicinal teas): www.traditionalmedicinals.com

US Wellness Meats (for grass-fed and humanely raised, beef, chicken, and lamb): www.grasslandbeef.com

Vital Choice (for wild, line-caught salmon, other high-quality seafood, and organic specialty foods): www.vitalchoice.com

National Grocery Chains and Online Markets

Local Harvest (immense directory to sources of locally grown organic food, plus an online catalogue for items not available locally): www.localharvest.org

Organic Provisions (online organic grocery): www.orgfood.com

Safeway (mainstream supermarket with its own line of organic food and produce): www.safeway.com

Sun Organic Farm (online organic market): www.sunorganic.com

Sunflower Farmers Markets (chain of supermarkets in the western United States, with a focus on natural and high-quality products): www.sunflowermarkets.com

Trader Joe's (nationwide grocery store with organic products): www.traderjoes.com

Whole Foods (the first certified organic supermarket in the United States): www.wholefoodsmarket.com

Farmers' Markets and Local Foods

Eat Well Guide (directory to local, sustainable, and organic farmers' markets, restaurants, stores, bakeries, and more): www.eatwellguide.org

Eat Wild (state-by-state directory of sources for local grass-fed meats, poultry, and dairy products): www.eatwild.com

Epicurious Seasonal Ingredients Map (for info on local produce that's ripe and in season your area at any given time): www.epicurious.com/articlesguides/seasonalcooking/farmtotable/seasonalingredientmap

Local Harvest (immense directory to sources of locally grown organic food, plus an online catalogue for items not available locally): www.localharvest.org

Organic Kitchen (resource guide with listings for organic markets, restaurants, farms, vineyards, and more): www.organickitchen.com

Real Time Farms (directory of local farmers and restaurants that use local foods, along with information on how food travels from field to plate): www.realtimefarms.com

US Department of Agriculture (nationwide farmers' market finder): apps.ams.usda.gov/FarmersMarkets

Environmental Resources

Collaborative on Health and the Environment and their initiatives on healthy aging: www.healthandenvironment.org and www.healthandenvironment.org/initiatives/healthy_aging

Environmental Working Group and their shopper's guide to pesticides in produce: www.ewg.org and www.ewg.org/foodnews

Monterey Bay Aquarium (for a list of sustainable seafood): www.montereybayaquarium.org/cr/seafoodwatch.aspx

Organic Center (for the latest science and news about organics): www.organic-center.org

Organic Trade Association (for information on organic foods): www.ota.com

Nutrition Resources

US Department of Agriculture Nutrient Data Laboratory (for nutritional databases on every food from apples to zucchini): www.nal.usda.gov/fnic/foodcomp

World's Healthiest Foods (for information on topics related to nutrition and health): www.whfoods.com

Bibliography

This bibliography presents just a small sampling of the hundreds of research articles consulted during the writing of this book.

Adeleye, I. A., et al. 2003. Antimicrobial activity of extracts of local cough mixtures on upper respiratory tract bacterial pathogens. *West Indian Medical Journal* 52(3):188–90.

Al-Howiriny, T., et al. 2003. Prevention of experimentally-induced gastric ulcers in rats by an ethanolic extract of "Parsley" *Petroselinum crispum*. *American Journal of Chinese Medicine* 31(5):699–711.

American Cancer Society. 2008. Quercetin. www.cancer.org/Treatment/TreatmentsandSideEffects/ComplementaryandAlternativeMedicine/DietandNutrition/quercetin.

Anderson, J. W. 2004. Whole grains and coronary heart disease: The whole kernel of truth. *American Journal of Clinical Nutrition* 80(6):1459–60.

Anderson, J. W., et al. 2011. Soy protein effects on serum lipoproteins: A quality assessment and meta-analysis of randomized, controlled studies. *Journal of the American College of Nutrition* 30(2):79–91.

Atta, A. H., et al. 2010. Hepatoprotective effect of methanol extracts of *Zingiber officinale* and *Cichorium intybus*. *Indian Journal of Pharmaceutical Sciences* 72(5):564–70.

Avena-Bustillos, R. J., et al. 2009. Effects of allspice, cinnamon, and clove bud essential oils in edible apple films on physical properties and antimicrobial activities. *Journal of Food Science* 74(7):M372–78.

Ban, J. O., et al. 2009. Anti-inflammatory and arthritic effects of thiacremonone, a novel sulfur compound isolated from garlic via inhibition of NF-kB. *Arthritis Research and Therapy* 11(5):R145.

Basu, A., et al. 2010. Berries: Emerging impact on cardiovascular health. *Nutrition Reviews* 68(3):168–77.

Bazzano, L. A., et al. 2003. Dietary fiber intake and reduced risk of coronary heart disease in US men and women: The National Health and Nutrition Examination Survey I Epidemiologic Follow-up Study. *Archives of Internal Medicine* 163(16):1897–904.

Bazzano, L. A., et al. 2011. Non-soy legume consumption lowers cholesterol levels: A meta-analysis of randomized controlled trials. *Nutrition, Metabolism, and Cardiovascular Diseases* 21(2):94–103.

Beydoun, M. A., et al. 2007. Plasma n-3 fatty acids and the risk of cognitive decline in older adults: The Atherosclerosis Risk in Communities Study. *American Journal of Clinical Nutrition* 85(4):1103–11.

Butler, L. M., et al. 2010. A vegetable-fruit-soy dietary pattern protects against breast cancer among postmenopausal Singapore Chinese women. *American Journal of Clinical Nutrition* 91(4): 10–13.

Cade, J. E., et al. 2007. Dietary fibre and risk of breast cancer in the U.K. Women's Cohort Study. *International Journal of Epidemiology* 36(2):431–38.

Calderón-Montaño, J. M., et al. 2011. A review on the dietary flavonoid kaempferol. *Mini Reviews in Medicinal Chemistry* 11(4):298–344.

Chithra, V., et al. 1997. Hypolipidemic effect of coriander seeds (*Coriandrum sativum*): Mechanism of action. *Plant Foods for Human Nutrition* 51(2):167–72.

Chrysohoou, C., et al. 2007. Long-term fish consumption is associated with protection against arrhythmia in healthy persons in a Mediterranean region—the ATTICA study. *American Journal of Clinical Nutrition* 85(5):1385–91.

Dhonukshe-Rutten, R. A., et al. 2003. Vitamin B_{12} status is associated with bone mineral content and bone mineral density in frail elderly women but not in men. *Journal of Nutrition* 133(3):801–7.

Dong, L., et al. 2010. 3,3'-Diindolylmethane attenuates experimental arthritis and osteoclastogenesis. *Biochemical Pharmacology* 79(5):715–21.

Ensminger, A. H. 1986. *Food for Health: A Nutrition Encyclopedia.* Clovis, CA: Pegus Press.

Erkkila, A., et al. 2004. Fish intake is associated with a reduced progression of coronary artery atherosclerosis in postmenopausal women with coronary artery disease. *American Journal of Clinical Nutrition* 80(3):626–32.

Fang, N., et al. 2006. Inhibition of growth and induction of apoptosis in human cancer cell lines by an ethyl acetate fraction from shiitake mushrooms. *Journal of Alternative and Complementary Medicine* 12(2):125–32.

Ferrarini, L., et al. 2011. Anti-proliferative activity and chemoprotective effects towards DNA oxidative damage of fresh and cooked Brassicaceae. *British Journal of Nutrition* 17:1–9.

Galeone, C., et al. 2009. Allium vegetable intake and risk of acute myocardial infarction in Italy. *European Journal of Nutrition* 48(2):120–23.

Goldberg, R. J., et al. 2007. Long-term survival after heart failure: A contemporary population-based perspective. *Archives of Internal Medicine* 167(5):490–96.

Graham, T., et al. 2012. The happiness diet. *Prevention* 64(1):52–59.

Griel, A. E., et al. 2007. An increase in dietary n-3 fatty acids decreases a marker of bone resorption in humans. *Nutrition Journal*, January 16, 6:2.

Guay, D. R. 2009. Cranberry and urinary tract infections. *Drugs* 69(7):775–807.

Gurrola-Diaz, C. M., et al. 2010. Effects of *Hibiscus sabdariffa* extract powder and preventive treatment (diet) on the lipid profiles of patients with metabolic syndrome. *Phytomedicine* 17(7):500–505.

He, J., et al. 1995. Oats and buckwheat intakes and cardiovascular disease risk factors in an ethnic minority of China. *American Journal of Clinical Nutrition* 61(2):366–72.

Higdon, J. 2003. Micronutrient Information Center: Choline. Linus Pauling Institute. http://lpi.oregonstate.edu/infocenter/othernuts/choline.

Higdon, J. 2005. Micronutrient Information Center: Indole-3-carbinol. Linus Pauling Institute. http://lpi.oregonstate.edu/infocenter/phytochemicals/i3c.

Hirano, R., et al. 2001. Antioxidant ability of various flavonoids against DPPH radicals and LDL oxidation. *Journal of Nutritional Science and Vitaminology* 47(5):357–62.

Hirata, F., et al. 1996. Hypocholesterolemic effect of sesame lignan in humans. *Atherosclerosis* 122(1):135–36.

Hitokoto, H., et al. 1980. Inhibitory effects of spices on growth and toxin production of toxigenic fungi. *Applied and Environmental Microbiology* 39(4):818–22.

Hosseinzadeh, H., et al. 2005. Protective effect of aqueous saffron extract (*Crocus sativus* L.) and crocin, its active constituent, on renal ischemia-reperfusion-induced oxidative damage in rats. *Journal of Pharmacy and Pharmaceutical Sciences* 8(3):387–93.

Houghton, P. S. 2003. Alternative treatment to Alzheimer's drug. Research presented at the British Pharmaceutical Conference in Harrogate, South Australia, September 15–17.

Howell, W. H., et al. 1997. Plasma lipid and lipoprotein responses to dietary fat and cholesterol: A meta-analysis. *American Journal of Clinical Nutrition* 65(6):1747–64.

Iconomidou, V. A., et al. 2008. Natural protective amyloids. *Current Protein and Peptide Science* 9(3):291–309.

Jenkins, D. J., et al. 2006. Almonds decrease postprandial glycemia, insulinemia, and oxidative damage in healthy individuals. *Journal of Nutrition* 136(12):2987–92.

Jenkins, D. J., et al. 2011. Effect of a dietary portfolio of cholesterol-lowering foods given at 2 levels of intensity of dietary advice on serum lipids in hyperlipidemia: A randomized controlled trial. *Journal of the American Medical Association* 306(8):831–39.

Jonnalagadda, S. S., et al. 2011. Putting the whole grain puzzle together: Health benefits associated with whole grains—Summary of American Society for Nutrition 2010 Satellite Symposium. *Journal of Nutrition* 141(5):1011S–22S.

Joseph, J. A., et al. 2000. Oxidative stress protection and vulnerability in aging: Putative nutritional implications for intervention. *Mechanisms of Ageing and Development* 116(2–3):141–53.

Joseph, J. A., et al. 2010. Blueberry supplementation improves memory in older adults. *Journal of Agricultural and Food Chemistry* 58(7):3996–4000.

Kalmijn, S., et al. 2004. Dietary intake of fatty acids and fish in relation to cognitive performance at middle age. *Neurology* 62(2):275–80.

Katayama, S., et al. 2011. Apricot carotenoids possess potent anti-amyloidogenic activity in vitro. *Journal of Agricultural and Food Chemistry* 59(23):12691–96.

Kontogianni, M. D., et al. 2007. Relationship between meat intake and the development of acute coronary syndromes: The CARDIO2000 case-control study. *European Journal of Clinical Nutrition* 62(2):171–77.

Kurl, S., et al. 2002. Plasma vitamin C modifies the association between hypertension and risk of stroke. *Stroke* 33(6):1568–73.

Lagouri, V., et al. 1996. Nutrient antioxidants in oregano. *International Journal of Food Science and Nutrition* 47(6):493–97.

Lahon, K., et al. 2011. Hepatoprotective activity of *Ocimum sanctum* alcoholic leaf extract against paracetamol-induced liver damage in albino rats. *Pharmacognosy Research* 3(1):13–18.

Lanou, A. J. 2011. Soy foods: Are they useful for optimal bone health? *Therapeutic Advances in Musculoskeletal Disease* 3(6):293–300.

Lin, Y., et al. 2008. Luteolin, a flavonoid with potential for cancer prevention and therapy. *Current Cancer Drug Targets* (7):634–46.

Liou, Y., et al. 2007. Decreasing linoleic acid with constant alpha-linolenic acid in dietary fats increases (n-3) eicosapentaenoic acid in plasma phospholipids in healthy men. *Journal of Nutrition* 137(4):945–952.

Liu, S., et al. 2003. Relation between changes in intakes of dietary fiber and grain products and changes in weight and development of obesity among middle-aged women. *American Journal of Clinical Nutrition* 78(5):920–27.

Marinou, K. A., et al. 2010. Differential effect of *Pistacia vera* extracts on experimental atherosclerosis in the rabbit animal model: An experimental study. *Lipids in Health and Disease* July 16, 9:73.

Mateljan, G. 2007. *The World's Healthiest Foods: Essential Guide for the Healthiest Way of Eating.* Seattle: George Mateljan Foundation.

McIntosh, M., et al. 2001. A diet containing food rich in soluble and insoluble fiber improves glycemic control and reduces hyperlipidemia among patients with type 2 diabetes mellitus. *Nutrition Review* 59(2):52–55.

McKay, D. L., et al. 2010 *Hibiscus sabdariffa* L. tea (tisane) lowers blood pressure in prehypertensive and mildly hypertensive adults. *Journal of Nutrition* 140(2):298–303.

Miccadei, S., et al. 2008. Antioxidative and apoptotic properties of polyphenolic extracts from edible part of artichoke (*Cynara scolymus* L.) on cultured rat hepatocytes and on human hepatoma cells. *Nutrition and Cancer* 60(2):276–83.

Miyazaki, Y., et al. 2005. Effects on immune response of antidiabetic ingredients from white-skinned sweet potato. *Nutrition* 21(3):358–62.

Mullin, G., et al. 2011. *The Inside Tract: Your Good Gut Guide to Great Digestive Heath.* New York: Rodale Press.

Murray, M., et al. 2005. *The Encyclopedia of Healing Foods.* New York: Atria Books.

National Oceanic and Atmospheric Administration. Sablefish. www.fishwatch.gov/seafood_profiles/species/cod/species_pages/sablefish.htm.

Oliff, H. S. 2010. Saffron extract shows promise for Alzheimer's disease in comparative trial *Herbal-Gram*, May–July 86:30–31.

Opalchenova, G., et al. 2003. Comparative studies on the activity of basil—an essential oil from *Ocimum basilicum* L.—against multidrug resistant clinical isolates of the genera *Staphylococcus*, *Enterococcus* and *Pseudomonas* by using different test methods. *Journal of Microbiological Methods* 54(1):105–10.

Orafidiya, L. O., et al. 2001. The formulation of an effective topical antibacterial product containing *Ocimum gratissimum* leaf essential oil. *International Journal of Pharmaceutics* 224(1–2):177–83.

Pandey, A., et al. 2011. Pharmacological screening of *Coriandrum sativum* Linn. for hepatoprotective activity. *Journal of Pharmacology and Bioallied Sciences* 3(3):435–41.

Paul, R., et al. 2011. Avocado fruit exhibits chemo-protective potentiality against cyclophosphamide induced genotoxicity in human lymphocyte culture. *Journal of Experimental Therapeutics and Oncology* 9(3):221–30.

Ping, H., et al. 2010. Antidiabetic effects of cinnamon oil in diabetic KK-Ay mice. *Food and Chemical Toxicology* 48(8–9):2344–49.

Puel, C., et al. 2005. Prevention of bone loss by phloridzin, an apple polyphenol, in ovariectomized rats under inflammation conditions. *Calcified Tissue International* 77(5):311–18.

Rainey, C. J., et al. 1999. Daily boron intake from the American diet. *Journal of the American Dietetic Association* 99(3):335–40.

Redman, C. 2002. Reap the goodness of red fruit. *Natural Health* 32(4):66–73.

Rocha-González, H. I., et al. 2008. Resveratrol: A natural compound with pharmacological potential in neurodegenerative diseases. *CNS Neuroscience and Therapeutics* 14(3):234–47.

Ruch, S. 2009. The power of greens. *Organic Gardening*, February–March, 56:64–69.

Scott, K. 2006. *Medicinal Seasonings: The Healing Power of Spices.* Cape Town, South Africa: Medspice.

Smiechowska, A., et al. 2008. Cancer chemopreventive agents: Glucosinolates and their decomposition products in white cabbage (*Brassica oleracea* var. capitata) [article in Polish]. *Postepy Hig Med Dosw* (online), April 2 62:125–40.

Srinivasan, K. 2007. Black pepper and its pungent principle—piperine: A review of diverse physiological effects. *Critical Reviews in Food Science and Nutrition* 47(8):735–48.

Thakkar, S. K., et al. 2008. Bioaccessibility of pro-vitamin A carotenoids is minimally affected by non pro-vitamin a xanthophylls in maize (*Zea mays* sp.). *Journal of Agricultural and Food Chemistry* 56(23):11441–46.

Tildesley, N. T., et al. 2003. *Salvia lavandulaefolia* (Spanish sage) enhances memory in healthy young volunteers. *Pharmacology, Biochemistry, and Behavior* 75(3):669–74.

Uma Devi, P. 2001. Radioprotective, anticarcinogenic, and antioxidant properties of the Indian holy basil, *Ocimum sanctum* (Tulasi). *Indian Journal of Experimental Biology* 39(3):185–90.

Valussi, M. 2011. Functional foods with digestion-enhancing properties. *International Journal of Food Sciences and Nutrition* 63(Suppl 1):82–89.

Van Dam, R. M., et al. 2006. Dietary calcium and magnesium, major food sources, and risk of type 2 diabetes in US black women. *Diabetes Care* 29(10):2238–43.

Vanharanta, M., et al. 2003. Risk of cardiovascular disease-related and all-cause death according to serum concentrations of enterolactone: Kuopio Ischaemic Heart Disease Risk Factor Study. *Archives of Internal Medicine* 163(9):1099–104.

Weil, A. 2006. Mushrooms for good health? Q & A Library. www.drweil.com/drw/u/QAA400053/are-mushrooms-good-for-your-health.html.

Wood, R. 1999. *The New Whole Foods Encyclopedia.* New York : Prentice-Hall Press.

Yamauchi, M., et al. 2011. Crocetin prevents retinal degeneration induced by oxidative and endoplasmic reticulum stresses via inhibition of caspase activity. *European Journal of Pharmacology* 650(1):110–19.

Index

EGCG (epigallocatechin
gallate), 27
Eggs, 26, 132
Black Bean Skillet Cakes with
Poached Eggs, 134–35
Curried Deviled Eggs, 173
Layered Frittata with Leeks,
Swiss Chard, and
Tomatoes, 132
organic, 130, 131
Elders, wisdom of, 3–5
Ellagic acid, 31
Endocrine system, 17–18
Enteric nervous system, 11, 57
Epigenetics, 9–10
Eritadenine, 32
Ethnic cuisines, ingredients for, 48
Eugenol, 21, 22
Eye health, 22–24, 26, 27

F
Farro with Kale-Basil Pesto, 121
FASS (fat, acid, salt, and sweet),
44–47
Fennel, 26
Chicken Magic Mineral Broth
2.0, 56
Magic Mineral Broth 2.0, 55
Shrimp Via My Ma, 143
Strawberry, Fennel, and
Arugula Salad, 91
Velvety Mediterranean
Gazpacho with Avocado
Cream, 58
Fiber, 12, 17, 28, 113
Fish. *See individual species*
Flat-Out Good Chicken, 148–49
Flavanols, 25
Flavor, balancing, 44–47
Flaxseeds, 206
Flexibility promoters, 36–37
Folate, 22, 28, 30
Folic acid, 16
Free radicals, 15
Frittata, Layered, with Leeks, Swiss
Chard, and Tomatoes, 132
Fucoidans, 28

G
Garbanzo beans. *See* Chickpeas
Garlic, 26, 64, 125
Chicken Magic Mineral
Broth 2.0, 56
Magic Mineral Broth 2.0, 55
roasted, 64
Vampire Slayer's Soup, 64

Gazpacho, Velvety Mediterranean,
with Avocado Cream, 58
Genes, effects of, 8, 9–10
Gershon, Michael, 11
Geyer, Cynthia, 19, 20, 104, 200
Ginger, 26–27
Glucobrassicin, 27
Glucosinolates, 23, 24
Glutathione, 15, 22, 30, 34, 82
Gluten-Free Blueberry Mini
Muffins, 164
Glycemic index, 18
Glycemic load, 18
Golden Roasted Cauliflower, 111
Good Mood Sardines, 135
Grains
gluten-free, 116, 160
whole, 116
See also individual grains
Greek Chicken Salad, 145
Greener Than Green Goddess
Dressing, 186
Greens, 95
Indian Greens, 97
Latin Kale, 95
Mediterranean Greens, 98
prepping, 95
Sweet-and-Sour Asian
Cabbage and Kale, 96
Tuscan Beans and Greens,
100–101
Green tea. *See* Tea
Gregg's Morning Protein
Shakes, 206
Gremolata, Many-Herb, 181
Guacamole, Minted, with
Pomegranate Seeds, 171
Gut. *See* Digestive system health

H
Halibut, 27
Roasted Halibut with Lime
and Papaya and Avocado
Salsa, 137
Southeast Asian Seafood
Stew, 75
Hartnell, Randy, 137, 139
Hazelnuts, Roasted Asparagus
Salad with Arugula and, 88
Heart health, 13–14, 21–32, 34,
37, 120
Heavy metals, 12, 113
Helicobacter pylori, 11–12
Hepburn, Katherine, 213
Herbs, 47–48, 50
Herby Turkey Sliders, 153

Hibiscus, 27
Hibiscus Pomegranate Cooler,
205
Raspberry Hibiscus Sorbet,
215
Homocysteine, 22, 27, 28, 30, 31,
33, 97
Honey, 27
Hot-and-Sour Sesame Soba
Noodles, 126
Hydration, 12, 198
Hydrochloric acid (HCl), 11
Hyman, Mark, 15

I
Immune system health, 15, 24, 28,
29, 33, 35
Indian Greens, 97
Indian ingredients, 48
Indonesian Drizzle, 183
Inflammation, 15, 21–25, 27, 28,
30–34, 111
Insanely Good Chocolate
Brownies, 221
Insulin, 13, 17–18, 109
Inulin, 22
Isothiocyanates, 34

J
Jicama
Mexican Cabbage Crunch, 86
sticks, 171
Joint health, 29, 32, 33
Julienne peelers, 84
Julie's "Spring Is Busting Out All
Over" Soup, 61

K
Kaempferol, 28, 34
Kale, 27
Kale-Basil Pesto, 121
Latin Kale, 95
Mediterranean Greens, 98
Sweet-and-Sour Asian
Cabbage and Kale, 96
Tuscan Beans and Greens,
100–101
Kebabs, Mediterranean, 150–51
Kidneys, 12
Kombu, 28, 100

L
Lamb Chops, Moroccan Mint, 154
Lassis, Mango, 208
Latin ingredients, 48
Latin Kale, 95

For my husband, Gregg, who adds so much to my life.

Copyright © 2013 by Rebecca Katz
Photographs copyright © 2013 by Leo Gong
Foreword copyright © 2013 by Andrew Weil, MD

All rights reserved.
Published in the United States by Ten Speed Press, an imprint of the Crown Publishing Group, a division of Random House, Inc., New York.
www.crownpublishing.com
www.tenspeed.com

Ten Speed Press and the Ten Speed Press colophon are registered trademarks of Random House, Inc.

Discovering Your Culinary GPS on page 43 was originally published in different form in *The Cancer-Fighting Kitchen* by Rebecca Katz published by Ten Speed Press, an imprint of the Crown Publishing Group, a division of Random House, Inc. in 2009.

Library of Congress Cataloging-in-Publication Data is on file with the publisher

ISBN 978-1-60774-294-4
eISBN 978-1-60774-295-1

Printed in China

Design by Chloe Rawlins
Food styling by Jen Straus
Prop styling by Christine Wolheim

10 9 8 7 6 5 4 3 2 1

First Edition